PATHOLOGY
INTEGRATED

EDUCATION AN   EARC

This i

To

A renew:

PATHOLOGY INTEGRATED

AN A–Z OF DISEASE AND ITS PATHOGENESIS

PETER M LYDYARD MSc PhD FRCPath
Professor of Immunology
Royal Free and University College Medical School, London, UK

SUNIL R LAKHANI BSc MBBS MD MRCPath
Reader and Honorary Consultant
Department of Histopathology, Royal Free and University College Medical School, London, UK

AHMET DOGAN MD PhD MRCPath
Clinical Lecturer
Department of Histopathology, Royal Free and University College Medical School, London, UK

JOHN M HOLTON BSc MB ChB PhD MRCPath
Senior Lecturer
Department of Medical Microbiology, Royal Free and University College Medical School, London, UK

KEITH G PATTERSON FRCP FRCPath
Consultant Haematologist
Department of Clinical Haematology, University College Hospital, London, UK

JOHN BOLODEOKU MBBS MSc DPhil MRCPath
Honorary Lecturer in Chemical Pathology
Department of Chemical Pathology, Royal Free and University College Medical School, London, UK

JOHN HL PLAYFAIR MB BChir PhD DSc
Emeritus Professor of Immunology
Royal Free and University College Medical School, London, UK

A member of the Hodder Headline Group
LONDON
Co-published in the USA by Oxford University Press, Inc., New York

First published in Great Britain in 2000
by Arnold, a member of the Hodder Headline Group,
338 Euston Road, London NWI 3BH

http://www.arnoldpublishers.com

Co-published in the United States of America by
Oxford University Press, Inc.,
198 Madison Avenue, New York, NY 10016
Oxford is a registered trademark of Oxford University Press

Arnold International Students' Edition published 2000. Arnold
International Students' Editions are low-priced un-abridged editions
of important textbooks. They are only for sale in developing
countries.

Whilst the advice and information in this book is believed to be true
and accurate at the date of going to press, neither the authors nor the
publisher can accept any legal responsibility or liability for any errors
or omissions that may be made. In particular (but without limiting
the generality of the preceding disclaimer) every effort has been made
to check drug dosages; however, it is still possible that errors have
been missed. Furthermore, dosage schedules are constantly being
revised and new side-effects recognized. For these reasons the reader
is strongly urged to consult the drug companies' printed instructions
before administering any of the drugs recommended in this book.

British Library Cataloguing in Publication Data
A catalogue record for this book is available from the British Library

Library of Congress Cataloging-in-Publication Data
A catalog record for this book is available from the Library of
Congress

ISBN 0 340 74063 9

ISBN 0 340 76067 2 (International Students' Edition)

1 2 3 4 5 6 7 8 9 10

Commissioning Editor: Fiona Goodgame
Project Editor: Catherine Barnes
Production Editor: Julie Delf
Production Controller: Iain McWilliams
Project Manager: Alison Nick
Cover designer: T. Griffiths

Typeset in 9.5/12 pt Sabon by
Scribe Design, Gillingham, Kent
Printed and bound in Malta

What do you think about this book? Or any other Arnold title?
Please send your comments to feedback.arnold@hodder.co.uk

PREFACE

Pathology – the study of disease processes – has traditionally been taught in a confusing variety of different ways. One can approach it through its underlying mechanisms: inflammatory, degenerative, neoplastic, and so on. Or it can be integrated into a system-based medical course: diseases of the kidney, liver, blood, etc. Yet another tradition views it through the eyes of hospital departmental specialties: clinical chemistry, haematology, histopathology, immunology, microbiology. All these methods have their disadvantages. A single clinical entity (e.g. myeloma, rheumatoid arthritis) may exemplify more than one disease process and frequently involves more than one body system, as well as teachers from more than one department. The result has been that for the student this vitally important subject often seems to lack the weight and focus of medicine, surgery, obstetrics and other components of the curriculum.

In this book we present a completely new approach, in which diseases are listed by name, alphabetically. Thus one can look up, for example, myeloma, without having to know whether it is considered as a disease of the blood or the bones or the serum proteins, whether it is an infection or a neoplasm, and whether it 'belongs' to the haematologists, clinical chemists, or immunologists. In this way the relevant information is available to the student whether or not he/she has covered the topic in lectures, and without the need to consult several advanced textbooks – a particular advantage in curricula where clinical problems are encountered early in the course.

About 90 common and important diseases have been given extended treatment, including a typical clinical case; these are the ones most likely to turn up in exams and will be valuable for revision. At the other end of the scale, some rare syndromes get no more than a definition. Relevant entries are cross-referenced. Symptomatology and treatment are given a brief mention where appropriate, but it should be stressed that this is not intended to be, and cannot replace, a textbook of medicine. The appendices at the end of the book provide useful lists (normal laboratory values, infectious organisms) plus aids to system-based revision.

P.M. Lydyard
S.R. Lakhani
A. Dogan
J.M. Holton
K.G. Patterson
J. Bolodeoku
J.H.L. Playfair

HOW TO USE THIS BOOK

To learn about a disease, first consult the main entry. An asterisk after a word in the text indicates a separate entry, which may be consulted if time permits. Entries listed at the end, after the icon (📄) should be looked up immediately; they are directly relevant and will amplify your knowledge of the main condition. For more leisurely follow-up, a short list of widely used textbooks is given below, together with further reading and some useful web sites.

When revising, e.g. before an exam, it would be wise to start with the core entries (listed on p. xiii), following up the icons, too. If concentrating on a particular organ or system, use the checklists in Appendix 3. Finally, if you have any difficulties or complaints, let the authors know!

OTHER RESOURCES TO USE WITH THIS BOOK

Textbook references

Bloom AL, Forbes CD, Thomas DP. *Haemostasis and Thrombosis*, 3rd edn. Edinburgh: Churchill Livingstone, 1994.

Chandrosoma P, Taylor CR. *Concise Pathology*, 3rd edn. Appleton & Lange, 1998.

Chapel M, Heaney HM. *Essentials of Clinical Immunology*, 4th edn. Oxford: Blackwell Science, 1999.

Cotran RS, Kumar V, Collins T. *Robbins' Pathologic Basis of Disease*, 6th edn. Philadelphia and London: WB Saunders, 1999.

Degos L, Linch DC, Liwenberg R. *Textbook of Malignant Haematology*. London: Martin Dunitz, 1999.

Henderson B, Wilson M, McNab R, Lax AJ. *Cellular Microbiology*. Chichester: Wiley, 1999.

Hoffbrand AV, Lewis SM, Tuddenham EGD. *Postgraduate Haematology*, 4th edn. Oxford: Butterworth Heinemann, 1999.

Kerr JB. *Atlas of Functional Histology*. St Louis: Mosby, 1998.

Lakhani SR, Dilly SS, Finlayson C. *Basic Pathology: an Introduction to the Mechanisms of Disease*, 2nd edn. London: Arnold, 1998.

Marshall W, *Clinical Chemistry*. Gower Medical Publishing, 1995.

Marshall WJ, Bangert SK. *Clinical Biochemistry (Metabolic and Clinical Aspects)*. Edinburgh: Churchill Livingstone, 1995.

Mims CA, Dimmock N, Nash A, Stephen J. *Mims' Pathogenesis of Infectious Disease*, 4th edn. New York and London: Academic Press, 1995.

Mims CA, Playfair JHL, Riott IM, Wakelin D, Williams R. *Medical Microbiology*. St Louis: Mosby, 1993.

Mollison PL, Engelfriet CP, Contreras M. *Blood Transfusion in Clinical Medicine*, 10th edn. Oxford: Blackwell Science, 1998.

Parums DV. *Essential Clinical Pathology*. Oxford: Blackwell Science, 1996.

Playfair JHL, Lydyard PM. *Medical Immunology for Students*, 2nd edn. Edinburgh: Churchill Livingstone, 2000.

Schaechter M, Engleberg NC, Eisenstein BI, Medoff G. *Mechanisms of Microbial Disease*. Baltimore: Williams & Wilkins, 1998.

Stevens A, Lowe J. *Pathology*. St Louis: Mosby, 1995.

Stites DP, Terr AJ, Parslow TG. *Basic and Clinical Immunology*, 8th edn. New York: Prentice-Hall International, 1994.

Thomas ED, Blume KG, Forman SJ. *Haematopoietic Cell Transplantation*, 2nd edn. Oxford: Blackwell Science, 1999.

Underwood JCE. *General and Systemic Pathology*, 2nd edn. Edinburgh: Churchill Livingstone, 1996.

Woolf N. *Pathology (Basic and Systemic)*. Philadelphia and London: WB Saunders, 1998.

Further reading

Barnes PJ. Chronic obstructive pulmonary disease: new opportunities for drug development. *Trends Pharmacol Sci* 1998; **19**(10): 415–23.

Beaser RS. Managing diabetes: current strategies. *J Am Optom Assoc* 1998; **69**(11): 711–25.

Bertagnolli MM, McDougall CJ, Newmark HL. Colon cancer prevention: intervening in a multistage process. *Proc Soc Exp Biol Med* 1997; **216**(2): 266–74.

Droller MJ. Bladder cancer: state-of-the-art care. *CA Cancer J Clin* 1998; **48**(5): 269–84.

Gressner AM. The cell biology of liver fibrogenesis – an imbalance of proliferation, growth arrest and apoptosis of myofibroblasts. *Cell Tissue Res* 1998; **292**(3): 447–52.

de Guia TS. Acute respiratory distress syndrome: diagnosis and management. *Respirology* 1996; **1**(1): 23–30.

Iadecola C, Ross ME. Molecular pathology of cerebral ischemia: delayed gene expression and strategies for neuroprotection. *Ann N Y Acad Sci* 1997; **835**: 203–17.

de Leeuw PW, Kroon AA. Hypertension and the development of heart failure. *J Cardiovasc Pharmacol* 1998; **32**(Suppl 1): S9–15.

MacKie RM. Incidence, risk factors and prevention of melanoma. *Eur J Cancer* 1998; **34**(Suppl 3): S3–6.

Mahadeva R, Lomas DA. Genetics and respiratory disease. 2. Alpha 1-antitrypsin deficiency, cirrhosis and emphysema. *Thorax* 1998; **53**(6): 501–5.

Nicholls MG, Richards AM, Agarwal MJ. The importance of the renin-angiotensin system in cardiovascular disease. *Hum Hypertens* 1998; **12**(5): 295–9.

Nyren O. Is *Helicobacter pylori* really the cause of gastric cancer? *Semin Cancer Biol* 1998; **8**(4): 275–83.

O'Hollaren MT. Update in allergy and immunology. *Ann Intern Med* 1998; **129**(12): 1036–43.

Orntoft TF, Wolf H. Molecular alterations in bladder cancer. *Urol Res* 1998; **26**(4): 223–33.

Pasquier F, Leys D. Why are stroke patients prone to develop dementia? *J Neurol* 1997; **244**(3): 135–42.

Perl DP, Olanow CW, Calne D. Alzheimer's disease and Parkinson's disease: distinct entities or extremes of a spectrum of neurodegeneration? *Ann Neurol* 1998; **44**(3 Suppl 1): S19–31.

Prusiner SB. The prion diseases. *Brain Pathol* 1998; **8**(3): 499–513.

Rosenberg L. Clinical islet cell transplantation. Are we there yet? *Int J Pancreatol* 1998; **24**(3): 145–68.

Sanders DS. The differential diagnosis of Crohn's disease and ulcerative colitis. *Baillière's Clin Gastroenterol* 1998; **12**(1): 1933.

Schiller JH, Cleary J, Johnson D. Lung cancer: review of the ECOG experience. Eastern Cooperative Oncology Group. *Oncology* 1997; **54**(5): 353–62.

Slominski A, Wortsman J, Nickoloff B, McClatchey K, Mihm MC, Ross JS. Molecular pathology of malignant melanoma. *Am J Clin Pathol* 1998; **110**(6): 788–94.

Southern SA, Herrington CS. Molecular events in uterine cervical cancer. *Sex Transm Infect* 1998; **74**(2): 101–9.

Web sites

http://cjp.com/blood/
http://dir.yahoo.com/Science/Biology/Microbiology/
http://medstat.med.utah.edu/WebPath/webpath.html
http://www.hslib.washington.edu/courses/blood/
http://www.immunology.com/

ABBREVIATIONS

5HIAA	5-Hydroxyindoleacetic acid
ACE	Angiotensin-converting enzyme
ACR	Acetylcholine receptor
ACTH	Adrenocorticotrophic hormone
ADA	Adenosine deaminase
ADP	Adenosine diphosphate
AFP	Alpha-fetoprotein
AICD	Activation-induced cell death
AIDS	Acquired immunodeficiency syndrome
AIHA	Autoimmune haemolytic anaemia
ALA	δ-Aminolaevulinic acid
ALL	Acute lymphoblastic leukaemia
ALP	Alkaline phosphatase
ALT	Alanine aminotransferase
AMA	Antimitochondrial antibodies
AML	Acute myeloid (myeloblastic) leukaemia
ANA	Anti nuclear antibodies
ANCA	Antineutrophil cytoplasmic antigen (c – cytoplasmic pattern; p – peri-nuclear pattern)
APA	Alkaline phosphatase
APTT	Activated partial thromboplastin time
ARA	American Rheumatology Association
ARC	AIDS-related complex
ARDS	Adult respiratory distress syndrome
AS	Ankylosing spondylitis
ASD	Atrial septal defect
ASO	Anti-streptococcal O antigen
AST	Aspartate aminotransferase
AT	Ataxia telangiectasia
BCC	Basal cell carcinoma
BCG	Bacillus Calmette–Guérin
BJP	Bence Jones protein (free immunoglobulin light chains)
BM	Basement membrane
BMR	Basal metabolic rate
BMT	Bone marrow transplant
BR	Bilirubin
BSE	Bovine spongiform encephalopathy
BU	Blood urea
cAMP	Cyclic adenosine monophosphate
CAPD	Chronic ambulatory peritoneal dialysis
CCDC	Consultant in Communicable Disease Control
CD	Cluster of differentiation
CDC	Centers for Disease Control
CEA	Carcinoembryonic antigen
CFTR	Cystic fibrosis transmembrane conductance regulator
CGD	Chronic granulomatous disease
CHAD	Cold haemagglutinin disease
CIN	Cervical intraepithelial neoplasia
CJD	Creutzfeldt–Jakob disease
CK	Creatinine kinase
CLL	Chronic lymphocytic leukaemia
CML	Chronic myeloid (granulocytic) leukaemia
CMML	Chronic myelomonocytic leukaemia, one of the myelodys-plasias
CMV	Cytomegalovirus
CNS	Central nervous system
CPK	Creatinine phosphokinase
CREST	Calcinosis–Raynaud–oesophageal dysmotility–sclerodactyly–telangiectasia
CRP	C-reactive protein
CSF	Cerebrospinal fluid
CT	Computerized axial tomography
CVA	Cerebrovascular accident
CVID	Common variable immunodefi-ciency
DAF	Decay-accelerating factor
DAT	Direct antiglobulin (Coombs) test
dsNA	Double-stranded nucleic acid
DI	Diabetes insipidus
DIC	Disseminated intravascular coagulation
DLE	Discoid lupus erythematosus
DM	Diabetes mellitus
DNA	Deoxyribonucleic acid
DTH	Delayed-type hypersensitivity
DVT	Deep venous thrombosis
EBV	Epstein–Barr virus
ECG	Electrocardiograph
ECHO	Enteric cytopathic swine orphan virus
EDTA	Ethylenediaminetetra-acetic acid
ELAM	Endothelial adhesion molecule
EMU	Early morning urine
EPO	Erythropoietin
ER	Oestrogen receptor
ERCP	Endoscopic retrograde cholan-giopancreatography
ESR	Erythrocyte sedimentation rate
ET	Essential thrombocythaemia, one of the myeloproliferative disorders

FAB	French-American-British. Method of morphologically classifying haematological malignancies
FAP	Familial adenomatous polyposis
FDPs	Fibrin degradation products
FEV	Forced expiratory volume
FNA	Fine needle aspiration
FSH	Follicle stimulating hormone
FT3	Free tri-iodothyronine
FT4	Free thyroxine
G6PD	Glucose-6-phosphate dehydrogenase
GABA	Gamma amino butyric acid
GAD	Glutamate decarboxylase
GBM	Glomerular basement membrane
G-CSF	Granulocyte colony-stimulating factor
GGT or γGT	Gamma glutamyltransferase
GH	Growth hormone
GN	Glomerular nephritis
GVH	Graft-versus-host
GVHD	Graft-versus-host disease
Hb	Haemoglobin
HBV	Hepatitis B virus
HCG	Human chorionic gonadotrophin
HCL	Hairy cell leukaemia
Hct	Haematocrit (packed cell volume)
HDN	Haemolytic disease of the newborn
HHV	Human herpes virus
HIV	Human immunodeficiency virus
HLA	Human leucocyte antigen
HNPCC	Hereditary non-polyposis colorectal cancer
HPLC	High-pressure liquid chromatography
HPV	Human papilloma virus
HS	Hereditary spherocytosis
HSV	Herpes simplex virus
HUS	Haemolytic uraemic syndrome
IAT	Indirect antiglobulin (Coombs) test
IC	Immune complexes
ICA	Islet cell antibodies
ICAM	Intercellular adhesion molecule
IDDM	Insulin-dependent diabetes mellitus
IFN	Interferon
IHD	Inherited metabolic disease
IL	Interleukin
IMB	Inherited metabolic disease
INR	International normalized (prothrombin) ratio; international ratio
ITP	Idiopathic thrombocytopenic purpura
ITU	Intensive care unit
IVDU	Intravenous drug user
JAS	Juvenile ankylosing spondylitis
JCA	Juvenile chronic arthritis
JRA	Juvenile rheumatoid arthritis
LAD	Leucocyte adhesion deficiency
LATS	Long-acting thyroid stimulator
LCR	Ligase chain reaction
LD	Lactate dehydrogenase
LDH	Lactate dehydrogenase
LH	Luteinizing hormone
LPS	Lipopolysaccharide
MAHA	Microangiopathic haemolytic anaemia
MAO-B	Monoamine oxidase-B
MCH	Mean corpuscular haemoglobin – the average amount of haemoglobin in the red cells
MCHC	Mean corpuscular haemoglobin concentration – this red cell index has been largely supplanted by the MCH in the identification of hypochromic anaemias
MCV	Mean (red) cell volume
MEA	Multiple endocrine adenomatosis
MEN	Multiple endocrine neoplasia
MG	Myasthenia gravis
MGUS	Monoclonal gammopathy of undetermined significance
MHC	Major histocompatibility complex
MPV	Mean platelet volume
MRI	Magnetic resonance imaging
MSH	Melanocyte-stimulating hormone
MSU	Midstream specimen of urine
NADPH	Nicotinamide adenine dinucleotide phosphate
NBT	Nitroblue tetrazolium
NHL	Non-Hodgkin lymphoma
NK	Natural killer
NOS	Nitric oxide synthetase
NP	Nucleoprotein
NS	Nodular sclerosing [Hodgkin disease]
NSAID(s)	Non-steroidal anti-inflammatory drug(s)
OAF	Osteoclast-activating factor
OMP	Outer-membrane protein
PAF	Platelet activating factor
PAS	Periodic acid Schiff
PBC	Primary biliary cirrhosis
PBG	Porphobilinogen
PBSC	Peripheral blood stem cells
PCR	Polymerase chain reaction
PCV	Packed cell volume (haematocrit)
PDA	Patent ductus arteriosus
PE	Pulmonary embolism
PGE	Prostaglandin E
Ph	Philadelphia chromosome

PID	Pelvic inflammatory disease	TSI	Thyroid-stimulating immunoglobulin
PIN	Prostatic intraepithelial neoplasia		
Plt	Platelet (count)	TT	Thrombin time
PMC	Pseudomembranous colitis	TT3	Total tri-iodothyronine
PML	Progressive multifocal leucoencephalopathy	TT4	Total thyroxine
		TTP	Thrombotic thrombocytopenic purpura
PMN	Polymorphonuclear (cell); neutrophil	UV	Ultraviolet
PNH	Paroxysmal nocturnal haemoglobinuria	VAD	Vincristine, Adriamycin and dexamethasone
PNP	Purine nucleoside phosphorylase	VAMP	Vesicle-associated membrane protein
PR	Progesterone receptor	VC	Vital capacity
PRV	Polycythaemia rubra vera (primary polycythaemia)	VDRL	Venereal disease-related lipid
PSA	Prostate specific antigen	VIP	Vasoactive intestinal polypeptide
PT	Prothrombin time	VMA	Vanillylmandelic acid
PTH	Parathyroid hormone	VSD	Ventricular septal defect
PTHrP	Parathyroid hormone-related protein	vWF	von Willebrand factor
		VZV	Varicella-zoster virus
PUO	Pyrexia of unknown origin	WAIHA	Warm autoimmune haemolytic anaemia
RA	Refractory anaemia – one of the myelodysplasias; rheumatoid arthritis		
		WBC	White blood cell (count)
		XLA	X-linked agammaglobulinaemia
RAEB	Refractory anaemia with excess of blasts		
RAEB-t	Refractory anaemia with excess of blasts in transformation (to AML)		
RARS	Refractory anaemia with ring sideroblasts, one of the myelodysplasias		
RAST	Radio-allergo-sorbent test (for IgE)		
RBC	Red blood cell (count)		
RDW	Red cell (size) distribution width – an electronic measurement of anisocytosis		
RNA	Ribonucleic acid		
RSV	Respiratory syncytial virus		
SAGM	Saline-adenine-glucose-mannitol		
SCID	Severe combined immunodeficiency		
SIADH	Syndrome of inappropriate antidiuretic hormone		
SIDS	Sudden infant death syndrome		
SLE	Systemic lupus erythematosus		
SS	Sjögren syndrome		
SSPE	Subacute sclerosing panencephalomyelitis		
TB	Tuberculosis		
TIA	Transient ischaemic attack		
TIBC	Total iron-binding capacity		
TNF	Tumour necrosis factor		
TSH	Thyroid-stimulating hormone		

Genus abbreviations

Aspergillus = A.
Bacillus = B.
Bacteroides = Bact.
Chlamydia = Ch.
Clostridium = Cl.
Corynebacterium = C.
Coxiella = Cox.
Entamoeba = Ent.
Escherichia = E.
Helicobacter = H.
Legionella = L.
Mycobacterium = M.
Neisseria = N.
Plasmodium = P.
Pseudomonas = Ps.
Rickettsia = R.
Salmonella = Salm.
Schistosoma = Schist.
Shigella = Sh.
Staphylococcus = Staph.
Streptobacillus = Str.
Streptococcus = Strep.
Trichomonas = T.
Trypanosoma = Try.
Yersinia = Y.

ACKNOWLEDGEMENTS

The authors would like to thank the following people for their help and advice.

CLINICAL ADVISOR
Dr Gerard S Conway
Consultant Endocrinologist and Honorary Senior Lecturer
UCL Hospitals NHS Trust and University College
London, UK

INTERNATIONAL ADVISORS ON CORE CONTENT

Professor L Blendis
Professor of Medicine
Tel Aviv University
Israel

Dr D MacGregor
Director of Anatomical Pathology
University of Melbourne
Australia

Dr J Cullen
Professor of Pathology
University of Toronto
Canada

Professor R Smallwood
Professor of Medicine
University of Melbourne
Australia

Professor M Khurshid
Professor of Pathology
The Aga Khan University
Pakistan

STUDENT ADVISORS

Emilia Moretto
Final year medical student
Royal Free and University College Medical School
London, UK

James Scurr
Final year medical student
Royal Free and University College Medical School
London, UK

GENERAL
We are also grateful to the following authors for granting permission to re-use artwork from their books:

N Browse, *An Introduction to the Symptoms and Signs of Surgical Disease*, 3rd edn. London: Arnold, 1997
J Curtis and G Whitehouse, *Radiology for the MRCP*. London: Arnold, 1998
T Evans and C Haslett, *Acute Respiratory Distress Syndrome*. London: Arnold, 1992
S Lakhani, S Dilly and C Finlayson, *Basic Pathology: an*
Introduction to the Mechanisms of Disease, 2nd edn. London: Arnold, 1998
D Lisle, *Imaging for Students*. London: Arnold, 1995
P Toghill, *Examining Patients*, 2nd edn. London: Arnold, 1994
M J Walsh and M H Asmi, *A Practical Guide to Echocardiography*. London: Arnold, 1996

The authors would also like to acknowledge colleagues for providing other figures and/or helpful advice in the preparation of some of the entries.
Professor David A Isenberg
Professor Michael W Fanger
Dr Frances Cowan
Dr Steve Chatters
Dr Meryl Griffiths
Dr Elizabeth Benjamin
Dr Gabriella Kocjan
Dr Janice Holton

CORE ENTRIES

Acquired immunodeficiency syndrome (AIDS)
Acromegaly
Acute lymphoblastic leukaemia
Acute myeloid leukaemia
Addison disease
Adult respiratory distress syndrome
Allergy
Alzheimer disease
Anaphylaxis
Antibody deficiency
Aplastic anaemia
Aspergillosis
Asthma
Bladder carcinoma
Blood transfusion reactions
Breast carcinoma
Brucellosis
Bullous skin diseases
Burkitt lymphoma
Cerebrovascular disease
Cervical carcinoma
Chronic granulomatous disease
Chronic lymphocytic leukaemia
Chronic myeloid leukaemia
Chronic obstructive airways disease
Cirrhosis
Coeliac disease
Colorectal carcinoma
Creutzfeldt-Jakob disease
Crohn disease
Cushing syndrome
Cystic fibrosis
Diabetes mellitus
Disseminated intravascular coagulation
Diverticulitis
Dysentery
Endocarditis
Extrinsic allergic alveolitis
Gastric carcinoma
Glandular fever
Glomerulonephritis
Gonorrhoea
Gout
Haemochromatosis
Heart failure
Hepatitis B infection

Herpes simplex encephalitis
Hodgkin disease
Hyperparathyroidism
Hypertension
Hypothyroidism
Idiopathic thrombocytopenic purpura
Legionnaires disease
Leprosy
Lung carcinoma
Malaria
Malignant melanoma
Malignant mesothelioma
Meningococcal meningitis
Multiple sclerosis
Myeloma
Myocardial infarction
Necrotizing fasciitis
Non-Hodgkin lymphoma
Osteoarthritis
Osteomyelitis
Pancreatitis
Parkinson disease
Pelvic inflammatory disease
Peptic ulcer
Pernicious anaemia
Phaeochromocytoma
Pneumococcal pneumonia
Porphyria
Primary biliary cirrhosis
Prostatic carcinoma
Pyelonephritis
Renal transplantation
Rheumatoid arthritis
Sarcoidosis
Sickle cell disease
Stem cell transplantation
Sudden infant death syndrome (SIDS)
Systemic lupus erythematosus
Thalassaemia
Thromboembolism
Thyrotoxicosis
Toxoplasmosis
Tuberculosis
Typhoid fever
Ulcerative colitis
Uveitis

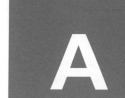

ABSCESS: A localized area of tissue destruction following an acute inflammatory reaction caused by micro-organisms, usually bacteria.

Aetiology and risk factors

Predisposing factors for abscess formation are trauma, often leading to haematoma formation, ischaemia, and the presence of a foreign body or blocked drainage from a viscus.

Usually an invading micro-organism lodges at the site, brought there by blood-borne spread or following trauma.

Organisms commonly forming abscesses include *Bacteroides fragilis*, *Streptococcus milleri* and *Staphylococcus aureus*, although many abscesses contain more than one bacterial species. Abscesses may also be caused by *Entamoeba histolytica* (see Amoebiasis).

Pathology

An abscess is the host's attempt to isolate the invading pathogen and confine the conflict to a restricted area of the body. By sequestering the invading pathogen in a fibrinous exudate, the normal clearing process is inhibited, leading ultimately to the formation of pus, walled off by the fibrin deposition and proliferation of fibroblasts. The pus is formed from the necrotic debris of host cells, including polymorphs and bacteria (Fig. A1). Many pus-forming bacteria produce enzymes that can contribute to abscess formation, e.g. by precipitation of fibrin (coagulase of *Staphylococcus aureus*), lysis of host cells (lipases, proteases or DNases of *Staph. aureus* or *Bact. fragilis*), destruction of polymorphs (leucocidins of *Staph. aureus*), disruption and destruction of organ architecture (collagenases, hylauronidases).

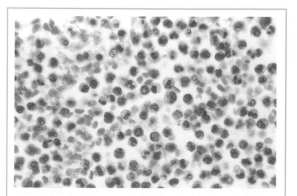

Fig. A1 Section of an abscess showing abundant polymorphonuclear leucocytes.

An abscess may present with systemic signs of acute inflammation such as a high, spiking temperature, pain, swelling, an elevated white count and acute phase proteins. There is regional lymphadenopathy. The specific presenting signs depend on the localization of the abscess. There may be few localizing signs other than pain and tenderness (e.g. liver abscess) or there may be loss of function (e.g. bone abscess) or signs of raised intracranial pressure and focal neurological signs (e.g. cerebral abscess). Complications include thrombophlebitis, septic emboli and septicaemia with septic shock. The management of abscesses is by surgical drainage and the appropriate anti-infective agent.

ACANTHOSIS NIGRICANS: A diffuse thickening of the skin with associated dark pigmentation, usually occurring in skin folds such as the axilla. It is associated with internal malignancy.

ACHALASIA: This results from a failure of smooth muscle to relax, particularly at the oesophago-gastric junction. It is due to degeneration of the ganglion cells within the oesophagus.

ACHONDROPLASIA: An autosomal dominant disorder leading, in heterozygotes, to abnormal development of the long bones and resulting in short stature. The head and trunk are not affected. Homozygotes do not survive.

ACOUSTIC NEUROFIBROMA: A benign tumour of acoustic nerves. It is a schwannoma rather than a neurofibroma; however, there are many similarities between the two. It may be sporadic or part of neurofibromatosis type II, in which case it may be bilateral.

 Neurofibromatosis

ACQUIRED IMMUNODEFICIENCIES: Immuno-deficiency diseases due to influences external to the immune system, e.g. immunosuppressive drugs, infections themselves, or other disease processes; also referred to as secondary immunodeficiencies.

 Immunodeficiency

A

ACQUIRED IMMUNODEFICIENCY SYNDROME (AIDS): An immunodeficiency disease caused by the human deficiency viruses HIV-1 and HIV-2.

Case

A 28-year-old man attending a clinic for sexually transmitted diseases had a 4-week history of painful perianal soreness. The doctor asked him about previous episodes and it transpired that he had had recurrences of the same complaint over a 2-year period but had not gone to his GP because it was not very painful and he was frightened of what the soreness might be related to. It further transpired that the patient had lost weight over the last few months and that he had painful swelling in his axillary regions. He had also noticed that his mouth was rather sensitive to hot drinks and complained of occasional headaches.

On examination, he was seen to have oral thrush (*Candida*) and leucoplakia and his perianal soreness was due to extensive herpes simplex infection. From the history and examination, the doctor felt that the patient had advanced HIV disease. He was counselled on the need for a blood test for HIV infection. Although previously reluctant, he now agreed to give a blood sample to be tested for antibodies to HIV and a CD4 count. He was asked to return to the clinic 3 days later for his results.

HIV-1 antibodies: +
WBC: 4.8 (3–11 × 10⁹/l)
CD4 × 10⁶/l: 80 (350–1200 × 10⁹/l)

A confirmatory antibody test was then sent. p24 antigen was detected in his serum and antibodies confirmed by Western blotting. The patient was then told that HIV infection had been confirmed by the laboratory tests. A further blood sample was taken to determine his HIV viral load (by PCR) and he was started on therapy. He was given oral aciclovir for his herpes, amphotericin lozenges for oral thrush, and co-trimoxazole as prophylaxis against *Pneumocystis carinii* pneumonia and reactivation of *Toxoplasma gondii*.

Aetiology and risk factors

AIDS is classified as a secondary/acquired immunodeficiency disease. It was recognized as a syndrome in mid-1981 in the USA as a result of an increase in reported cases of pneumocystis infection, but the aetiological agent was not identified as human immunodeficiency virus (HIV) until 2 years later. HIV is an RNA virus and two major strains have been identified which can cause AIDS: HIV-1 and HIV-2. There are many accompanying indicator

Table A1 Indicator diseases for AIDS

Herpes simplex (HSV)	*Pneumocystis carinii* pneumonia	Cytomegalovirus
Tuberculosis	Atypical myco-bacterial infection	Cryptosporidiosis
Cerebral toxoplasmosis	Non-Hodgkin lymphoma	Kaposi sarcoma

diseases and the most common are shown in Table A1.

In later stages of the disease, the blood CD4+ T-cell count is severely reduced and the Centers for Disease Control and Prevention (CDC) in the USA now defines AIDS as having < 200 × 10⁶/l of CD4+ T-cells irrespective of an indicator disease. Patients with HIV disease are classified by the CDC (Fig. A2) according to whether they have acute HIV

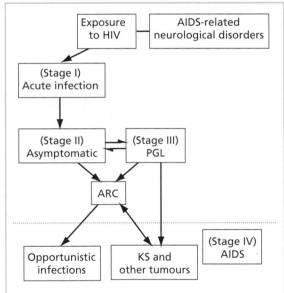

Fig. A2 Clinical spectrum of HIV infection and staging. ARC, AIDS-related complex; KS, Kaposi sarcoma; PGL, persistent generalized lymphadenopathy.

infection (stage I), are asymptomatic (stage II), have persistent generalized lymphadenopathy (stage III) or an AIDS-indicator disease (stage IV). The mode of transmission is via body fluids, especially blood, blood products, and semen. It is also transmitted through cervical secretions, tears, saliva and breast milk. Sexual intercourse is still the commonest route of transmission. Preparations of factor VIII for haemophilic patients were a major source of infection until the products were eventually tested for the virus and coagulation factor concentrates were treated by heat and detergent to inactivate

HIV. Vertical transmission is also common (14–30%), although it can be considerably reduced with antiretroviral therapy.

Pathology

The initial response of patients to HIV resembles that to other viruses. A primary response results in production of IgM antibodies, which convert to IgG (seroconversion) within a few weeks. There are several stages to the development of 'full-blown AIDS' (see Fig. A2) and it may take between 2 and 10 years. Some patients seem to progress even more slowly and these 'long-term non-progressors' may provide clues to the exact mechanism of progression and possible ways to prevent it.

The main target of HIV is the CD4 T-cell, but other important immune cells are infected since they also possess low amounts of the surface viral receptor CD4 itself. The virus binds to CD4 through one of its surface proteins (gp 120) and through one of a number of associated chemokine receptors, e.g. CCR5. Different strains of virus have been shown to infect one type of cell rather than another due to the different chemokine co-receptors, which are required for the virus to penetrate into a particular cell. Lack of infection in high-risk individuals can be explained by lack of expression of a particular chemokine receptor and by inhibition of HIV replication by chemokines (e.g. RANTES – regulated upon activation, normal T-cell expressed and secreted chemokine). It is thought that infection of cells other than T-cells, e.g. macrophages and dendritic cells, may control the progression of the disease. HIV infection of the CD4 T-cells leads to a progressive loss of these cells from the circulation, which in turn leads to depression of cell-mediated immunity and infections by opportunistic infections normally controlled by T-cell responses. Both CD4 and CD8 responses are affected. The patient described had a chronic herpes infection but other common presenting infections include mycobacteria and CMV (see Table A1). *Pneumocystis carinii* is another infectious organism (normally controlled by T-cells) that results in pneumonia and patients frequently die of this pulmonary complication. *Candida* infection (oral thrush) as seen in our patient is also common.

These secondary infections are mainly intracellular but other infections can also occur because CD4+ T-cells are pivotal cells, important for many other immune cells to function (see Fig. A3).

The mechanisms by which CD4 T-cells are depleted in HIV infection are not completely understood. HIV might have a weak cytopathic effect leading to direct cytolysis, but it seems that the CD4 T-cell lymphopenia is the result of the virus predis-

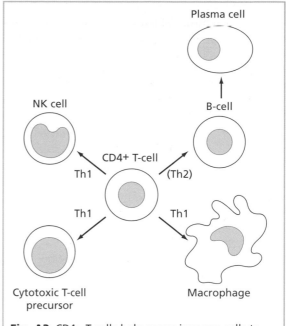

Fig. A3 CD4+ T-cells help many immune cells to function.

posing the cell to commit suicide when stimulated by antigen or making it a target for a classical cytotoxic CD8+ T-cell-mediated response.

There are still some aspects of pathology that are unclear in AIDS. Autoantibodies to MHC class II are often found but their role in pathogenesis is uncertain. The generalized lymphadenopathy, as the result of generalized follicular hyperplasia, seems to be due to polyclonal activation of B-cells in the lymph nodes, probably as the result of immune complexes of antibodies and HIV attached to the follicular dendritic cells. The lymphadenopathy explains the uncomfortable axillary swelling reported by our patient. The reason for the association of non-Hodgkin lymphoma with HIV infection is unclear but might be due to T-cell immunodeficiency. In support of this, patients treated with anti-T-cell therapy for transplantation have also been shown to have an increased incidence of non-Hodgkin lymphoma. Some patients with sexually acquired HIV disease develop Kaposi sarcoma. The aetiological agent for this is believed to be a herpes virus (HHV-8), suggesting that this might also be under the control of T-cell-mediated immunity.

In addition to immunological abnormalities, HIV-infected patients also show haematological abnormalities such as thrombocytopenia, which may be due to infection of the bone marrow progenitor cells. HIV infection of microglial cells can lead to neuropathological changes.

A

Management

At initial diagnosis the patient should receive drugs to treat his opportunistic infections, such as amphotericin for candida and aciclovir for perianal herpes. He should be started on prophylaxis against pneumocystis pneumonia and reactivation of *Toxoplasma gondii* with co-trimoxazole, as well as aggressive anti-HIV therapy.

The field of antiretroviral therapy is developing rapidly. The aim of treatment is to minimize viral replication. Current recommendations are to start patients on a combination of (at least) three antiretroviral drugs, for example:

- zidovudine (nucleoside analogue – inhibits reverse transcriptase)
- didanosine (DDI, nucleoside analogue – inhibits reverse transcriptase)
- indinovir (protease inhibitor – specifically inhibits assembly of the virus).

By using three drugs which inhibit viral replication by different routes, it is hoped to minimize development of resistance to the therapeutic agents. This treatment should reduce HIV viral load to undetectable levels (the limit of detection of current assays is < 50 copies per ml) which in turn leads to a sustained rise in CD4 T-cell count.

Patients need to be regularly monitored by measuring HIV viral load and CD4 T-cell count so that treatment failure can be detected. Any opportunistic infections should be treated. Clearly, an effective prophylactic vaccine to prevent viral acquisition is the long-term goal.

 Immunodeficiency; non-Hodgkin lymphoma; Kaposi sarcoma; Opportunistic infections

---

ACROMEGALY: Overgrowth of the extremities in adults as a result of an excessive amount of growth hormone (GH) in the blood.

Case

A 55-year-old man presented at the clinic with complaints of frequent headaches and excessive sweating. He also noticed that he was drinking a lot of fluids and urinating more frequently, and he thought his feet and hands were growing as he had had to go up one size with his gloves and shoes.

On examination, the facial texture was coarse, with prominent supraorbital ridges and a broad nose (Fig. A4). His hands were spade-like in appearance and blood pressure was 190/110 mmHg.

Laboratory investigations revealed a serum sodium of 140 mmol/l, potassium 3.5 mmol/l and glucose (fasting) 10.0 mmol/l. A moderate amount of glucose was present in his urine.

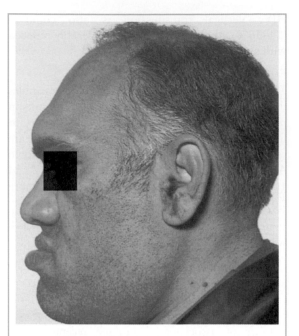

Fig. A4 Appearance of a patient with acromegaly. A heavy head with a prominent nose, chin and lips. (Reproduced with permission from Browse NL. *An Introduction to the Symptoms and Signs of Surgical Disease*, 3rd edn. London: Arnold, 1997)

A diagnosis of acromegaly was considered and further tests were requested, including a glucose tolerance test plus growth hormone and a CT scan. In addition, the visual fields were evaluated, which revealed a bitemporal hemianopia.

The results of the oral glucose tolerance test are shown in Table A2.

Table A2 Results of oral glucose tolerance test

Time (min)	Serum glucose (mmol/l)	Serum growth hormone (mU/l)
0	7.8	23
30	14.0	19
60	15.1	23
90	13.6	24
120	12.8	21

CT scan revealed a mass in the pituitary fossa with suprasellar extension.

Aetiology and risk factors

Excessive amounts of growth hormone are produced in GH-secreting tumours in the pituitary. In acromegaly, the diagnosis is usually suspected before any specific tests are requested. By the time the clinical diagnosis is made the systemic effects are significant.

Pathology

This patient's symptoms, signs and laboratory findings are the results of exposure to excessive amounts of GH. The somatic effect of excessive GH on the skin and subcutaneous tissue results in enlarging hands and feet, producing the typical 'spade-like' hands. In addition, there is coarsening of facial features and an oily skin. Other somatic effects include hypertension, cardiomegaly and the prominence of the supraorbital ridges and nose.

The local effects of the growing tumour in the pituitary presented in this patient with frequent headaches and bitemporal hemianopia. This was confirmed by the CT scan, which showed suprasellar extension of the tumour and compression of the optic chiasma.

The biochemical findings are due to the elevated and non-suppressible serum GH levels. The oral glucose tolerance test in this patient showed a non-suppressible GH, despite the glucose load. In normal individuals given a glucose load, GH is suppressed to very low levels. In addition, the oral glucose tolerance test also confirmed that the patient was diabetic. This is not surprising as he gave a history of polyuria, his serum glucose concentration was high, and there were moderate amounts of glucose in his urine. Diabetes is seen in about 10% of acromegalics.

Management

The mainstay of treatment is to reduce the excessive GH production from the tumour by surgery (trans-sphenoidal) supplemented by external irradiation, plus dopamine agonists.

ACTINOMYCOSIS: An infection with *Actinomyces* spp. (Gram-positive rods) which occurs mainly in the cervicofacial region but may occur anywhere in the body, particularly in association with intrauterine contraceptive device and appendicectomy scars.

Aetiology and risk factors

Infection is endogenous, as *Actinomyces* are part of the normal flora of the oropharynx, vagina and gastrointestinal tract. The organism is introduced into the tissue following mucosal trauma, e.g. dental surgery, and proliferates in the tissue.

Pathology

Actinomycosis is the host's attempt to isolate the invading pathogen and confine the conflict to a restricted area of the body. By sequestering the invading pathogen in a fibrinous exudate, the normal clearing process is inhibited, leading ultimately to the formation of pus, walled off by the

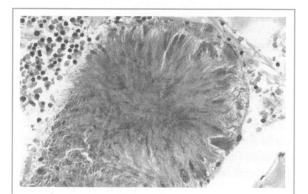

Fig. A5 Section of a 'sulphur' granule with surrounding inflammatory cells.

fibrin deposition and proliferation of fibroblasts. The pus is formed from the necrotic debris of host cells, including polymorphs and bacteria. The host mounts an acute pyogenic inflammatory reaction to the organism, leading to erythema, pain and swelling. As the infection becomes chronic, multiple draining sinuses are formed (see Mycetoma), discharging 'sulphur granules' to the surface of the skin (Fig. A5) and there is considerable fibrosis giving the indurated lesions a hard 'wooden' feel. Histologically the sulphur granules (microcolonies of the actinomycete) are surrounded by neutrophils and are walled off by fibrosis to produce a multi-loculated abscess. The organism may invade adjacent bone and occasionally haematogenous spread may occur to solid organs (e.g. the brain) or aspiration may occur to produce pulmonary disease.

Clinically the patient may present with an indurated swelling in the region of the oropharynx or abdominal scar with a fever and peripheral leucocytosis: weight loss, productive cough and haemoptysis if disease involves the lungs; intra-abdominal abscess following involvement of the gastrointestinal tract or cervix. Laboratory diagnosis is by histology and isolation of the organism and treatment is with penicillin for several months.

ACUTE BRONCHITIS: Acute inflammation of the trachea and bronchi caused mainly by viruses and some bacteria, e.g. *Streptococcus pneumoniae*, *Mycoplasma pneumoniae*.

ACUTE INFLAMMATION: See inflammation.

ACUTE LYMPHOBLASTIC LEUKAEMIA: A clonal proliferation of primitive lymphoblasts infiltrating bone marrow and blood.

A

Case

A 12-year-old schoolboy presented with a fortnight's history of mouth ulcers and aching joints. He had not been able to cycle because of his arthralgia and his mother had noted him to be unusually pale. He had also noticed occasional bruises and small red spots on his feet. There was no significant previous medical or family history. He had two sisters aged 10 and 13 who were well. On examination he had a fever of 39°C. Bruising was noted on his left arm and anterior chest and purpura on his feet. Numerous 1 cm lymph nodes were palpated in both axillae, groins and neck, but there was no palpable enlargement of liver or spleen. In the chest radiograph (Fig. A6) there was an upper mediastinal mass suggestive of thymic enlargement. The lung fields were clear.

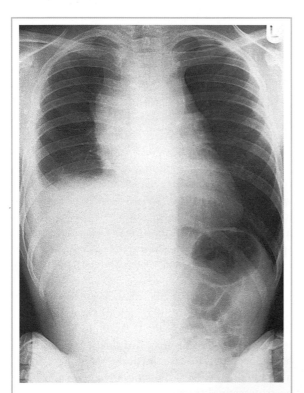

Fig. A6 Chest radiograph showing enlargement of the upper mediastinum due to a thymic mass.

The blood count showed:

WBC 133.0 × 10⁹/l
RBC 4.49 × 10¹²/l; Hb 11.6 g/dl; Hct (ratio) 0.344
MCV 90.5 fl; MCH 30.5 pg
MCHC 33.6 g/dl; RDW 14.0 %
Plt 24 × 10⁹/l
Differential: neutrophils 12%, lymphocytes 64%, monocytes 3%, blasts 21%.

A bone marrow aspirate showed gross hypercellularity, with reduced numbers of megakaryocytes and 95% blast cells with scanty erythroid and myeloid precursors. The blast cells showed negative staining for peroxidase. Five per cent of blast cells stained positively for PAS and the majority showed polar positivity with acid phosphatase. The bone marrow morphology is demonstrated in Figs. A7–A9. Immunological surface marker analysis by flow cytometry showed the blast cells to be positive for CD2, CD5, CD7 and Tdt (terminal deoxynucleotidyl transferase). Karyotype analysis of 20 Giemsa-banded metaphases showed normal chromosomes.

He was started on allopurinol, and a Hickman central venous catheter was inserted under general anaesthetic and with platelet transfusion cover.

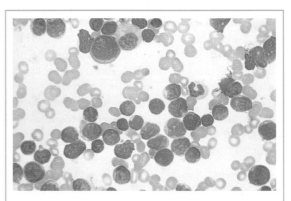

Fig. A7 Lymphoblasts in bone marrow aspirate.

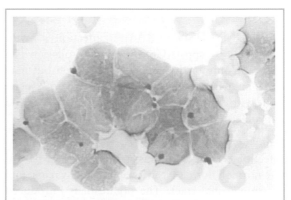

Fig. A8 Periodic acid Schiff (PAS) stains carbohydrate material in lymphoblasts red. Such positivity is characteristic of ALL and helps distinguish the disease from acute myeloid leukaemia (AML).

He started chemotherapy with vincristine and prednisolone. After 48 hours of chemotherapy, electrolytes showed: sodium 135, potassium 6.0,

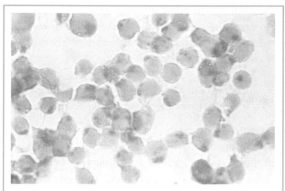

Fig. A9 Polar staining for the enzyme acid phosphatase is a characteristic finding in T-cells. This investigation has largely been replaced by immunological detection of T-cell antigens by flow cytometry.

bicarbonate 21, urea 14.8. Blood count showed a white cell count of 20.1. The electrolyte abnormalities settled with continuing intravenous hydration (3 litres daily). Further chemotherapy was administered through a peripheral vein according to the Medical Research Council Acute Lymphoblastic Leukaemia ALL97 protocol.

When blast cells had disappeared from the blood, a lumbar puncture was performed, with normal CSF findings. A bone marrow aspirate 4 weeks after presentation showed remission. Three months after presentation his stepfather developed shingles. Antibody titres indicated that the patient was not immune to varicella/zoster, so he was given an injection of zoster immunoglobulin.

After three courses of intensification chemotherapy, the patient was treated with 18 months of lower dose maintenance chemotherapy given as an outpatient. In addition he had a course of intrathecal methotrexate injections.

Aetiology and risk factors

Acute lymphoblastic leukaemia is the commonest malignant disease of childhood. After the age of 10 the incidence decreases with age until after the sixth decade when the incidence again increases. The best prognosis is found in patients between the ages of 1 and 10 years.

Most cases are sporadic and not associated with known aetiological factors. An inherited predisposition, though reported in a few families, is extremely rare and parents should be reassured that other siblings are most unlikely to suffer from the same disease. Periodically time–space clusters of

Table A3 Important cytogenetic abnormalities found in haematological malignancies

(a) Found mainly in lymphoid malignancies		
Cytogenetic abnormality	**Found in**	**Effect on prognosis (compared with average for that disease)**
Hyperdiploid	More than 47 chromosomes. Childhood ALL	Better
t(1;19)	Childhood pre-B-ALL	Worse
t(4;11)	Childhood ALL in infants age <1 year	Worse
t(8;14)	B-cell ALL and Burkitt lymphoma	Worse
t(14;18)	Follicular lymphoma – found in 3/4 cases	A diagnostic characteristic
(b) Found mainly in myeloid malignancies		
t(9;22)	Philadelphia chromosome found in chronic myeloid leukaemia and a small proportion of cases of acute myeloid and lymphoblastic leukaemia	A diagnostic characteristic in CML. Worsens prognosis in ALL and AML
t(15;17)	Acute promyelocytic leukaemia (M3) – better prognosis than average provided the patient does not die of disseminated intravascular coagulation during remission induction	Better
t(8;21)	AML with some evidence of differentiation (M2)	Better
inv(16)	Inversion of the long arm of chromosome 16. Found in acute myelomonocytic leukaemia (AML M4) with marrow eosinophilia (M4Eo)	Better
Abnormalities of chromosomes 5 and 7	Myelodysplasia and secondary acute myeloid leukaemia	Worse

acute lymphoblastic leukaemia and related diseases are reported in the UK and abroad. One much-publicized cluster occurred close to the Sellafield nuclear reprocessing plant in Cumbria, UK. It is likely that the increased incidence of ALL in this area is related to an unknown infectious or environmental factor other than radiation as similar clusters have been reported from other countries, nowhere near nuclear facilities.

Marrow cytogenetic abnormalities are found in a high proportion of cases of ALL and chromosome damage is likely to be aetiologically related to its development. The detection and characterization of these cytogenetic abnormalities is important because they act as markers of the disease, being absent in remission. They may also carry prognostic significance (Table A3), which dictates clinical treatment. One of the most powerful treatments for acute leukaemia is bone marrow transplantation* but this carries higher risks than conventional chemotherapy and should only be employed in poor prognosis cases at high risk of relapse. Such a case would be ALL with Philadelphia chromosome, a cytogenetic abnormality most commonly found in chronic myeloid leukaemia*.

Pathology

The white cell count is higher than that usually found in a reactive lymphocytosis. There is a high count of blast cells, which are not found in the blood in normal circumstances. This is associated with anaemia and thrombocytopenia due to impairment of marrow function by blast cell infiltration. Mouth ulcers are common in patients with decreased numbers of neutrophils in the blood. Bone pain and arthralgia are common in patients with malignant marrow infiltration and bone tenderness may be found on examination when pressing firmly on the sternum with the flat of the hand.

The blood electrolytes are normal at presentation, but after initial chemotherapy a minor degree of tumour lysis syndrome occurs. This is due to the release of various cytoplasmic constituents from tumour cells that are very sensitive to the cytotoxic effects of chemotherapy. Tumour lysis may be found in poorly differentiated lymphoproliferative disorders, particularly when associated with a high tumour bulk. The release of phosphate from within cells combines with and removes calcium and release of potassium causes hyperkalaemia. Breakdown of large amounts of nucleic acid results in hyperuricaemia. Sometimes, release of tissue thromboplastin from damaged tumour cells may cause disseminated intravascular coagulation*. Tumour lysis syndrome can be prevented by hydra-

tion before chemotherapy and premedication with the xanthine oxidase inhibitor allopurinol. In patients at high risk, a graded start to chemotherapy may then be made.

Classification of ALL

Normal lymphocytes may be classified as T-lymphocytes or B-lymphocytes. Malignant lymphoid cells may be similarly classified by immunological methods. Most cases of childhood lymphoblastic leukaemia are of early B-cell lineage – pre-B-cell ALL. Historically, one of the first antigens to be reliably detected on ALL blast cells was the common ALL antigen. In the 'cluster of differentiation' (CD) antigen classification system this is CD10. More than 90% of cases of childhood ALL express the CD10 antigen. In the case described, the blast cells are of T-cell lineage, and express antigens such as CD2 and CD5. T-cell disease carries a worse prognosis than pre-B-cell ALL. This may in part be because cases of T-ALL have a higher blast cell count in the blood at presentation. Table A4 shows some of the CD antigens commonly used in the immunological classification of acute leukaemias.

Table A4 Cluster of differentiation (CD) markers used in the diagnosis of acute leukaemia

B-cell markers	T-cell markers	Myeloid markers
CD10	CD2	CD13
CD19	CD5	CD33
CD20	CD7	CD34

B-cell ALL is the rarest of the immunological subtypes and has characteristic morphological, immunological and cytogenetic features. In conventionally stained smears, the blast cells of B-ALL have characteristic deep blue staining cytoplasm and prominent clear cytoplasmic vacuoles. These cells are identical to those found in Burkitt tropical lymphoma*. The cytogenetic abnormality usually consists of a translocation between chromosomes 8 and 14. B-ALL carries a relatively poor prognosis.

Sanctuary disease in ALL

In early chemotherapy trials for the treatment of ALL it was found that lymphoblasts could be cleared from blood and bone marrow but patients would relapse with nervous system disease. The central nervous system, testes and eyes are 'sanctuary sites' where chemotherapy may not penetrate. To prevent this, injections of some chemotherapeutic agents are given directly into the cerebrospinal fluid by lumbar puncture. Some patients also have cranial radiotherapy.

Management

Supportive treatment with red cell transfusions, platelet transfusions and antibiotics for neutropenic sepsis is important. Chemotherapy treatment is divided into three phases: induction, consolidation and maintenance. Induction chemotherapy, given over about a month, usually results in a remission, when the blood and bone marrow go back to normal appearances. Without further consolidation chemotherapy most patients would relapse. Most patients with ALL then have an extended period of 1–2 years of maintenance chemotherapy, given at low doses as an outpatient. Patients with relapsed or poor prognosis disease may be treated by bone marrow transplantation. Treatment of the CNS has been referred to above. Approximately three-quarters of cases of childhood ALL may be cured by chemotherapy, but cure is less likely in adults.

ACUTE MYELOID (MYELOBLASTIC) LEUK-AEMIA: A clonal proliferation of primitive myeloid cells infiltrating bone marrow and blood.

Case

A 33-year-old man attended at his local A&E department complaining of nosebleeds and blood blisters in his mouth. These had been troubling him intermittently for the last week. On examination he was noted to have purpura of the lower limbs and a fever of 38°C. A blood count and coagulation screen were performed:

WBC 29.0 × 10⁹/l
RBC 4.59 × 10¹²/l; Hb 13.6 g/dl; Hct (ratio) 0.385
MCV 85 fl; MCH 30.1 pg
MCHC 35.2 g/dl; RDW 13.3 %
Plt 12 × 10⁹/l
Differential: neutrophils 5%, lymphocytes 14%, myelocytes 1%, promyelocytes 63%, blasts 17%.

Because of his bleeding problems, coagulation studies were also performed with the following results:

Prothrombin time 12 seconds (control 12 seconds)
APTT 35 seconds (control 32 seconds)
Thrombin time 17 seconds (control 12 seconds)
Fibrinogen degradation products 2.5 mg/l (normal <2.5)
Fibrinogen titre 1 in 16 (normal 1 in 32 or higher).

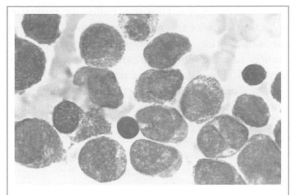

Fig. A10 Bone marrow aspirate in acute promyelocytic leukaemia showing hypergranular promyelocytes some of which have characteristic dumb-bell shaped nuclei and Auer rods.

The presence of blast cells in the blood suggested a diagnosis of acute leukaemia so a bone marrow aspirate was performed (Fig. A10). This was grossly hypercellular, with reduced numbers of megakary-ocytes; 40% of nucleated cell were blasts, and 50% hypergranular promyelocytes. Sudan black staining showed numerous Auer rods (Fig. A11). The appearances were of acute myeloid leukaemia with partial differentiation to promyelocytic forms (acute promyelocytic leukaemia – FAB type M3). Cytogenetic studies on bone marrow cells showed a reciprocal translocation involving chromosomes 15 and 17 – t(15;17).

The patient was treated with combination chemotherapy of daunorubicin, cytosine arabi-noside and etoposide, with allopurinol and the synthetic vitamin A analogue ATRA (all-*trans* retinoic acid) as a differentiation-inducing agent. After his first course, he developed a pancytopenia with a hypoplastic marrow and no evidence of leukaemic infiltration. Blood transfusion and

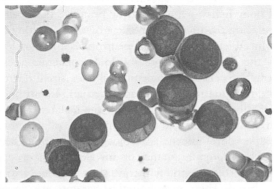

Fig. A11 Myeloblasts containing Auer rods in the blood of a patient with AML, FAB type M1.

A

platelet support was required. Following remission induction he was treated with a second course of the same drugs as consolidation therapy. Two months later he relapsed, again with promyelocytic forms in the blood. A second remission was induced with a combination of idarubicin and high-dose cytosine arabinoside chemotherapy. Tissue typing of his two siblings showed that his younger brother was an HLA match and after a second remission was induced he was referred to a transplant centre for bone marrow transplantation*.

Aetiology and risk factors

Acute myeloid leukaemia (AML) is associated with abnormal proliferation and failure of differentiation of myeloid precursors. The underlying defect appears to lie within DNA. In AML a frequently detected abnormality is a point mutation within the *ras* oncogene. This codes for a family of proteins that control cellular division, differentiation and apoptosis. If Ras protein is injected into resting cells it induces DNA synthesis, as if the cell was entering an active phase of division. Normal cells depend on stimulation by cytokine growth factors to prevent them dying in an organized fashion termed apoptosis*. The expression of Ras proteins in some cell lines prevents apoptosis on withdrawal of cytokine stimulation. The cause of mutations in the *ras* oncogene is unclear but may be chemical, viral or radiation induced. Not all cases of AML have mutations affecting the *ras* oncogene and it is likely that several mechanisms may result in the genesis of AML. The majority of cases of AML have structural defects of the chromosomes, visible by microscopy, which may be prognostically useful, as discussed below.

The pre-leukaemic condition myelodysplasia eventually progresses to AML, though it may not do so for a number of years.

Pathology

Acute leukaemia is characterized by the infiltration of bone marrow and blood by primitive blast cells, replacing the normal bone marrow and resulting in reduced levels of red cells, neutrophils and platelets in the blood. In acute myeloid leukaemia these primitive cells may sometimes show a small degree of differentiation which may be recognized morphologically. In this case many of the leukaemic cells have differentiated to the promyelocyte stage before further development was blocked. Sometimes the visible differentiation may be down one of the recognized developmental pathways such as monocyte or erythroid. These morphological variants are classified by the French-American-British (FAB) morphological classification (see below).

In acute myeloid leukaemia of all types, a crystallization of the normal myeloid cytoplasmic granules may be found as thin stick-like structures in the cytoplasm of the myeloid blast cells termed Auer rods. These are not found in acute lymphoblastic leukaemia. They are particularly common in FAB types M2 and M3. In acute promyelocytic leukaemia, they may clump together to form bundles termed faggots.

Another common feature of acute promyelocytic leukaemia is disseminated intravascular coagulation*, particularly during induction chemotherapy, although the patient considered above had only modest abnormalities of his thrombin time and plasma fibrinogen concentration. Chemotherapy disrupts the abnormal promyelocytes, releasing their procoagulant granules. These activate the coagulation and fibrinolytic systems, with worsening thrombocytopenia and prolongation of all coagulation tests. Vigorous support with transfusions of platelets and fresh frozen plasma is often required during induction chemotherapy of promyelocytic leukaemia, and excessive fibrinolysis should be blocked by anti-fibrinolytic drugs such as tranexamic acid.

The French-American-British classification of AML

- M0: acute myeloid leukaemia undifferentiated. No morphological feature to distinguish it from ALL. Cytochemistry or analysis of immunological surface markers will be required.
- M1: acute myeloid leukaemia with recognizable myeloid features such as Auer rods.
- M2: acute myeloid leukaemia with a few cells differentiating to the promyelocyte stage. There is an association with the good-prognosis translocation t(8;21).
- M3: acute promyelocytic leukaemia. Many Auer rods are usually seen, and there is a good-prognosis cytogenetic translocation t(15;17).
- M4: myelomonocytic leukaemia. A mixture of granulocyte and monocyte precursors is present in the bone marrow, which may be identified by morphology, cytochemistry, and immunological surface markers.
- M5: pure monocytic leukaemia. The blast cells stain for non-specific (monocyte) esterase and express the monocyte antigen CD14. Clinically these patients may have tissue infiltration by monoblasts, causing hypertrophy of the gums and enlargement of liver, spleen and lymph nodes, which is unusual in other varieties of AML.
- M6: acute erythroleukaemia. Some of the blast cells are erythroid precursors.

• M7: acute megakaryoblastic leukaemia.
As with any morphological grouping, the FAB classification is subjective and there will be some intermediate cases.

Management
As with acute lymphoblastic leukaemia, chemotherapy treatment is divided into induction and consolidation phases, though there is no proven role for maintenance chemotherapy in AML. Many of the chemotherapeutic drugs used in ALL are also used in AML, though steroids are not of proven benefit in AML. Central nervous system leukaemia is rare in AML, so intrathecal chemotherapy is not routinely employed. Supportive treatment with red cell transfusion, antibiotics for infection during phases of neutropenia and platelet transfusion support are vitally important. Bone marrow transplantation provides a powerful, though risky, method of treatment and there are many international trials in progress to define its role.

Patients with good prognosis AML may be cured with chemotherapy only. Such patients may be identified by cytogenetic means as t(8;21), t(15;17) and inv16 are known to be associated with a good prognosis. The response to the first course of chemotherapy is also related to prognosis, patients in marrow remission before their second course of chemotherapy tending to do better. Some cytogenetic abnormalities are associated with a worse prognosis, such as the presence of a t(9;22) (Philadelphia chromosome), loss of chromosomes 7 or 5 and complex cytogenetic abnormalities. These patients would have bone marrow transplant in first remission if they are young enough, fit enough and have a suitable donor.

ACUTE TUBULAR NECROSIS: The most common cause of renal failure, characterized by abnormal renal function as a result of destruction of tubular epithelial cells. Causes include ischaemia and drug toxicity.

 Renal failure

ADDISON DISEASE: A condition resulting from a deficiency of adrenocortical hormones.

Case
A 30-year-old lady was brought into casualty in a coma. Her friends said that she had been feeling unwell for some time and had had bouts of vomiting and nausea.

On examination, she was pale and dehydrated. There was evidence of hyperpigmentation noticed in her axillae, perineum and mouth (Fig. A12). Her

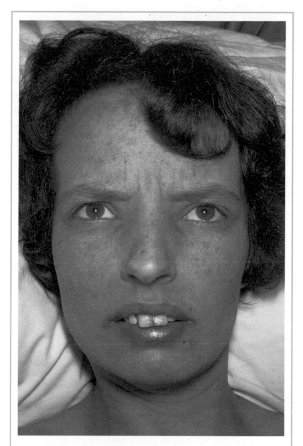

Fig. A12 Patient with Addison disease showing skin pigmentation. (Reproduced with permission from Toghill, PJ (ed.) *Examining Patients. An Introduction to Clinical Medicine*. London: Edward Arnold, 1995)

blood pressure was 90/50 mmHg. Blood tests revealed a sodium 116 mmol/l, potassium 5.6 mmol/l, glucose 2.0 mmol/l (random) and urea 19 mmol/l.

While in casualty, the senior house officer decided to perform a short Synacthen test (ACTH stimulation test). Her cortisol levels were measured, and the results became available later (see Table A5).

Based on her symptoms, a diagnosis of Addison disease was made, and this was confirmed by the inadequate cortisol response to ACTH.

Table A5 Synacthen test results

Time after ACTH (min)	Serum cortisol (nmol/l)
0	90
30	110
60	120

Aetiology and risk factors

A reduction in circulating glucocorticoids produced by the adrenal gland can arise acutely or chronically. The causes of Addison disease can be divided into three main categories: acute, chronic and drugs (Table A6). Meningitis is a common cause of acute adrenal insufficiency in children, whilst in the elderly, the cause is more likely to be autoimmunity or a chronic disease such as tuberculosis. As with

Table A6 Categories of Addison disease

Acute	Chronic	Drugs
Adrenal haemorrhage	Autoimmune	Metyrapone
Infections – meningitis	Infections – tuberculosis, histoplasmosis, cryptococcosis	Amino-glutethimide
Anticoagulant therapy	Haemochromatosis	Ketoconazole
Adrenal vein thrombosis	Metastatic tumour	
Surgery	CAH Steroid therapy	

other autoimmune endocrine diseases, there is an association with HLA-B8 and DR3. A high prevalence of other autoimmune diseases such as Hashimoto thyroiditis*, hypothyroidism*, insulin-dependent diabetes mellitus* are associated with autoimmune-related Addison disease. Autoantibodies to several adrenal antigens are found and also autoantibodies to steroid 21-hydroxylase p450 are found in most autoimmune patients with Addison disease.

Pathology

The symptoms, signs and laboratory findings that the patient presented are the result of exposure to lower than normal amounts of cortisol.

The biochemical manifestations of reduced cortisol are reduced gluconeogenesis and reduced mineralocorticoid activity, which result in a low blood sugar, increased salt excretion and potassium retention in the renal tubules, giving rise to the hypoglycaemia, hyponatraemia and hyperkalaemia seen in this patient. In addition, serum chloride is decreased and there is an acidosis.

The reduced amount of cortisol results in an increase in ACTH release from the pituitary. This is co-released with a β-lipoprotein, which is hydrol-

ysed to β-melanocyte-stimulating hormone (MSH). This results in the marked pigmentation observed in the axillae, perineum and oral cavity of this patient.

The hypotension observed in this patient arises as a consequence of the loss of myocardial contractility, diminished vascular tone and contraction of blood volume, which are enhanced by the action of cortisol. The increased urea resulted from dehydration and reduced renal perfusion.

The diagnosis of Addison disease is relatively simple to make. The short Synacthen test is performed and in this patient the 30 min (110 nmol/l) and 60 min (120 nmol/l) cortisol levels do not suggest an adequate response, even though there is an increase compared to the basal value (90 nmol/l). The normal response would be a rise of 180 nmol/l from the basal value. In this patient, the adrenals failed to increase plasma cortisol in response to a standard dose of ACTH.

Management

Treatment is with glucocorticoid (cortisol) replacement. Fludrocortisone is also necessary to correct the mineralocorticoid deficiency.

ADENOCARCINOMA: A malignant tumour of glandular tissue.

 Breast carcinoma; Colorectal carcinoma; Lung carcinoma

ADENOMA: A benign tumour of glandular epithelium. The malignant counterpart is adenocarcinoma. Adenomas may be solid, papillary or polypoid, and in some cases multiple.

 Polyp; polyposis

ADENOMATOUS POLYPOSIS COLI: An autosomal dominant disorder in which patients develop hundreds of polyps in the colon with subsequent transformation into colorectal carcinoma.

Aetiology and risk factors

The disease is due to an inherited germline mutation in the adenomatous polyposis coli (APC) gene, which is on chromosome 5q21.

Pathology

Patients with inherited defects in the APC gene develop numerous adenomatous polyps throughout the colon (Fig. A13). It is inevitable that one of these adenomas will transform into a malignant tumour (Fig. A14). A large proportion of non-familial colorectal carcinomas also show mutations in the APC gene.

A

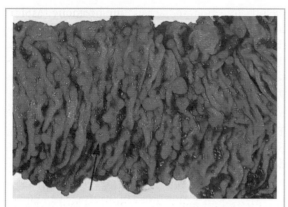

Fig. A13 Large bowel with numerous polyps in patient with familial adenomatous polyposis. (Reproduced with permission from Lakhani SR, Dilly SA, Finlayson CJ. *Basic Pathology*, 2nd edn. London: Arnold, 1998)

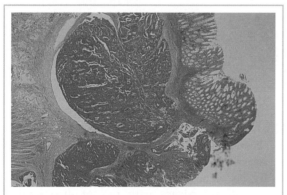

Fig. A14 Invasive adenocarcinoma of colon.

Management

This comprises resection of the colon harbouring the polyps. If surgical removal is not carried out, the patient will present with an invasive cancer. Close follow-up and genetic counselling is also offered to the patients.

 Adenoma; Colorectal carcinoma

ADENOSINE DEAMINASE DEFICIENCY: An enzyme deficiency of the DNA salvage pathway leading to severe combined immunodeficiency. Adenosine deaminase (ADA) catalyses the conversion of adenosine to inosine and deoxyadenosine into deoxyinosine in the purine pathway; ADA deficiency leads to accumulation of dATP which is toxic to lymphoid stem cells. Its relief was the first example of successful 'gene therapy'.

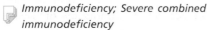 *Immunodeficiency; Severe combined immunodeficiency*

ADULT RESPIRATORY DISTRESS SYNDROME: A syndrome caused by diffuse alveolar capillary damage with resultant respiratory failure and later multisystem failure. Other names include 'shock lung' and 'diffuse alveolar damage' (DAD).

Case

A 75-year-old man was admitted to hospital with uncontrolled bleeding following a tooth extraction. He had had a tooth removed that afternoon but the bleeding had failed to stop. His tooth socket was packed with gauze and haematological and biochemical investigations were arranged. Chest radiograph was reported as normal.

Blood tests showed:

Hb 12.0 g/l
WCC 8 × 10⁹/l
Platelets 40 × 10⁹/l
Coagulation screen normal
Biochemistry normal.

He was transferred to the ward where he was transfused with platelets. Later that evening, he started to complain of feeling unwell and short of breath. Examination revealed tachycardia, tachypnoea and a blood pressure of 100/70 mmHg. Auscultation revealed evidence of mild cardiac failure. He was treated with a diuretic and had regular monitoring. The next day his condition had deteriorated with increasing dyspnoea. He became cyanosed and his blood gases showed him to be hypoxic. Chest radiograph showed dense consolidation (Fig. A15). He was transferred to the

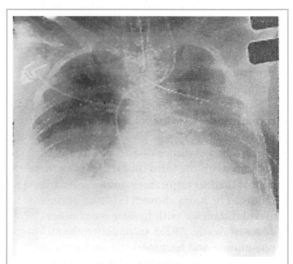

Fig. A15 Chest radiograph showing dense consolidation in the lower lobes. (Reproduced with permission from Evans T, Haslett C. *Acute Respiratory Distress Syndrome*. London: Arnold, 1992)

Intensive Care Unit. Despite intubation and artificial ventilation, he failed to show improvement and over the next 48 hours, his condition continued to deteriorate. He had a cardiac arrest and was certified dead. A postmortem examination was carried out the next day.

Postmortem findings The postmortem conclusions were:

- respiratory system: both lungs were heavy and congested. Slicing revealed intra-alveolar haemorrhage and patchy bronchopneumonia. Histological examination of the lungs confirmed the presence of bronchopneumonia but in addition, alveolar spaces contained hyaline membranes and hyperplasia of type II pneumocytes (Fig. A16). Occasional alveolar spaces were replaced by fibrous tissue.

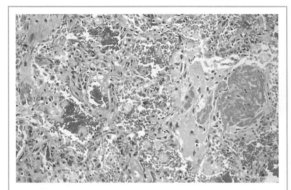

Fig. A16 Histological section of the lung showing haemorrhage and hyaline membranes within alveolar spaces.

- lymphoreticular system: he had enlarged para-aortic lymph nodes which on slicing revealed a homogeneous, pale, cut surface. Histology confirmed a diagnosis of non-Hodgkin lymphoma. The bone marrow was extensively replaced by tumour.
- comment: the bleeding diathesis was caused by marrow failure secondary to metastatic disease. He also had evidence of pneumonia and this, together with the intra-alveolar haemorrhage contributed to respiratory failure and cardiac failure. The lungs showed evidence of diffuse alveolar damage with hyaline membranes.
- cause of death: ARDS secondary to bronchopneumonia and haemorrhage secondary to disseminated lymphoma.

Aetiology and risk factors

ARDS is the final manifestation of damage to alveolar capillary walls due to a host of causes. These include infection and sepsis, drug toxicity, aspiration of gastric contents, air and fat emboli, radiotherapy, trauma and fracture, uraemia, pancreatitis, disseminated intravascular coagulation and inhalation of irritant gases including high concentrations of oxygen.

Pathology

The case illustrated here is unusual in terms of presentation; however, patients who develop ARDS do present with a variety of symptoms. Since the main underlying pathology is diffuse damage to capillary walls, a wide range of disorders can potentially result in this life-threatening situation. Once capillary damage occurs, fluid leaks out into alveolar spaces and the lungs become heavy, red and congested. Intra-alveolar oedema compromises the respiratory function further, which in turn can have profound effects on the cardiac and systemic systems. The leakage from capillaries results in a fibrin-rich fluid and this, together with the remnants of the dead epithelial cells (lipids and cytoplasm), leads to the characteristic hyaline membranes seen in ARDS. There is a reactive hyperplasia of type II pneumocytes. Oxygen, which is used to treat the hypoxia, may itself perpetuate the disorder and patients with severe ARDS eventually become resistant to oxygen therapy.

The presence of bronchopneumonia and metastatic disease conspires to worsen the ARDS, directly by further damage within the lung and indirectly by the bleeding tendency with risk of disseminated intravascular coagulation (DIC) in the patient. Once ARDS is established, there is a risk of cardiac failure and renal failure and unless the spiral into systemic failure is halted, death becomes inevitable.

A similar histological picture in the lungs is also seen in hyaline membrane disease in the newborn. Note, however, that whereas ARDS results from damage to capillary walls, hyaline membrane disease is due to a lack of surfactant.

Management

The key to management is the treatment of the underlying condition such as bronchopneumonia or withdrawal of drugs that may be toxic. Supportive treatment with oxygen may become necessary to treat the hypoxaemia. Patients may also require artificial ventilation while attempts are made to break the vicious cycle set up, leading to multi-system failure.

 Bronchopneumonia; Disseminated intravascular coagulation, Lymphoma

AGRANULOCYTOSIS: A condition of severe neutropenia, often associated with fever and stomatitis or other pyogenic infection. It may occur as an idiosyncratic reaction to drugs such as carbimazole or rarely as an autoimmune phenomenon. It may be a predictable response to cytotoxic drugs or radiotherapy, in which case thrombocytopenia is usually also present.

ALCOHOLIC LIVER DISEASE: In patients who consume large amounts of alcohol over a long period, liver disease may manifest as fatty liver, acute hepatitis, chronic liver disease, or cirrhosis*.

Fatty liver is a common early manifestation of excessive alcohol intake, characterized by fat globules accumulating within the hepatocyte; this causes diffuse enlargement of the hepatocytes and the condition is reversible if the patient stops drinking alcohol. **Acute alcoholic liver disease** (hepatitis) is characterized by focal lytic necrosis of hepatocytes with neutrophil infiltration of the sinuosoids and hepatocytes, cholestasis and sclerosis around the central venule. In addition, there are Mallory bodies in the cytoplasm of the hepatocytes. **Chronic alcohol liver disease** is a result of repeated insult from alcohol and results in necrosis, progressive fibrosis in the centrizonal region of the liver and some distortion of liver architecture and regeneration; this condition may be reversible. In **cirrhosis** of the liver, there is ongoing hepatocyte necrosis, extensive fibrosis, nodules of regenerating hepatocytes, loss of normal liver architecture and irreversible damage.

The clinical presentation depends on the type of liver disease. In fatty liver the presentation is hepatomegaly with liver function tests showing mild abnormalities, e.g. elevation of the aminotransferases and γ-glutamyltransferase. In acute hepatitis, the presentation is acutely with fever, jaundice, tender hepatomegaly and ascites. In very severe cases, encephalopathy and death may occur. Laboratory tests reveal increased liver enzymes (aminotransferases and γ-glutamyltransferase), bilirubin, alkaline phosphatase and prothrombin time. In chronic alcohol liver disease and cirrhosis, the clinical manifestations are of insidious onset and are jaundice, mild tender hepatomegaly, splenomegaly, palmar erythema, spider telangiectasia, hormonal disturbances, variceal bleeding, encephalopathy, coagulopathy and ascites. Hepatoma is a complication in about 10% of patients.

Cirrhosis; Fatty liver; Macrocytic anaemia

ALKAPTONURIA: A rare autosomal recessive disorder which occurs as a result of a deficiency in the enzyme homogentisic acid oxidase. This results in the accumulation of homogentisic acid and its metabolites in collagen (dermis, ligaments, tendons, etc.) and cartilage (nose, ear, larynx, etc.). All these areas become black and radiopaque and the urine darkens on exposure. Clinical symptoms (arthritis) appear in the weight-bearing joints and may be severely debilitating, resulting in juvenile osteoarthrosis.

ALLERGY: Allergy, atopy, and type I hypersensitivity are nearly synonymous terms. Strictly speaking, type I hypersensitivity refers to harmful immune responses associated with overproduction of specific IgE and mast cell degranulation, atopy refers to the predisposition to such conditions, whereas the resulting diseases are termed 'allergic'.

Case

An 18-year old schoolboy performed less well in his June exams than expected because of almost continuous watering of his nose and eyes, with episodes of repeated sneezing and blocked nose requiring frequent application of decongestant drops. The previous summer, on holiday in California, he had had a bad attack of wheezing, but this had not recurred. His mother was 'allergic to cats'. His GP diagnosed hay fever and referred him to an allergist, who skin tested him and detected an immediate response to pollen. His chest radiographs, blood count and blood chemistry were normal, but his serum IgE was markedly raised at 610 IU/ml (normal 3–150). Allergic rhinitis (hay fever) was confirmed and he was prescribed sodium cromoglycate nasal inhalation and eye drops, which kept the condition under control. Now a medical student, he additionally uses a corticosteroid spray at exam time.

Aetiology and risk factors

About one individual in six displays allergic responses to some foreign antigen ('allergen') and as many as one in three are positive on skin testing. Allergies to foods (e.g. eggs, milk) may develop before the age of 2, but those to inhaled antigens come on a few years later. A family history is very common, and the response to particular allergens is linked to particular HLA-DR alleles. There is also evidence for a gene (11q13) controlling the tendency to overproduce IgE. Some of the commonest allergens are shown in Table A7.

Pathology

The underlying pathology in all atopic diseases is similar. Specific IgE is formed against one or more allergen, and binds to mast cells and/or basophils;

A

Table A7 Some common allergens

Plant pollens	Animals products	Foodstuffs	Other
Rye	House dust mite (faeces)	Eggs	Fungal spores
Timothy	Non-biting midges	Milk	Moulds
Ragweed	Cat dander	Shrimp/prawns	
Russian thistle	Dog dander	Cod	
Alder	Horse dander	Nuts (peanuts)	
Silver birch	Bee venom		
Hazel	Wasp venom		
Japanese cedar			

further contact with the allergen causes the mast cells to degranulate, releasing molecules that increase local vascular permeability. Note that these molecules may have more than one physiological effect (Table A8).

Table A8 The major products of degranulating mast cells and their effects

Product	Effects
Inflammatory activator Histamine	Vasodilation and vascular permeability
Platelet activation factor (PAF)	Microthrombi
Tryptase	Activates C3
Kininogenase	Generates kinins which cause vasodilation and oedema
Chemoattractants Cytokines, e.g. IL-5, TNFα and IL-8	Affect neutrophils, eosinophils and basophils
Leukotriene B4, PAF	basophils
Spasmogens Histamine	Bronchial smooth muscle contraction
Prostaglandin D2	Mucosal oedema and mucus secretion
Leukotriene C4 and D4	

The actual symptoms depend on where this process takes place. In the case described above it would have been limited to the nasal and ocular mucous membranes. In allergic asthma*, which accounts for about 60% of all asthma, the mucus lining of the airways is the main target, with hyper-

secretion of mucus and constriction of the bronchi, resulting in wheezing, shortness of breath and a sticky cough. Reactions in the skin lead to urticaria*, whilst reactions in the gut wall lead to food allergy, with pain, vomiting and diarrhoea. When the allergen reaches the blood in large amounts (e.g. bee venom or penicillin in susceptible subjects) the symptoms may be systemic and severe with circulatory shock*, which may even be fatal; this is known as anaphylaxis*.

Management

This depends on the location. Hay fever is usually well controlled by intranasal cromoglycate and/or steroids, together with avoidance of allergen where possible.

 Anaphylaxis; Asthma

ALPORT SYNDROME: A form of hereditary nephritis, associated with nerve deafness and eye disorders, including cataracts and corneal dystrophy.

ALVEOLAR PROTEINOSIS: A disease of unknown aetiology, characterized by diffuse pulmonary infiltrates on x-ray. Histologically there is accumulation within alveolar spaces of a granular, PAS-positive material that contains lipid. It may become chronic but does not lead to fibrosis.

ALVEOLITIS: Inflammation of alveolar walls.

 Pneumoconiosis

ALZHEIMER DISEASE: A degenerative condition of the cerebral cortex leading to dementia.

Case

While attending the surgery for a common cold, a lady mentioned to the doctor that her 66-year-old husband had started to get forgetful and appeared to have bouts of depression. He had retired as a university professor the previous year and the symptoms were put down to 'coming to terms with retirement from academic life'. Three years later, the doctor met the gentleman at the shopping arcade. The man did not recognize the doctor and became agitated by the meeting. Two years later, his wife came to see the doctor because his memory loss had become severe and he was failing to recognize members of his own family. The memory loss combined with his mood change and depression meant that on two occasions, he had failed to come back from his walk and the police had to be alerted to find him.

The doctor arranged for a formal examination by a neurologist and psychiatrist who concluded that he had short memory deficit and personality change as a result of dementia. Over the next 2 years he became progressively worse with loss of sphincter control. He died in hospital following a chest infection. A postmortem examination was carried out.

> **Postmortem examination** Examination confirmed the presence of bilateral bronchopneumonia. The rest of the systemic examination was unremarkable apart from the central nervous system. His brain weighed 1050 g and showed marked atrophy of the cerebral cortex (Fig. A17). Slicing the brain revealed compensatory dilatation of the cerebral ventricles. Histological examination of the section from the cortex revealed numerous neuritic plaques, neurofibrillary tangles and features of an amyloid angiopathy (Fig. A18).
> Conclusion: features consistent with Alzheimer disease.

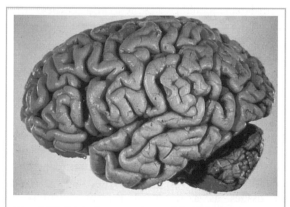

Fig. A17 Brain from patient with Alzheimer disease showing marked cerebral atrophy.

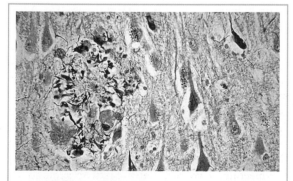

Fig. A18 Histological section of the brain on silver stain, showing the classical neurofibrillary tangles of Alzheimer plaque.

Aetiology and risk factors

Most cases are sporadic and the pathogenesis remains unclear although it is postulated that it may represent a disorder of the processing of amyloid precursors. Family history is recognized as a risk factor. People with Down syndrome who survive beyond 40 years of age inevitably develop Alzheimer disease.

Pathology

The symptoms are related to the loss of cerebral cortical tissue as a result of atrophy. The characteristic features are the presence of neurofibrillary tangle and plaques. The tangles represent bundles of filaments, which are present within the cytoplasm of cortical neurons, and these occasionally show a classical 'flame-shaped' appearance. They are by no means specific for Alzheimer disease and may also be seen in Parkinson disease and in supranuclear palsy; hence, they may represent an end result of a number of different processes. Neuritic plaques have a central amyloid core composed of Aβ protein. This may be the link with Down syndrome since this protein is coded for by a gene on chromosome 21. Amyloid angiopathy is a result of deposition of abnormal amyloid protein in the vessel walls.

Whilst all these features point to the diagnosis of Alzheimer disease, they are not specific and the diagnosis rests on a correlation of clinical and pathological findings. The histopathological features are also seen to a variable extent in brains of elderly individuals who do not have the clinical manifestations described above.

Management

No treatment is currently available that either halts the progress of or cures the disease, so management is supportive.

 Dementia; Down syndrome; Parkinson disease

AMNIONITIS: Acute inflammation of the amniotic sac and amniotic fluid which can be caused by a number of different bacteria, commonly group B *Streptococcus* and *Listeria monocytogenes*.

AMOEBIASIS: A disease caused by the protozoan *Entamoeba histolytica*, which can range from mild diarrhoea to severe dysentery with fever, blood, and mucus.

Aetiology and risk factors

The organism is acquired by faeco-oral spread due to poor sanitation, eating faecally contaminated vegetables or by sexual practices. *Ent. histolytica* has two forms, the trophozoite and the cyst; the latter, being resistant to adverse environmental conditions, is responsible for transmission.

Pathology

The trophozoite of *Ent. histolytica* binds to the colonic mucus and epithelial cells. Colonic cells and polymorphs are lysed by the trophozoite (rather like a giant macrophage attacking bacteria), possibly by pore-forming toxins. Contact with the matrix proteins induces the trophozoite to release cysteine proteases, which degrade collagen, laminin, etc. Cell death and disruption of the matrix proteins eventually result in the characteristic flask-shaped colonic ulcers with symptoms of dysentery (bloody diarrhoea) (Fig. A19). The lysis of polymorphs also releases lysosomal contents, which further aggravate the host damage. There is little inflammatory infiltrate in the mucosae between the ulcers.

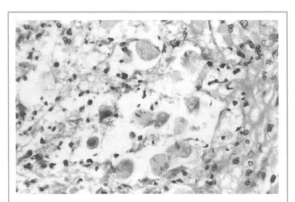

Fig. A19 Amoebic colitis containing numerous amoeba at the base of an ulcer.

The patient presents with fever, weight loss, right upper quadrant pain and tenderness, and an enlarged liver. There is peripheral neutrophilia with elevated conjugated bilirubin, alkaline phosphatase, liver transaminases, and acute phase proteins. Rarely, amoebiasis may present as a skin ulcer or as an amoeboma (a granulomatous reaction) resembling a colonic adenoma. Complications of intestinal amoebiasis are perforation and invasion and dissemination of the amoeba to give rise to abscesses typically in the liver, lung or brain. Diagnosis is made by serology and by demonstration of the trophozoites or cysts in the faeces. Treatment is with a nitroimidazole. Diloxanide, chloroquine and tetracycline are also used.

AMYLOIDOSIS: An extracellular deposition of the proteinaceous material amyloid.

Aetiology and risk factors

Amyloidosis may be localized or systemic. It is often a reactive process secondary to systemic inflammatory disorders but may also occur in patients with

Table A9 Pathogenesis of amyloidosis

Disorder	Amyloid fibril	Related serum protein
Systemic		
Immune dyscrasia	AL	Ig light chains
Reactive systemic	AA	SAA
Neuropathic type 1	ATTR	Transthyretin
Non-neuropathic	AA	SAA
Haemodialysis associated	Aβ2m	β2-Microglobulin
Senile	Ascl	Atrial natriuretic peptide
Localized		
Cerebral (Alzheimer, Down)	Aβ2	APP
Endocrine related	AE	Calcitonin, Islet amyloid peptide, etc.
Plasmacytoma	AL	Ig light chain
Cutaneous	AD	? Keratin

APP, amyloid precursor protein; SAA, serum amyloid associated.

plasma cell malignancies, on haemodialysis, or with endocrine tumours (see Table A9).

Pathology

The term 'amyloid' was coined by Virchow because of the reaction of this material to iodine and sulphuric acid, indicating a 'starch like' substance.

The organs affected by amyloidosis become enlarged and firm compared with normal tissues. Although non-toxic in itself, amyloid causes damage to tissues as a result of pressure atrophy or ischaemia. The presence of the material in glomeruli or heart muscle can also affect the normal function of these tissues. Organs commonly affected include the heart, kidneys, joints, skin and soft tissues (Fig. A20).

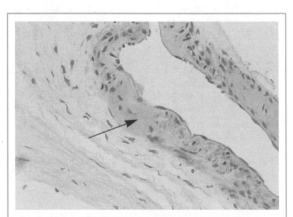

Fig. A20 Extracellular amyloid deposition in blood vessel. (Reproduced with permission from Lakhani SR, Dilly SA, Finlayson CJ. *Basic Pathology*, 2nd edn. London: Arnold, 1998)

On light microscopy amyloid appears similar in all tissues; however, it is a heterogeneous material with many different chemical compositions and hence aetiologies.

The pathogenesis of amyloidosis is far from clear but is believed to be fundamentally due to the production of amyloid proteins through catabolism of precursor molecules. These precursor molecules may result from an excess production, a reduced excretion or production of an abnormal form of the protein (Table A9).

Management
This is of the underlying disorder. There is no treatment for established amyloidosis.

 Dementia; Down syndrome; Myeloma; Osteomyelitis; Rheumatoid arthritis

ANAEMIA: A reduction in the concentration of circulating haemoglobin. The normal haemoglobin level varies with age, neonates having a physiological polycythaemia with a haemoglobin concentration between 14 and 20 g/dl. This drops rapidly during the first week of life. Children have lower haemoglobin levels than adults and women have lower levels than men.

Aetiology and risk factors
Anaemia may be classified by cause (e.g. pernicious anaemia*) but often this is not known when a low haemoglobin is first recognized. Anaemia may also be classified as underproduction of red cells (e.g. haematinic deficiency) or loss of red cells (haemolysis or bleeding). Classification by red cell size is the most popular and useful method (Table A10). Macrocytic anaemias are associated with an increase in mean red cell volume (MCV); in normocytic anaemias the MCV is normal and in microcytic anaemias it is low. Each variety of anaemia is associated with various causes of anaemia, listed in Table A10.

Table A10 Classification of anaemia by red cell size

Microcytic	Normocytic	Macrocytic
Iron deficiency	Acute haemorrhage (after physiological compensation by haemodilution)	Vitamin B12 deficiency
Thalassaemia	Chronic renal failure (lack of erythro-poietin)	Folic acid deficiency
	Anaemia of chronic disease (Usually normo-cytic, sometimes microcytic)	Severe haemolysi (young cells are large cells)

Pathology
The decreased concentration of circulating haemoglobin will result in tissue hypoxia unless physiological compensations are made. Shortness of breath on exertion is a common presenting symptom. Cardiac output is increased by an increase in heart rate and stroke volume. Elderly patients may develop ankle oedema or other evidence of cardiac failure. An awareness of the heart beating (palpitations) may be a symptom of anaemia, and increased blood flow in the inner ear may cause tinnitus of a pulsatile nature. Pallor is a useful, but not very specific, sign of anaemia. When anaemia is very severe, tissue hypoxia may result, one manifestation being the appearance of retinal haemorrhages.

One of the physiological compensations for chronic anaemia is an increase in the level of the red cell enzyme 2,3-diphosphoglycerate (2,3-DPG). One of the effects of increasing concentrations of this enzyme is a shift to the right of the oxygen dissociation curve. This means that oxygen is more easily released from haemoglobin to hypoxic cells. Stored banked blood has low levels of 2,3 DPG and levels are restored to normal a day or two after transfusion. The clinical consequence is that patients transfused for the correction of anaemia may not feel the full benefit of the transfusion immediately. Physiological compensation takes time, so anaemia is better tolerated if slow in onset.

Management
The cause of the anaemia must be diagnosed and treated. Red cell transfusion provides a rapid method of correcting anaemia in severe cases.

ANAPHYLACTOID REACTION: An anaphylaxis-like reaction not mediated by IgE.

Anaphylactoid and anaphylactic reactions are identical in presentation. A list of known causes of anaphylactoid reactions is shown in Table A11 (see over). The mechanisms by which mast cells are activated to release histamine in these cases are mostly unknown.

 Allergy; Anaphylaxis

ANAPHYLAXIS: A systemic clinical syndrome resulting from IgE-mediated mast cells and basophil degranulation.

Case
A 72-year-old man was driving to his local supermarket when he felt a sharp pain on his ankle. He had been stung by a large bee and noticed that the sting was now rather painful. A few minutes later,

Table A11 Causes of anaphylactoid reactions

Treatments
    Gammaglobulin: aggregates activate complement
    leading to induction of anaphylatoxins C3a,C4a and
    C5a which directly activate mast cells

Drugs: non-steroidal anti-inflammatory
    Aminopyrine
    Aspirin
    Fenoprofen
    Ibuprofen
    Indomethacin
    Mefenamic acid
    Naproxen
    Tolmetin
    Zomepirac

Drugs: opiates
    Codeine
    Meperidine
    Morphine

Diagnostics
    Iodinated contrast medium for radiography

Additives
    Mannitol

Others
    Curare
    Tubocurarine

Conditions
    Exercise: activation of mast cells through endorphins?
    Emotional stress
    Overheating (rare)

Table A12 Some common causes of anaphylaxis

Foodstuffs	Drugs	Insect venoms
Peanuts	Penicillin	Bees
Nuts	Other antibiotics	Wasps
Fish (shellfish)	Vitamins	
Egg whites		
Sesame seeds		
Sunflower seeds		

year) and commoner with certain allergens such as antibiotics (notably penicillin), foodstuffs, plant and animal proteins and pharmacological agents (see Table A12). What determines susceptibility to developing type I hypersensitivity to certain antigens is unknown but clearly it has some genetic basis. It may also be, in part, the result of a breakdown in regulation of the immune response, leading to abnormally high levels of IgE production.

Anaphylactoid reactions, resulting from mast cell degranulation not mediated by IgE, can also occur. These result from the induction of the anaphylatoxins C3a and C5a by some blood products such as immunoglobulins and some therapeutic and diagnostic substances which probably act directly by stimulating mast cells to degranulate (see Anaphylactoid reactions*).

Pathology
As with all allergic reactions, mast cell degranulation results in production of histamine and other pharmacological agents. In the case of anaphylaxis, systemic release of these mediators cause rapid changes in blood pressure (hypotension) and these may be experienced first in peripheral capillaries. Later, this gives rise to vascular collapse, leading to fainting and pulmonary insufficiency resulting in increased respiratory rate. Itching, angioedema, bronchial obstruction and wheezing, and abdominal pain are common features of the anaphylactic attack. Respiratory obstruction and prolonged shock are the major causes of death.

Management
In the case of antigens known to produce anaphylaxis, care should be taken to avoid contact with them, e.g. penicillin, peanuts. The rapid administration of adrenaline s.c. or i.m. is the essence of treatment. In the above case, on visiting his GP, the patient was given an 'EpiPen' to self-administer adrenaline in an emergency following another bee sting.

 Allergy; Hypersensitivity

he started to feel an itching sensation in several parts of his body. He became rather alarmed, and since his local hospital was a couple of minutes away he went immediately to the outpatient department. By the time he arrived he was feeling very faint. He saw a nurse and told him about the sting. By now he was very short of breath and collapsed. His breathing was very rapid and he was wheezy. The nurse administered adrenaline intramuscularly. He soon regained consciousness but was kept under observation for 2 hours until his respiratory rate had returned to normal and was discharged with advice to see his GP about the incident. He had the classical symptoms of anaphylaxis.

Aetiology and risk factors
Anaphylaxis is the result of the systemic effects of excessive mast cell degranulation. It can occur as the sequel to sensitization with any of the antigens which can give rise to allergy (type I hypersensitivity). Thus any patient who is allergic is potentially at risk for developing anaphylaxis. However, anaphylaxis is very rare (less than 1 per million per

ANENCEPHALY: A congenital defect resulting in malformation of the cranial vault, with either small or missing cerebral hemispheres.

A

ANEURYSM: A localized dilatation of a blood vessel or the heart.

Aetiology and risk factors
Aneurysms may result from developmental abnormalities (berry aneurysms) or may arise secondary to atheroma, hypertension, vasculitis or myocardial infarction.

Pathology
Berry aneurysms are developmental abnormalities, which result in a defect in the media of the cerebral vessels at sites of bifurcation. Rupture leads to intracranial haemorrhage. The most common types of aneurysms arise due to atherosclerotic disease. The abdominal aorta is a common site. Damage to the wall due to deposition of the lipid plaques leads to weakening and dilatation. Rupture leads to fatal intraperitoneal haemorrhage. Hypertension may also exacerbate the atherosclerotic damage. Patients with hypertension are also at risk of bleeding from micro-aneurysms within the cerebral vessels. Aneurysms of the proximal aorta are classically seen in syphilitic aortitis, now fortunately rare. Myocardial infarction can lead to weakening of the ventricular wall, leading to aneurysm formation (Fig. A21).

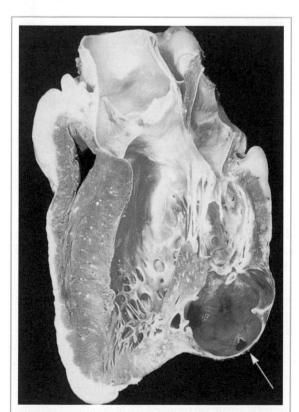

Fig. A21 Sagittal section through the left ventricle showing a cardiac aneurysm. (Reproduced with permission from Lakhani SR, Dilly SA, Finlayson CJ. *Basic Pathology*, 2nd edn. London: Arnold, 1998)

Dissection of the aorta is also referred to as a dissecting aneurysm, although it is not a true aneurysm as defined above.

Complications of aneurysm formation include rupture and haemorrhage, which may be fatal. Cardiac aneurysms may be the site for thrombus formation and hence systemic embolism*.

Management
Patients with aneurysms of the heart may have to be anticoagulated to prevent thrombosis. Cerebral aneurysms are usually asymptomatic until they bleed and at that stage, either the patient is kept stable until recovery, or emergency surgical intervention is contemplated to ligate the aneurysm. Elective surgery is performed for large abdominal aneurysms.

 Cerebrovascular disease; Hypertension; Myocardial infarction; Syphilis

ANGIOEDEMA: See Complement deficiencies; Urticaria.

ANGIOMA: A benign tumour of blood vessels, also called a haemangioma.

ANGIOSARCOMA: A malignant tumour of blood vessels.

 Sarcoma

ANKYLOSING SPONDYLITIS: A chronic inflammatory arthritis mainly affecting the spine and sacroiliac joints, commonest in young men and almost invariably associated with HLA-B27.

Presentation is usually with low back pain, stiffness and limitation of movement, and the disease may progress to ankylosis of the spinal joints ('bamboo spine', Fig. A22). Other joints may be affected and episodes of uveitis are common. The absence of autoantibodies, including rheumatoid factor, in the serum leads to the inclusion of AS in the group of seronegative arthritides*. Apart from a raised ESR and serum IgA, routine investigations are generally normal, but more than 90% of patients are HLA-B27 positive (compared with 7% of the general population). This may be due to 'mimicry' between HLA-B27 and an antigen from the intestinal bacterium *Klebsiella pneumoniae*, but the complete pathogenesis is not understood.

The incidence is 1–4 per 1000, with a 3:1 male:female ratio. Onset is rare before 15 or after 40. Management includes physiotherapy and anti-inflammatory drugs.

 Arthritis; Reiter disease; Seronegative arthritides

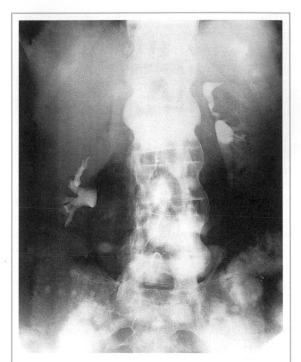

Fig. A22 Intravenous urogram showing 'bamboo spine' associated with ankylosed sacroiliac joints. (Reproduced with permission from Curtis J, Whitehouse G. *Radiology for the MRCP*. London: Arnold, 1998)

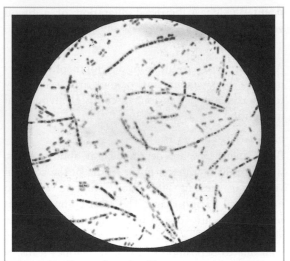

Fig. A23 The anthrax bacillus.

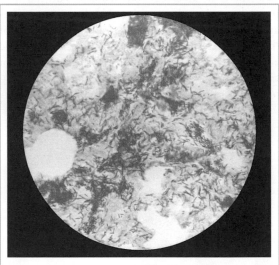

Fig. A24 The anthrax bacillus in lung tissue.

ANTHRAX: An infection caused by *Bacillus anthracis*, usually acquired from animals (see Zoonosis).

Aetiology and risk factors

There are two forms of the disease, cutaneous anthrax ('malignant' pustule) and a rapidly fatal pneumonia (wool-sorters' disease). In the UK the disease used to be an occupational hazard of dock-workers who handled infected animal hides and acquired the cutaneous form of the disease and mill-workers who acquired the pulmonary form of the disease following carding and spinning of infected wool. The organism can be found in the soil in many areas of the world and has recently been found in the fabric of King's Cross station in London, due to the use of infected hides in the construction of the building. The organism is a favourite one for use in biological weapons and the first anthrax bomb was developed by Professor Fildes (microbiologist) and biochemists at the then Middlesex Hospital Medical School and Courtauld Institute of Biochemistry (now part of UCLMS) in 1938–39. The device was exploded on Gruinard Island off the coast of Scotland in 1942–43 but testing was stopped after some crofters on the mainland died of pulmonary anthrax.

Pathology

The organism is a Gram-positive spore-forming bacillus with an anti-phagocytic capsule (Figs A23, A24).

B. anthracis produces a toxin whose precise action is not known; however, there is inhibition of phagocytic function and cell necrosis results, accompanied by disturbances of the capillary circulation, leading to extravasation of plasma and erythrocytes. The cutaneous form of the disease presents as an erythematous papule, which becomes vesicular and develops into a black eschar of necrotic tissue surrounded by pronounced oedema. There is regional lymphadenopathy. The organism may disseminate and the patient may develop a severe fatal pneumonia in which case the organism may be spread by the respiratory route. In the pneumonic phase there is severe shortness of breath and haemoptysis. The prominent oedema and extravascular erythrocytes occurring in the lungs explain the clinical findings of the pulmonary presentation. The cutaneous manifestations can be treated with penicillin but the pulmonary presentation is rapidly fatal despite antibiotics, hence its use as a weapon of biological warfare. A vaccine does exist but its efficacy is in doubt.

ANTIBODY DEFICIENCY: this occurs in a spectrum of diseases where antibodies are either absent (agammaglobulinaemia) or present in low amounts (hypogammaglobulinaemia), leading to an increased susceptibility to infection.

Case

A 30-year-old bank clerk attended his GP clinic with a 2-week history of a chesty cough. He had twice been admitted to hospital over the past 3 years with bronchopneumonia. It also transpired that he had suffered from sinopulmonary infections and occasional bouts of diarrhoea since childhood. He also complained of aching wrist joints but had put that down to recent heavy computer usage. There was no history of recurrent infections in his family and his parents, younger brother and sister were healthy. He was diagnosed as having pneumonia and *Haemophilus influenzae* was isolated. The GP also thought that with his history he should have some immunology tests carried out, so a blood sample was taken for antibody levels, specific antibodies and lymphocyte counts. His WBC was normal, as was his lymphocyte count (both T- and B-cells). He had low levels of IgG and IgA but normal levels of IgM (Table A13).

Table A13 Immunoglobulin levels (g/l) in antibody deficiency

IgM	IgA	IgG (total)	IgG1	IgG2	IgG3	IgG4
0.8	0.2	2.5	1.9	0.3	0.2	0.1

He had no serum anti-hepatitis B antibodies, even though he had been vaccinated for a trip abroad 6 months earlier. He was also negative for antinuclear antibodies and rheumatoid factor. He was asked to have a jejunal biopsy and on analysis this proved to contain the protozoan *Giardia lamblia*. The patient was diagnosed as having common variable immunodeficiency (CVID) with complicating *Giardia* infection. He was started on regular intravenous normal human immunoglobulin for his hypogammaglobulinaemia and treated for his *Giardia* infection.

Aetiology and risk factors

The type of immunodeficiency reported here is commonly associated with arthropathy and it is important to establish that this is not rheumatoid in nature, since CVID is also associated with some autoimmune diseases. Patients with antibody deficiencies have a 10–200-fold increase in incidence of malignant disease. Although CVID can be acquired, the majority of cases (80%) result from a primary defect in B-cell maturation. In this case, the B-cells developed normally into IgM-producing plasma cells but not into IgG or IgA plasma cells. This defect is mediated by failure of the B-cells to respond appropriately to T-cell signals.

Pathology

Table A14 (see over) shows a comparison of the antibody/B-cell deficiencies and the cellular /molecular mechanisms responsible for them.

Management

The stable treatment for antibody deficiencies is human immunoglobulin produced from pooled serum (free of HIV, HepB and HepC) given every 2–4 weeks. Where the specific gene affected is known, there may be a future for gene therapy.

 Hypogammaglobulinaemia; Immunodeficiency

APLASTIC ANAEMIA: A pancytopenia (low counts of red cells, white cells and platelets) in the blood associated with a hypoplastic (empty) bone marrow

Case

A 30-year-old woman visited her GP with her third respiratory infection in 4 months. He noted that she was pale and had a fever of 38.5°C. Her throat was sore and there were multiple haemorrhagic ulcers on the buccal mucosa. He referred her for a blood count:

WBC 1.3 × 10⁹/l
RBC 2.58 × 10¹²/l; Hb 8.9 g/dl; Hct (ratio) 0.261
MCV 101.2 fl; MCH 34.6 pg
MCHC 34.1 g/dl; RDW 15.2 %
Plt 21 × 10⁹/l.
Differential white cell count:
neutrophils 28% = 0.36 × 10⁹/l
lymphocytes 70% = 0.91 × 10⁹/l
monocytes 2% = 0.02 × 10⁹/l.

Table A14 Antibody deficiencies and mechanisms responsible

Disease	Description	Site of defect
X-linked agammaglobulinaemia (XLA; Bruton disease)	Recurrent pyogenic infections usually begin 5–6 months of age; B-cells absent from blood; very low IgG, other Igs absent; normal numbers of pre-B-cells in the BM; mostly males affected	XLA gene on long arm of X chromosome; identified as B-cell tyrosine kinase (*btk*). Its role is not currently understood but probably is involved in early B-cell signalling
Common variable immunodeficiency (CVID)	Often seen in 2nd–3rd decades of life; susceptible to pyogenic infections; M:F = 1:1; often have intestinal *Giardia*; commonly associated with HLA-B8 and DR3	B-cell fails to mature into plasma cells due to defects in T-cell signalling to B-cells
Immunodeficiency with increased IgM (hyper-IgM syndrome)	Recurrent pyogenic infections in early life; no IgG or IgA but high levels of IgM; may form autoantibodies to platelets and tissue antigens	Defect in B-cell switch to IgG and IgA B cells; in 70%, defect in CD40 ligand expressed by T-cells; the rest ? a defect in CD40 on B cells. X-linked recessive inheritance
IgA deficiency	Often asymptomatic; most common primary immunodeficiency, 1/700 in Caucasians; may develop immune-complex diseases; 20% of patients show associated IgG2/IgG4 deficiencies, these have recurrent pyogenic infections	Failure of B-cells to terminally differentiate into IgA plasma cells
IgG subclass deficiency	One or more of the IgG subclasses is deficient; recurrent bacterial infections; IgG2 deficients fail to respond to poly-saccharide antigens; sometimes associated with IgA deficiency or ataxia telangiectasia	Failure of B-cells to terminally differentiate into IgG subclass plasma cells
Transient hypogamma-globulinaemia of infancy	Pyogenic infections in babies; delay in production of the babies' own antibodies when maternal antibodies have been catabolized (6 months)	B-cells normal but they seem to lack help from CD4+ T cells; mostly IgG affected

Admission to hospital was arranged, where she started broad-spectrum intravenous antibiotic treatment and received red cell and platelet transfusions. A bone marrow aspirate and trephine biopsy were performed (see Figs A25, A26).

Aetiology and risk factors

The commonest cause of bone marrow hypoplasia is as a predictable response to radiotherapy and chemotherapy treatment of cancer. The bone marrow will usually recover after a few weeks and

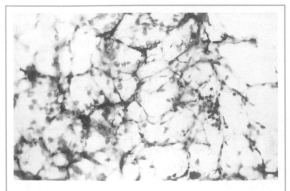

Fig. A25 Low power view of a bone marrow particle from a patient with aplastic anaemia. Instead of haemopoietic precursor cells, there is replacement with empty fat cells – the 'string vest' sign.

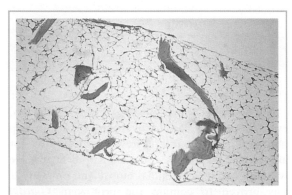

Fig. A26 H&E stained section of bone marrow trephine biopsy in aplastic anaemia. The narrow space in between the bone trabeculae is devoid of haemopoietic cells.

supportive treatment with red cell and platelet transfusions with antibiotic treatment of infections is required until it does. Aplastic anaemia may also be seen after exposure to radiation or a toxic chemical such as benzene.

Aplastic anaemia may be seen as an idiosyncratic reaction to drugs such as phenylbutazone or gold therapy for rheumatoid arthritis. It is important to take a careful drug history from patients with aplastic anaemia.

Some viruses, particularly those that cause hepatitis, may damage the bone marrow stem cells as well as the liver hepatocytes, causing a severe aplastic anaemia.

Fanconi anaemia is a rare congenital aplastic anaemia in which the pancytopenia and hypoplastic bone marrow are associated with stunted growth, skeletal abnormalities and other congenital anomalies. There is increased fragility of the patient's chromosomes, and spontaneous chromosome breaks are seen. This may explain the predisposition to malignancy that patients with Fanconi anaemia have.

When aplastic anaemia is not associated with one of the causes listed above, it is termed idiopathic. Most cases of idiopathic aplastic anaemia represent an autoimmune attack against the patient's stem cells, though it may be difficult to prove this in an individual case. In some cases populations of T-suppressor lymphocytes have been found in blood or bone marrow that suppress normal bone marrow growth *in vitro*. More convincing has been the good response of patients to immunosuppressive therapy with antilymphocyte globulin and other immunosuppressive agents.

Pathology
The finding of a grossly hypoplastic bone marrow without other haematological pathology led to a diagnosis of aplastic anaemia in this case. Slight macrocytosis is common in this disorder and measurements of blood folate and B12 levels were normal.

Management
Supportive Anaemia is corrected by red cell transfusions as required. Thrombocytopenia associated with bleeding is treated by platelet transfusions. Febrile neutropenia is managed by aggressive antibiotic and antifungal treatment, as appropriate. Inevitably problems with long-term supportive management will arise. These include the development of antibodies against HLA antigens on transfused platelets, leading to febrile transfusion reactions and relative loss of beneficial effect of platelet transfusion. Repeated red cell transfusion leads to iron overload, with damage to endocrine organs, myocardium and liver. Infections with

organisms such as methicillin-resistant *Staphylococcus aureus* and vancomycin-resistant *Enterococcus* are difficult to treat. Chronic neutropenia and antibiotic treatment predispose to superadded fungal infections such as *Aspergillus* and *Monilia*. For these reasons most cases of severe aplastic anaemia will have treatment to try to restore bone marrow function in addition to supportive measures.

Stimulation of residual bone marrow function Many of the haemopoietic growth factors that control bone marrow activity, such as granulocyte colony stimulating factor (G-CSF), have been cloned and are available for clinical use. These have a limited role to play in improving neutrophil counts in aplastic anaemia by stimulating residual bone marrow precursors and improving white cell function. Unfortunately, these growth factors tend to stimulate only the proliferation of the committed precursors, and not the most primitive of stem cells. Anabolic steroids such as oxymetholone also result in some improvement of bone marrow function in mild cases.

Immunosuppression In cases of idiopathic aplastic anaemia the autoimmune attack against the bone marrow, stem cells can be suppressed by treatment with antilymphocyte globulin, cyclosporin and high-dose steroids, allowing the regrowth of normal marrow and restoration of blood counts. Until this treatment takes effect, the patient will be even more immunosuppressed and at risk of infections.

Bone marrow transplantation This provides fresh bone marrow from a matched sibling donor. The conditioning treatment to 'empty' the bone marrow prior to the transfusion of fresh donor stem cells is not as stringent as in transplantation for leukaemia, as the bone marrow is already empty and there are no malignant leukaemia cells to be got rid of. Usually, high doses of immunosuppressive drugs such as cyclophosphamide are given without total body radiation. Nevertheless, marrow transplant in aplastic anaemia is a risky treatment and only used in severe cases in young patients who are likely to survive the procedure. Most patients will not be lucky enough to have a matched sibling available for donation.

APOPTOSIS: A form of programmed cell death which is important for removal of unwanted cells and thus the maintenance of normal tissue homeostasis. Apoptosis is essential in normal development (e.g. limb formation) and is characterized by nuclear fragmentation and 'cell blebbing'. Early events in many cell types result in a change in surface membrane lipids, leading to rapid uptake by phagocytic cells. There is also activation of proteolytic

A

enzymes (called caspases) that digest proteins associated with DNA and cut the DNA into regular-sized pieces. Many molecules are involved in inducing, activating, and inhibiting this process. These include the proto-oncogene c-*myc* and the inhibitory protein BCL2. Apoptosis normally occurs as the result of diminished levels of growth factors and or as an innate cell programme (e.g. in neutrophils). In contrast to necrosis, the apoptotic mechanism of cell death leads to minimal or no inflammation – a process characteristic of tissue damage caused by trauma or microbial infection. Many cells die by apoptosis as part of their natural history and failure of this process is likely to result in the production of tumours. Many tumours have elevated levels of BCL2. Breakdown in the delicate balance between cell survival and apoptosis has been implicated in the pathogenesis of some rheumatic diseases such as rheumatoid arthritis. Immune cells such as NK cells or cytotoxic T-cells induce apoptosis of virus-infected cells. This 'activation-induced cell death' (AICD) has also been implicated in the pathogenesis of a number of autoimmune diseases.

APPENDICITIS: Acute inflammation of the appendix.

Aetiology and risk factors
The commonest cause of acute appendicitis is obstruction of the lumen due to faecolith, or more rarely, worms or tumour.

Pathology
Appendicitis mainly occurs in young people but can be encountered at any age. Patients present with periumbilical pain, which then localizes to the right lower quadrant. There may be associated fever and nausea. A raised white cell count may also be seen on haematological examination.

Obstruction leads to distension of the appendix, which compromises the vascular supply, leading to ischaemic injury. This allows bacterial overgrowth, which adds to the inflammatory response. If the inflammation is transmural, it leads to inflammation of the serosal (peritoneal) lining and hence signs of peritonitis with abdominal pain and guarding. Rupture of the appendix will cause a widespread peritonitis, which is a surgical emergency. Other complications include peritoneal abscess, hepatic abscess and septicaemia.

Management
This involves surgical removal of the inflamed appendix.

 Abscess; Inflammation

ARNOLD–CHIARI MALFORMATION: An abnormality of the brain stem and cerebellum. It leads to downward misplacement of the cerebellum, vermis and tonsils through the foramen magnum. It is associated with hydrocephalus.

ARTERIOLOSCLEROSIS: This refers to proliferative and hyaline changes seen within small arteries and arterioles.

Aetiology and risk factors
The principal aetiological factor in arteriolosclerosis is hypertension.

Pathology
Hyaline and hyperplastic arteriolosclerotic changes are different from atheroma* since, unlike atherosclerotic plaques, they do not have an increase in lipid. They principally affect the media of the arteries and arterioles.

Hyaline arteriolosclerosis tends to occur in the elderly and in patients with diabetes. There is deposition of homogeneous pink material within

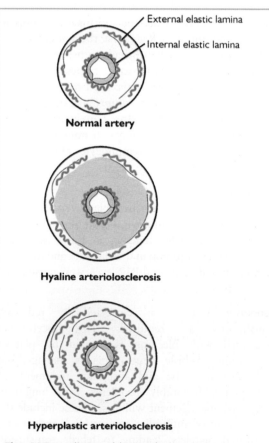

Fig. A27 Hyaline and hyperplastic arteriolosclerosis. (Reproduced with permission from Lakhani SR, Dilly SA, Finlayson CJ. *Basic Pathology*, 2nd edn. London: Arnold, 1998)

the media. This leads to narrowing of the blood vessels. The material is probably the result of an increase in extracellular matrix, which is produced by smooth muscle cells and due to leakage of plasma components.

Hyperplastic arteriolosclerosis is usually seen in patients with a severe and chronic increase in blood pressure. There is thickening of the media of the blood vessels with a concentric proliferation of smooth muscle cells. There may also be fibrinoid necrosis of the blood vessels (Fig. A27).

Management
Management comprises treatment of the underlying disorder, i.e. hypertension or diabetes.

 Diabetes; Hypertension

ARTERITIS: Inflammation of arteries.

Aetiology and risk factors
These can be broadly divided into two major categories, infectious agents and immunological mechanisms. Infections include *Neisseria gonorrhoeae*, syphilis and herpes virus. Vasculitis as a result of immunological mechanisms is diverse in its nature and includes Henoch–Schonlein purpura, lupus vasculitis, Goodpasture syndrome, Wegener granulomatosis, Churg–Strauss syndrome and polyarteritis (see separate entries). A number of other disorders for which the underlying mechanism is unclear, e.g. giant cell (temporal) arteritis*, lead to vasculitis.

Pathology
Injury to blood vessels (vasculitis) is seen in a number of different diseases and clinical settings. The terms arteritis, vasculitis and angiitis are essentially synonymous. As mentioned above, the two major groups of disorders leading to vasculitis are infections and immunological mechanisms. It is clearly important to distinguish between these two as the treatment and management of patients with these two different disorders is distinct. For example, steroid therapy, which may be used to treat immunological disorders, would exacerbate an infection.

The pathogenesis of vasculitis in infections is either a direct result of damage to the vessel wall or secondary to immune mechanisms, generally related to the deposition of immune complexes within the vessel wall.

Management
This can be broadly divided into two approaches: immunosuppresive therapy for immune-mediated vasculitis and antibiotics or antiviral therapy for infectious vasculitis.

 Churg–Strauss disease; Henoch–Schönlein purpura; Herpes simplex encephalitis; Syphilis; Systemic lupus erythematosus; Vasculitis; Wegener granulomatosis

---

ARTHRITIS: Inflammation of joints.

 Osteoarthritis; Rheumatoid arthritis

ASBESTOSIS: A lung disorder caused by exposure to asbestos.

Aetiology and risk factors
Asbestos exposure may be an occupational hazard as this material was used as lagging in the construction industry and in old buildings.

Pathology
Exposure to asbestos has been linked to the production of pleural plaques, lung fibrosis, bronchial carcinoma and mesothelioma. The type of disorders encountered depends on the concentration, size, and shape of the asbestos fibres. There are two distinct forms; the serpentine and amphibole. It is the amphiboles that are responsible for the pleural plaques and pleural mesothelioma. As in the other pneumoconioses*, asbestos interacts with macrophages and parenchymal cells within the lung. Macrophages are activated and try to ingest the fibres, which leads to release of chemical mediators that eventually lead to lung fibrosis. Within the lung there is diffuse pulmonary interstitial fibrosis and asbestos bodies may also be seen (Fig. A28). Fibrosis from asbestos exposure is not distinguishable from that caused by other pneumoconioses. Pleural plaques are the most common manifestation of exposure to asbestos, consisting of dense collagen. They are seen commonly over the anterior and posterolateral aspects of the parietal pleura. They are uncommon in patients who have not been exposed to asbestos. Bronchial carcinoma and malignant mesothelioma* are also complications of

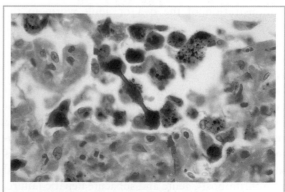

Fig. A28 Brown asbestos bodies in lung.

asbestos exposure, the risk of bronchial carcinoma being increased about five times, and that of mesothelioma over a thousand times compared with normal populations. Cigarette smoking increases the risk of bronchial carcinoma but not that of mesothelioma.

Management

The management is symptomatic. Once bronchial carcinoma or mesothelioma has occurred, the patient is usually treated with either surgery or combined surgery and chemotherapy. Pleural effusions can be drained and pleural plaques can be resected. Malignant mesothelioma is very resistant to treatment and patients inevitably die within the short period of time.

Lung carcinoma; Malignant mesothelioma

ASCARIASIS: Infection with the intestinal nematode *Ascaris lumbricoides*. Fertilized eggs are passed in the faeces and undergo a developmental stage in moist soil to become embryonated eggs, which are the infective stage. After ingestion of the egg, the larvae hatch out in the intestine, penetrate the intestinal wall, and are carried by the bloodstream to the lungs. From the lungs the larvae move into the trachea and bronchi, across the epiglottis and into the oesophagus. The larvae become sexually mature worms in the intestine and fertilized eggs are released with the faeces. Clinically the patients may present with pulmonary symptoms when the larvae invade the lungs, e.g. bronchospasm, fever and urticaria accompanied by peripheral eosinophilia. The chest radiograph will show diffuse shadows and eosinophils are present in the sputum. This condition is called **tropical eosinophilia**. The adult worm may also cause gastrointestinal symptoms of diarrhoea and abdominal colic. Complications include pancreatitis, cholecystitis and intestinal obstruction caused by worms blocking the pancreatic and biliary ducts and intestinal lumen. Laboratory diagnosis is by demonstration of the ova or adult worm in the faeces. Treatment is with mebendazole, levamisole or pyrantel.

ASCITES: The accumulation of extracellular fluid in the peritoneal cavity. There are a number of mechanisms that contribute to the formation of extracellular fluid, such as sodium retention as a result of secondary hyperaldosteronism, hypoalbuminaemia, and portal hypertension. Hepatic causes include cirrhosis, Budd–Chiari syndrome, portal vein thrombosis, acute and subacute hepatic failure. Non-hepatic causes include metastatic neoplasms, right-sided heart failure, constrictive pericarditis, tuberculous and bacterial peritonitis, and pancreatic disease. The protein concentration of the fluid is estimated to determine whether it is an exudate or transudate (see Effusion for definition).

ASPERGILLOSIS: Infection with the fungus *Aspergillus* spp.

Case

A 25-year-old leukaemic patient had undergone a bone marrow transplant (BMT) when some few days after the transplant he developed a temperature. There were no focal signs. The patient was given broad-spectrum antibiotics and initially the temperature resolved, although after 4 days it returned.

Radiology: A chest radiograph showed areas of consolidation in both lung fields.
Microbiology: Sputum culture yielded *Aspergillus fumigatus* as seen in Fig. A29.

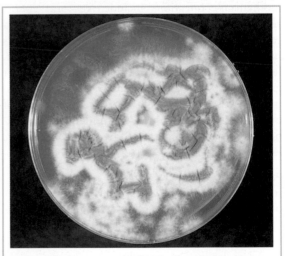

Fig. A29 Culture of *Aspergillus fumigatus*.

Aetiology and risk factors

Aspergillus is a mould that is commonly found in the environment. There are several species but *A. fumigatus* and *Aspergillus niger* are the ones commonly associated with infection. *Aspergillus* spores are very commonly detected in the air, particularly around building works. The spores, which are about 3 μm in diameter, are inhaled and are small enough to lodge in the alveoli of the lungs.

Pathology

The primary cellular defences against *Aspergillus* are the pulmonary macrophages and neutrophils. Immunocompromised individuals are prone to infection following inhalation, particularly if they are neutropenic. The inhaled spores germinate to produce hyphae and invade the lung tissue, including the cartilage and blood vessels, producing haemorrhagic necrosis. This may lead to haemoptysis which can be fatal. Dissemination of the fungus can lead to infection in the skin to give a haemorrhagic folliculitis or in the brain to give signs of a space-occupying lesion. In both skin and brain, as in the lungs, the hyphae invade and destroy the tissues.

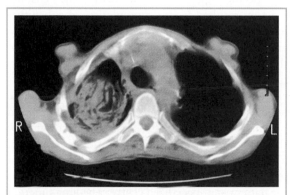

Fig. A30 CT scan showing aspergilloma in upper lobe of right lung. (Reproduced with permission from Curtis J, Whitehouse G. *Radiology for the MRCP.* London: Arnold, 1998)

In addition to invasive pulmonary disease, *Aspergillus* infection can give rise to invasive disease in the sinuses (rhinocerebral aspergillosis) or external auditory meatus and from there invade contiguous structures. *Aspergillus* can also colonize a pulmonary cavity to produce a fungal ball in the lung, called an aspergilloma (Fig. A30), for example in association with a tuberculous cavity. Invasion of associated blood vessels may also give rise to fatal haemoptysis. Finally, *Aspergillus* can colonize the bronchopulmonary tree or sinuses, producing an allergic reaction with elevated IgE, fleeting pulmonary shadows and eosinophilia. This may lead to permanent lung damage.

Diagnosis is difficult and serology (antibody or antigen detection) is poorly predictive of disease in invasive pulmonary disease although useful in aspergilloma. Isolation of the fungus in the sputum is also poorly predictive of disease as the fungus is common in the environment. The usefulness of PCR detection is still to be evaluated.

Management
Management is with amphotericin or an azole such as itraconazole or voriconazole. Surgery may be indicated for aspergilloma.

ASTHMA:
Also known as reversible obstructive airway disease, asthma is a disease characterized by narrowing of the bronchial airways and difficulty with expiration.

Case
A 14-year-old boy attended his GP clinic complaining of a 2-month history of coughing, wheezing and shortness of breath. It was often worse at night and his chest felt 'tight' in the morning. He had had eczema as a child. A family history revealed that his mother had suffered from hay fever as a child and had bouts of allergic rhinitis. The family had recently acquired a new puppy for his younger sister. On examination he showed fatigue and expiratory wheeze in both lungs on auscultation. A peak expiratory flow rate test showed that he was below normal for his height and age. A sputum sample was taken to test for lung infection but was negative; however, many eosinophils were noted. A blood test revealed normal haemoglobin levels but an increased white cell count, mainly due to eosinophilia. His immunoglobulin levels were normal for his age except for IgE, which was elevated.

WBC 14.2 × 10⁹/l
Eosinophils 1.3 × 10⁹/l
IgE 320 KU/l

On returning to his GP, he was given skin prick tests for common allergens. He was positive for house dust mite allergen (*Dermatophagoides pteronyssinus*) and dog antigen but negative for most grasses, cat and food antigens. He was diagnosed as having allergic asthma.

Aetiology and risk factors
Asthma is a worldwide problem, thought to be caused by bronchial hypersensitivity and affecting 5–7 % of people in Europe and the USA respectively, with the number of cases rising. It is more common in children than adults, with a peak age onset of less than 5 years of age. Many people still die from asthma and it is likely that many of these deaths are preventable. There appear to be many precipitating factors in Asthma (Table A15). It is estimated that up to 60% of all asthma is allergic (type 1, extrinsic asthma), the remainder (type 2, intrinsic) being of unknown cause.

Diagnosis of asthma in later life is often more difficult when a patient has chronic bronchitis as the result of smoking.

There appears to be a genetic predisposition for the development of asthma but it is complex. Some studies have suggested that if one parent has

Table A15 Precipitating factors in asthma

Specific antigens
  Seasonal, e.g. pollens – grass and tree
  Perennial, e.g. house dust mite, cat and dog dander
  Occupational
  Industry
    Plastics, e.g. isocyanates
    Chemical, e.g. chlorides
    Electrical, e.g. soldering flux
    Textiles, e.g. cotton dust
    Carpentry, e.g. wood dust
    Bakers, e.g. flour, grain
    Veterinary, agricultural, e.g. urine, serum and
    animal dander
    Laboratory workers

Non-antigen specific
  Upper respiratory tract infections
  Smoking
  Exercise
  Cold air
  Laughter
  Paint or chemical fumes
  Drugs, e.g. beta-blockers
  Stress

asthma, the chance of an offspring developing the disease is 1:6. There is slight preponderance of males over females in early onset disease.

Pathology

This young boy had all the signs that his asthma was of immunological origin and mediated by inhaled antigens of house dust mite (antigen in mite's faeces) and dog dander. An elevated level of serum IgE together with positive skin prick tests for house dust mites and dog dander indicates the role of specific IgE in pathogenesis. The ensuing reaction resulted from degranulation of subepithelial mast cells through binding of the inhaled antigens passing across the mucosal epithelium of the bronchus. These mast cells will have been 'sensitized' with IgE antibodies produced on previous encounters with the antigens (type 1, immediate hypersensitivity). Preformed and newly synthesized pharmacological mediators result in narrowing of the bronchus through smooth muscle contraction. This can be shown with 'bronchial provocation tests' where the antigen is carefully administered to the patient at a specialized centre. The lung function measured shows an immediate bronchoconstriction

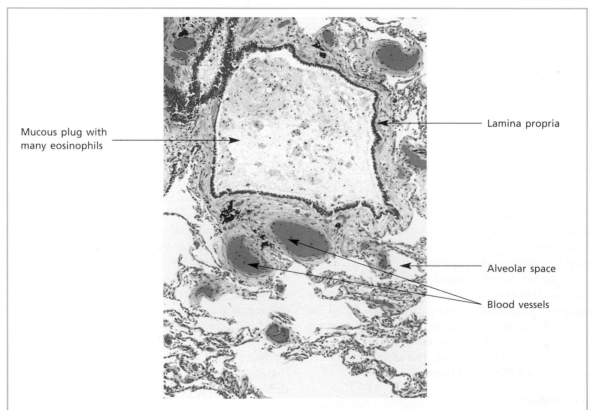

Fig. A31 Postmorten sample of lung of patient with asthma. Note the large mucous plug in the airway. (Courtesy of Dr Julie Crow and Professor Len Poulter)

with a return to baseline within a few minutes. With chronic stimulation, T-cells play a role (type IV hypersensitivity) leading to more intense inflammation with oedema and the formation of mucous plugs (Fig. A31).

The eosinophilia measured in the blood and sputum is probably due to cytokines secreted by T-cells and mast cells during chronic antigenic stimulation. Non-specific and specific predisposing factors might lead to an 'asthma attack' in a patient with chronic airway inflammation. Other mechanisms of bronchial hyper-reactivity include alterations in autonomic nervous control, abnormalities of Ca^{2+} flux and damage to epithelial 'tight junctions'.

Management
In the case of known antigens which induce asthma, care should be taken to reduce the exposure to the relevant antigen (avoidance). In the case described, the GP advised the patient's mother that she should frequently vacuum the mattress (home of the house dust mite) and furniture and carpets (dog dander) to reduce the source of antigen. Acute asthma attacks are treated with β-agonists, e.g. salbutamol in a nebulizer and sodium cromoglycate, which stabilize mast cells and inhibit degranulation. Corticosteroids are given orally and via a nebulizer.

 Allergy; Hypersensitivity

ATAXIA TELANGIECTASIA: A childhood disease characterized by ataxia, telangiectasia and immunodeficiency.

Clinical onset occurs by 2–6 years of age and the child presents with ataxia (wobbly gait), telangiectasia (dilated capillaries) of the eyes and skin and recurrent sinopulmonary infections. Ataxia telangiectasia (AT) is an autosomal recessive trait. About 70% of patients have IgA deficiency and some IgG2 and IgG4 deficiency. There is variable T-cell deficiency. Chromosome breaks are found at sites of T-cell receptor and immunoglobulin heavy chain genes. Cells from these patients show an increased susceptibility to the effects of ionizing irradiation and there is a defective gene coding for a protein involved in DNA repair. There is an increased risk of leukaemia, lymphomas and, in women, breast carcinoma.

 Immunodeficiency

ATHEROMA: A plaque composed of a fibrous cap covering a soft, yellow, lipid centre. It is found in the arterial intima and is a hallmark of atherosclerosis.

ATOPY/ATOPIC: Atopy is an inherited tendency to respond immunologically to common naturally occurring ingested and inhaled allergens with overproduction of IgE antibodies. Atopic is the term used to describe those individuals (at least 10–15% in the general population) who have this tendency, expressed as allergic diseases such as asthma, eczema, hay fever, urticaria and food allergy.

ATYPICAL PNEUMONIA: A term signifying pneumonia that does not present in the 'typical' fashion of pneumococcal pneumonia*.

Aetiology and risk factors
Atypical pneumonias are caused by a number of different agents: *Mycoplasma pneumoniae*, *Coxiella burnetii* (Q fever – see Rickettsial disease), *Chlamydia psittaci*, *Chlamydia pneumoniae* (see Chlamydial disease) and *Legionella pneumophila* (see Legionnaires disease).

Pathology
Mycoplasma organisms attach to respiratory epithelial cells and may have a direct toxic action on the cells. Initially cilial action is inhibited which is then followed by desquamation of the epithelium. The inflammation primarily involves the bronchi, bronchioles and peribronchial tissue. Infection may be associated with the production of cold agglutinins directed against the I antigen on the surface of erythrocytes, although autoantibodies to other organs, e.g. the heart and brain, may also be induced. The Coombs test may be positive and the patient may develop haemolytic anaemia. The presence of cold agglutinins may also be related to the presentation of Raynaud disease* that some patients show. Other complications include Stevens–Johnson syndrome*, polyarthralgia, myocarditis and the Guillain–Barre syndrome*.

Other causes of atypical pneumonia are shown in Table A16.

***Ch. psittaci* (psittacosis)** In addition to the pneumonia, which can range from a mild influenza-like illness to severe pneumonia, there

Table A16 Other causes of atypical pneumonia

Organism	Disease	Transmission	Vector
Chlamydia psittaci	Psittacosis	Inhalation of contaminated dust	Infected birds
Chlamydia pneumoniae		Droplet infection	Infected humans
Coxiella burnetii	Q fever	Inhalation of contaminated dust; ingestion of contaminated milk	Infected animals

A

may be splenomegaly and evidence of hepatitis. Complications include myocarditis, arthritis and encephalitis.

Ch. pneumoniae Often produces epidemics of a mild pneumonia or flu-like illness. Pharyngitis and hoarseness may be prominent.

Cox. burnetii (Q fever) Infection can range from a mild flu-like illness to a severe pneumonia. Complications include chronic infection, such as granulomatous hepatitis, and endocarditis.

The pneumonia in these infections presents with malaise, fever, non-productive cough, shortness of breath and sometimes myalgia. A chest radiograph shows diffuse mottling, usually around the hilar or in the bases of the lungs.

Laboratory diagnosis is usually by serology and management is with erythromycin or tetracycline.

AUTOIMMUNITY; AUTOIMMUNE DISEASE; AUTOANTIBODIES:
Autoimmunity is the reaction of the immune system against 'self' antigen(s); autoimmune diseases are the pathological consequence of autoimmunity; and autoantibodies are the antibodies produced against self antigens found in several autoimmune diseases.

Aetiology and risk factors
Tolerance to self antigens is normally acquired during lymphopoiesis (central tolerance) or in the peripheral tissues of the body by a variety of mechanisms (peripheral tolerance), but mostly through anergy. Autoimmunity results from the breakdown of tolerance to self antigens. In many cases this leads to autoimmune diseases which affect up to 7% of the population. The mechanisms leading to breakdown in tolerance are generally unknown but a number have been suggested (Table A17), mainly from experiments in animals. It can be seen that at least some of the autoimmune diseases are probably mediated through responses to microbes.

Autoimmune diseases can affect many different organs/tissues of the body but are conventionally classified on the basis of whether one or several organs are targeted by the autoimmune response. We thus talk of a spectrum of autoimmune diseases with, at one end, those diseases with a single target organ (organ-specific diseases) to the other end where the target is several organs/tissues (non-organ-specific). Autoantigens in the non-organ-specific diseases tend to be common to several cell types and are usually intracellular components (Table A18). The distinction, however, is far from perfect and in polyendocrine autoimmune diseases and primary biliary cirrhosis, more than one gland is affected.

Table A17 Possible mechanisms for the breakdown of self-tolerance

Cross-reactive microbial antigens	Microbes have antigenic shapes and amino acid sequences that are similar to self and can stimulate self-reactive lymphocytes
Polyclonal activation:	Some microbes, e.g Epstein–Barr virus, stimulate B-lymphocytes, independently of their programmed specificity to secrete antibodies; self-reactive anergic B-cells will also be stimulated to produce autoantibodies
Aberrant antigen presentation	Self antigens are not normally presented to CD4 T-cells since they require HLA class II and this molecule is restricted to only a few specialized antigen presenting cells. Other cells, e.g. thyroid epithelial cells, may be made to express HLA class II and present self antigens, e.g. via cytokines induced by microbes
Release of sequestered antigens	Lymphocytes with specificity for sperm and lens proteins are not eliminated during lymphopoiesis since these proteins do not pass through the primary lymphoid organs. In mumps orchitis, sperm antigens are released into the circulation and cause autoantibodies to be produced. In addition, trauma releases lens proteins to which autoantibodies are produced (sympathetic ophthalmia)
Regulatory abnormalities	The normal immune system is regulated through cell interactions and defects in the molecules involved in these reactions can give rise to autoimmunity, e.g. fas (CD95), cytokines

Pathology
In some of the organ-specific diseases, the specific autoantibodies are directly pathogenic, as shown by transfer of the mother's disease via IgG across the placenta to the newborn and to experimental animals after injection; examples are myasthenia gravis, autoimmune haemolytic anaemia, Graves disease, pernicious anaemia and the bullous skin diseases. In other diseases (both organ and non-organ), the autoantibodies are of diagnostic significance and some can act as indicators of disease progression.

The mechanisms of tissue damage in autoimmune diseases are essentially those described for hypersensitivity* reactions. Generally speaking, the

Table A18 Autoimmune diseases and autoantigens

Disease	Antigen(s)
Organ-specific diseases	
Hashimoto thyroiditis	Thyroid peroxidase, thyroglobulin/T4
Pernicious anaemia	Intrinsic factor
Insulin-dependent diabetes mellitus (IDDM)	β-Cells in the pancreas (GAD, tyrosine phosphatase)
Addison disease	Adrenal cortical cells (ACTH receptor and microsomes)
Autoimmune haemolytic anaemia	RBC membrane antigens
Graves disease	TSH receptor
Pemphigus	Epidermal keratinocytes
Bullous pemphigoid	Basal keratinocytes
Guillain–Barré syndrome	Peripheral nerves (gangliosides)
Polymyositis	Muscle (histidine tRNA synthetase)
Non-organ-specific diseases	
Systemic lupus erythematosus	Double-stranded DNA, nuclear antigens
Chronic active hepatitis	Nuclei, DNA
Scleroderma	Nuclei, elastin nucleoli, centromeres, topoisomerase 1
Primary biliary cirrhosis	Mitochondria (pyruvate dehydrogenase complex E2)
Rheumatoid arthritis	IgG (rheumatoid factor, connective tissues, collagen)
Ankylosing spondylitis	Vertebral
Multiple sclerosis	Brain/myelin basic protein
Sjögren syndrome	Exocrine glands, kidney, liver, thyroid
Several organs affected	
Goodpasture syndrome	Basement membrane of kidney and lung (type IV collagen)
Polyendocrine	Multiple endocrine organs (hepatic – cytochrome p450; intestinal – tryptophan hydroxylase)

organ-specific diseases are mediated through type II, IV or V (Graves disease) mechanisms. The non-organ-specific diseases are mainly mediated through type III mechanisms, resulting from immune complex deposition in the skin (vasculitis) and vascular system, especially in the kidneys as in SLE and other forms of glomerulonephritis*. By contrast, in Goodpasture syndrome, renal damage is caused by antibodies to basement membrane, which is a type II response.

It is known that T-cells are involved in the aetiology of autoimmune diseases (i.e. they are required for production of autoantibodies) and are probably also involved in the pathogenesis (type IV) of at least some diseases, e.g. IDDM and probably rheumatoid arthritis (RA).

Management

Most therapy is directed towards treating the chronic inflammation. Steroids are commonly used and in some cases removal of the autoantibodies by plasmapheresis is of value. A reliable way to induce specific tolerance has not yet been found.

AVIUMOSIS: A disseminated infection with *Mycobacterium avium*, occurring mainly in AIDS patients.

 Mycobacteriosis

B

BACILLARY ANGIOMATOSIS: A disease caused by *Bartonella henselae* or *Bartonella quintana* and found mainly in patients with AIDS. The patient presents with reddish-purple papules on the skin, resembling verruca peruana (Oroya fever*) or Kaposi sarcoma (see AIDS). The organism can be seen in histological sections of the tissue when stained appropriately. In addition to the more clinically obvious angiomatous skin lesions, the disease can present in any organ and when affecting the liver it is called peliosis hepatis. In this case the liver contains a variable number of blood-filled cystic spaces. Alternatively, parenchymatous disease can present as a necrotizing granuloma similar to cat-scratch disease*. Diagnosis is by histology and detection of the organism by culture or the polymerase chain reaction. Serology may also be useful. Treatment is with tetracycline or erythromycin.

BACTERIAL VAGINOSIS: A disturbance of the normal flora of the vagina with a change in pH and proliferation of some organisms, principally *Mobiluncus* and *Gardnerella vaginalis*. This polymicrobial overgrowth leads to an offensive grey vaginal discharge and dysuria. The vaginal wall does not appear inflamed but is covered with a glistening film of secretions. There are few polymorphs in the discharge. The condition may

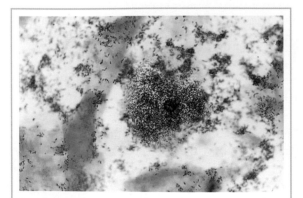

Fig. B1 Clue cell showing adherent Gram-positive bacilli.

lead to complications in pregnant women. It is diagnosed clinically by an offensive fishy smell caused by trimethylamine, particularly if the vaginal discharge is alkalinized with potassium hydroxide. Also diagnostic are the presence of 'clue cells' – epithelial cells with abundant adherent Gram-positive bacilli (*Gardnerella*; Fig. B1).

Bacterial vaginosis is usually treated with metronidazole.

BALANTIDIASIS: Gastrointestinal infection with *Balantidium coli*, probably acquired from animals, e.g. pigs, causing an illness ranging from watery diarrhoea to severe colitis.

BARE LYMPHOCYTE SYNDROME: An immunodeficiency disease resulting from the lack of expression of HLA class I and/or II genes. When MHC class II genes are not expressed, CD4+ T-cells fail to develop; when MHC class I genes are not expressed there is defective cytotoxic T-cell function and increased susceptibility to virus infections.

 Immunodeficiency

BARRETT OESOPHAGUS: A metaplastic change which results in transformation of the squamous epithelium of the lower oesophagus to a columnar glandular epithelium.

Aetiology and risk factors
The metaplastic changes may either be congenital or acquired as a result of reflux of acid from the stomach. This may occur over a background of a hiatus hernia.

Pathology
As a result of chronic injury due to reflux oesophagitis, the distal squamous epithelium is replaced by metaplastic columnar epithelium. Patients usually have a history of symptoms related to reflux, with chest pain and heartburn. The recurrent reflux oesophagitis with inflammation and ulceration leads to a replacement of the squamous epithelium by a more robust mucin-secreting gastric type of columnar epithelium. This metaplastic epithelium may be focal and not necessarily in continuity with the columnar epithelium of the stomach.

It is important to follow patients with Barrett oesophagus as the glandular epithelium within the oesophagus is prone to develop dysplastic changes. Patients with Barrett oesophagus have an increased risk (30–40×) of developing adenocarcinoma.

Management
This may be medical, aimed at reducing the acid reflux within the oesophagus, or surgical. Patients

with known Barrett oesophagus are followed up regularly to check for dysplastic changes.

 Gastric carcinoma; Oesophageal carcinoma

BARTONELLOSIS: Diseases caused by the genus *Bartonella*, which includes trench fever (*Bartonella*, previously *Rochalimaea quintana*), Oroya fever (*Bartonella bacilliformis*); bacillary angiomatosis (*Bartonella henselae*); cat-scratch disease (*Bartonella henselae*) and peliosis hepatis (*Bartonella henselae*).

BASAL CELL CARCINOMA (BCC): A low-grade malignant tumour arising from the basal cells of skin exposed to the sun.

Aetiology and risk factors

The most common risk factor is chronic sun exposure with damage to the skin. BCC may also arise as part of the rare Gorlin syndrome, and it is commoner in patients with defects of DNA repair, such as xeroderma pigmentosum.

Pathology

Patients usually present with an ulcerating lesion on the skin, which has been exposed to the sun, for example the head and neck area. The tumour is usually ulcerated with rolled pearly borders and dilated blood vessels (telangiectasia) at the margins of the lesion. Histologically the tumour is composed of islands of basaloid cells with a

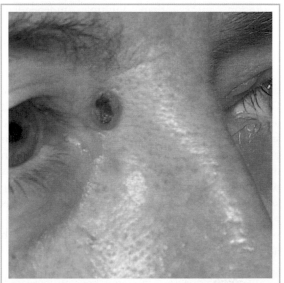

Fig. B2 A pigmented basal cell carcinoma. (Reproduced from Browse NL. *An Introduction to the Symptoms and Signs of Surgical Disease*, 3rd edn. London: Arnold, 1997)

palisaded border. Mitotic activity is usually brisk. Without complete excision, the tumour tends to recur locally. It is very unusual for this tumour to metastasize (Fig. B2).

Management

The management of these lesions is surgical with complete excision. Incomplete excision leads to local recurrence.

 Malignant melanoma; Squamous cell carcinoma

BEHÇET SYNDROME: A disease of unknown aetiology in which patients have recurrent ulcers within the oral mucosa and genital tract. Eye disease in the form of uveitis* may also be present. Other clinical manifestations include erythema nodosum, arthralgia and kidney disease.

BEJEL: A non-venereal disease of the skin, mucosa and bone caused by *Treponema pallidum* var. *endemicum*. Also called endemic syphilis.

 Treponematosis

BENCE JONES PROTEIN: Free monoclonal immunoglobulin light chains that have been filtered by the glomeruli and excreted in the urine of some patients with B-cell lymphomas and plasma cell neoplasms.

BENIGN MONOCLONAL GAMMOPATHY: See Monoclonal gammopathy of undetermined significance.

BERGER DISEASE: See IgA nephropathy.

BERI BERI: See Vitamin deficiencies.

BILHARZIA: Old terminology for schistosomiasis*.

BILIARY ATRESIA: A failure of development of either part or all of the biliary tree, resulting in jaundice. It may be either intrahepatic or extrahepatic.

BIRD FANCIER'S DISEASE: A form of extrinsic allergic alveolitis* triggered by the droppings of pigeons, hens and other domestic birds. Symptoms include fever, cough, and dyspnoea, which may progress to interstitial pulmonary fibrosis.

BLACKWATER FEVER: Haemoglobinuria due to haemolysis occurring in malaria.

 Malaria

BLADDER CARCINOMA: A malignant tumour arising from the transitional epithelium of the bladder.

Case

A 58-year-old man presented to his GP with blood-stained urine. He did not experience any pain on passing urine or have any other symptoms. He had been well and was not taking any medication. On direct questioning, he admitted to smoking 30 cigarettes per day but denied taking alcohol.

On examination, apart from haematuria, there was nothing significant to find. He was referred to the urologist.

At the hospital, a cystoscopy was performed. This showed a polypoid cauliflower-like lesion within the bladder measuring 1 cm in diameter. The tumour was excised and sent for histological examination.

> Histology: The specimen comprises a grade II (moderately differentiated) papillary transitional cell carcinoma with invasion of the superficial and deep lamina propria. Muscle is included but is not involved with the tumour (G2pT1) (Figs B3, B4).

Aetiology and risk factors

Risk factors include exposure to chemical carcinogens, e.g. β-naphthylamine, cigarette smoke, infection with *Schistosoma*, drug treatment with cyclophosphamide and, less convincingly, ingestion of coffee.

Pathology

Bladder carcinoma arises from the transitional epithelium and most carcinomas are therefore transitional cell carcinomas. Occasionally, squamous cell carcinoma (following squamous metaplasia due to chronic irritation or infection with schistosomiasis) and adenocarcinomas may be encountered. The tumours classically present with painless haematuria. The tumours may be unifocal or multifocal. It was believed that multifocal tumours were a result of a 'field effect' of carcino-

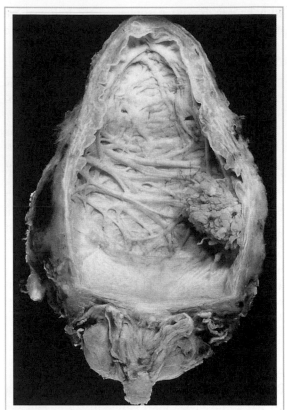

Fig. B4 Macroscopic picture of a cystectomy specimen showing bladder carcinoma.

gen exposure but recent work using chromosome X-linked inactivation methodology indicates that the different foci are monoclonal. This suggests that multifocal tumours are a result of tumour cell migration rather than multiple independent neoplastic proliferations.

Transitional cell carcinomas may be polypoid or flat and may be *in situ* (non-invasive) or invasive. They all have a tendency to recur. The prognosis depends on the grade and stage of the tumour. The G2pT1 is shorthand for the grade and stage. G2 means grade 2 (moderately differentiated). The stage is depicted as a p value. pT1 refers to invasion of lamina propria without involvement of the main muscle layer. Once it involves muscle, it is staged as pT2 and involvement of the full depth of the muscle layer (which may be difficult to assess on biopsy) is pT3. Patients with grade I tumours have a 98% 10-year survival, in contrast to grade III tumours which have a 40% 10-year survival.

Management

The main treatments available are surgical excision, intravesical chemotherapy or immune therapy (BCG).

 Schistosomiasis

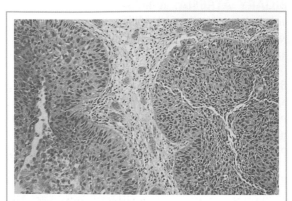

Fig. B3 Histological section showing a transitional cell carcinoma of the bladder.

BLASTOMYCOSIS: A systemic infection with the dimorphic fungus *Blastomyces dermatitidis* which is endemic in the Eastern half of North America, Africa and the Middle East. The fungus is inhaled as conidia (spores) from the environment and may cause an acute pulmonary infection resembling influenza, a chronic pulmonary infection with cough, fever, weight loss and pulmonary cavitation resembling tuberculosis, or disseminated disease affecting the liver, bone or particularly the skin. Diagnosis is by histology and isolation of the fungus. The treatment is usually with amphotericin or itraconazole.

BLOOD TRANSFUSION REACTIONS: These may be immune reactions caused by blood group incompatibility, allergic reactions to blood or its additives, infections acquired from the blood, or other untoward clinical consequence.

Case

A 60-year-old woman attended the day unit on a monthly basis for the transfusion of red cells for the correction of anaemia associated with chronic myelodysplasia. Four days after her last transfusion she telephoned to say that she had turned yellow and had had a recurrence of her symptoms of anaemia.

On examination she was noted to be jaundiced and pale, without other abnormalities. She had been transfused on a total of three occasions for her myelodysplasia and had had no children.

Her blood count showed a haemoglobin of 5 g/dl with a modest leucopenia and thrombocytopenia, which had been a consistent feature of her myelodysplasia since diagnosis. Biochemistry investigations confirmed an elevated bilirubin of 80 mmol/l. Further biochemical investigation confirmed that the elevated bilirubin was mostly unconjugated. Urine testing was positive for urobilinogen, negative for bilirubin.

The direct antiglobulin test was positive. Screening the patient's plasma for the presence of atypical red cell antibodies showed the presence of anti-Jk^a (Kidd) antibodies. The pretransfusion plasma was still available and it was re-screened for atypical red cell antibodies, with negative results. The empty blood packs were also retrieved and the red cells from the bleed lines typed for their Kidd antigen. Two out of three of the units transfused were found to be positive for Jk^a antigen. A diagnosis of delayed haemolytic transfusion reaction was made.

Aetiology and risk factors

The presence of naturally occurring anti-A and anti-B red cell antibodies can be predicted from the patient's ABO blood group. Atypical red cell antibodies are usually, but not exclusively, produced by exposure to red cells having different red cell subgroups such as Rhesus, Kell or Lewis by previous blood transfusion or transplacental bleed. These immunizing events may result in the production of red cell antibodies, which may cause a haemolytic transfusion reaction. Screening for atypical red cell antibodies involves incubating a mixture of donor red cells and recipient plasma. In the event of incompatibility this may result in a visible agglutination of red cells. To detect incompatibilities due to an IgG (non-agglutinating) antibody, an indirect antiglobulin test is performed. This detects antibodies from the recipient's serum that have coated the donor's red cells.

Pretransfusion testing includes ABO and Rhesus grouping of the donor and recipient, screening the recipient's plasma for the presence of atypical red cell antibodies, and mixing the donor's red cells with recipient's serum to look for immunological evidence of incompatibility. These precautions make serious haemolytic transfusion reactions a rare event. When they do occur they are usually due to a clerical error, when blood has been taken from or given to the wrong recipient due to incorrect patient identification. The plasma is removed from most donor units to make other blood products such as fresh frozen plasma and replaced with a red cell preserving solution such as SAGM (saline-adenine-glucose-mannitol). Thus effectively only red cells, not plasma, are given in a blood transfusion.

Pathology

In this case, pretransfusion compatibility testing was negative. In retrospect, however, it is likely that she had been immunized by a previous Jk^a-positive red cell transfusion and the administration of further red cells bearing this antigen resulted in a memory response with rapid production of antibodies that cause a delayed haemolytic reaction. This haemolysis was mostly extravascular, with antibody-coated red cells being removed from the circulation by the spleen and phagocytes of the reticuloendothelial system. In immediate haemolytic transfusion reactions the haemolysis is mostly intravascular, with free haemoglobin in the plasma and urine.

Haemolytic transfusion reactions are fortunately rare. Other unwanted side-effects of blood product administration include:

- transmission of blood-borne virus infection. All blood donations in the UK are tested for hepatitis B antigen, hepatitis C antibody and HIV antibody. Sufficient units are tested for CMV antibody to provide CMV-negative blood for immunocompromised recipients such as premature neonates or the recipients of organ transplants. Because of the theoretical risk of transmission of new variant Creutzfeld–Jakob disease by lymphocytes in blood from donors incubating the disease, leucocytes have been removed from blood by filtration since November 1999.

- production of alloantibodies against red cell, white cell and platelet antigens. Fortunately the development of red cell antibodies such as those in the case described is relatively rare. All patients should be screened for the presence of atypical red cell antibodies before transfusion by incubating their serum with a mixture of test red cells bearing the majority of common red cell antigens. If this antibody-screening test is negative then a sample of the actual donor red cells is mixed with the recipient's serum as a final compatibility test before transfusion. Evidence of incompatibility is shown by agglutination of the red cells, visible haemolysis, or antibody coating which may be detected by the antiglobulin test. Antibodies against HLA antigens on dead white cells and platelets in the blood may cause febrile non-haemolytic reactions. These may be minimized by leucocyte depletion of the blood units.
- bacterial infection from infected units. Approximately 0.1% of all blood products are contaminated by bacteria at the time of transfusion. Fortunately the incidence of symptomatic septicaemia in recipients is much less than this, thanks to the ability of the recipient's immune system to remove non-pathogenic bacteria from the circulation. In tropical countries, malaria* and other blood-borne infections may also be transmitted by transfusion.
- circulatory overload due to sudden increase in blood viscosity precipitating cardiac failure. In the elderly or those with cardiac impairment, transfusion of red cells should be given with caution, particularly in cases of megaloblastic anaemia. Plasma-reduced ('packed') red cells rather than whole blood should always be given for the correction of anaemia. Diuretic drugs may be given with the blood. A unit of red cells may be transfused over 4–6 hours. In cases of haemorrhage, transfusion is given more rapidly to correct hypotension.

Some unwanted effects of transfusion are related to the volume of blood transfused, being most commonly seen after massive transfusion, defined as the transfusion of more than the patient's blood volume in less than 24 hours. These include:

- coagulopathy. Stored banked blood contains insignificant levels of effective coagulation factors. When large volumes are transfused, particularly to operative and bleeding patients, a coagulopathy may result. In such patients coagulation screening tests and platelet count should be performed and fresh frozen plasma and platelet concentrate transfused as appropriate.
- hypothermia. When large volumes of blood, which is stored at 4°C, are transfused, an in-line 37°C blood warmer should be employed to prevent hypothermia.
- hyperkalaemia. The ion pump in the red cell membrane is inactive at refrigerator temperatures and sodium leaks into the red cells whilst potassium leaks out. This causes a relatively high potassium concentration in the suspending medium. With modern anticoagulants this is not a major problem except for patients who already have elevated plasma potassium, such as those with renal failure.
- citrate toxicity. The transfusion of large volumes of citrate anticoagulant may result in hypocalcaemia in the recipient. As with hyperkalaemia this is a rare problem with modern anticoagulants. It is most commonly seen in patients connected to the cell separator, when peri-oral tingling is the most common initial symptom. Administration of calcium gluconate by slow intravenous injection will usually alleviate the symptoms.

Management

Awareness of the unwanted effects of transfusion of blood products should prompt a careful review of the need for transfusion. Autologous transfusion, where the patient donates blood prior to operation, minimizes the risks of transfusion-transmitted infection and circumvents immunization against foreign red cell, white cell and platelet antigens. Blood in a suitable anticoagulant may be kept in the blood bank refrigerator for up to 5 weeks. Assuming weekly donation, 5 units can be collected for operation, which is enough for many elective orthopaedic operations such as hip replacement. Immediate haemolytic transfusion reactions may be associated with shock, acute renal failure and disseminated intravascular coagulation*. In such cases the transfusion must be stopped and i.v. fluids (for hypertension) or blood products (for DIC) given as required.

BONE MARROW FAILURE: Underproduction of red cells, white cells and platelets, as a result of bone marrow disease or treatment with radiotherapy or myelosupressive drugs. Deficiency of these cells may result in anaemia, infections and bleeding.

📄 *Aplastic anaemia.*

BONE MARROW TRANSPLANTATION: See Stem cell transplantation.

BORDETELLA: See Whooping cough.

BORNHOLM DISEASE: Usually caused by Coxsackie virus B presenting with acute pain in the chest or abdomen due to myositis. There may be an associated sore throat, fever and peri- or myocarditis.

BOTRIOMYCOSIS: A chronic bacterial (e.g. *Staphylococcus aureus*) infection of skin or subcutaneous tissue presenting as an indurated area with sinuses discharging pus.

BOTULISM: A toxicosis caused by *Clostridium botulinum*.

Aetiology and risk factors
Clostridium botulinum is an anaerobic Gram-positive spore-forming bacillus that is found in the environment and animal intestines. Disease is acquired by eating food contaminated with the toxin and has been linked to home-preserved vegetables, canned fish and contaminated yoghurts. Because the organism produces spores which are heat resistant, they may survive inadequate food processing and may germinate in the anaerobic environment of canned food to produce the toxin which is then ingested.

Pathology
The toxin is a peptidase whose target is the various proteins of the neurotransmitter vesicle exocytosis complex. These are proteins found on the vesicle containing the neurotransmitter (in this case acetylcholine) and on the presynaptic cleft membrane which are involved in receptor binding of the neurotransmitter-containing vesicle and ultimate release of the neurotransmitter into the synaptic cleft (Fig. B5).

The net effect of inhibiting acetylcholine release at the motor end plate and autonomic ganglia is to prevent muscular contraction which leads to a flaccid paralysis (characteristic of botulism), dizziness and a dry mouth. Typically the cranial nerves are affected first, leading to diplopia and dysarthria. With time, respiratory paralysis occurs. Diagnosis can be confirmed by detection of the

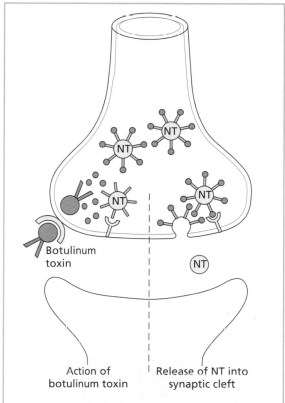

Fig. B5 Diagram showing action of botulinum toxin. NT, neurotransmitter.

toxin in the patient's blood and electromyography. Management includes respiratory support and antitoxin, although it should be given early as toxin binding is irreversible. Botulism may also occur following contamination of a wound or in infants where the organism may be found in the intestine and produces toxin *in situ*. This latter has been associated with infants being given contaminated honey. Botulinum toxin may also be given as treatment for strabismus or torticollis and cosmetically to obliterate wrinkles on the forehead.

BOWEN DISEASE: Full thickness dysplasia of the squamous epithelium or *in situ* carcinoma of the skin, without evidence of invasion through the basement membrane.

📄 *Dysplasia.*

BREAST CARCINOMA: A malignant tumour arising from the secretory (luminal epithelial) cells of the breast duct–lobular unit.

Case
A 56-year-old lady presented to the clinic with a 4-month history of a lump in her left breast. Her screening mammogram done 2 years previously

was normal. She had no other symptoms and no past medical history of note. Her mother died of breast cancer at the age of 55 and a sister, who is 46, had also been diagnosed recently with breast cancer. On examination, she had a 2 cm hard mass in her left breast, which was fixed to the skin, and erythema was noted around the nipple. No masses were palpable in the axilla. Her routine haematological and biochemical blood tests were normal. Mammography showed a spiculated mass with microcalcification suspicious of malignancy (Fig. B6).

Fine needle aspiration (FNA) cytology showed groups of pleomorphic cells with individual malignant cells in the background, graded C5 (Fig. B7). She underwent a mastectomy and axillary clearance.

The histopathological report was as follows. The specimen was sliced to reveal a 2 cm irregular firm, gritty mass. It was well clear of all margins. The

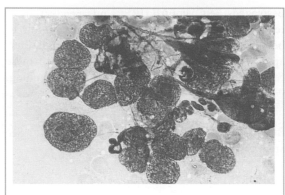

Fig. B7 FNA of breast showing hypochromatic nucleoli and nuclear pleomorphism in keeping with breast carcinoma.

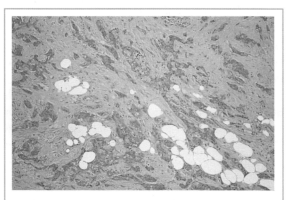

Fig. B8 Histological section showing a diffusely infiltrating invasive breast carcinoma.

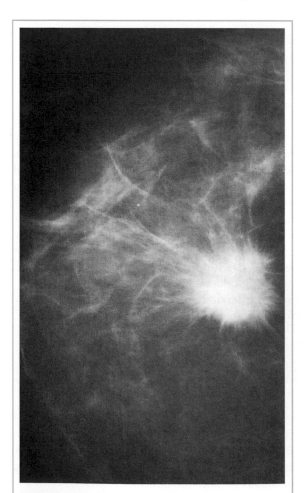

Fig. B6 Mammogram showing a spiculated mass consistent with a breast carcinoma. (Reproduced with permission from Lisle DA. *Imaging for Students*. London: Arnold, 1996)

nipple showed erythematous changes around the areola. Microscopical examination showed an *in-situ* and invasive ductal carcinoma grade III (Fig. B8) measuring 2.2 cm in maximum dimension. The nipple showed evidence of Paget disease. The tumour had been completely excised. Three of 13 lymph nodes in the axilla were involved by tumour. Oestrogen and progesterone receptor (ER & PR) status was positive. After surgery, her case was reviewed at the combined clinical, radiology and pathology meeting and she was advised to have local radiotherapy to the breast and axilla and chemotherapy.

Aetiology and risk factors

Approximately 5% of breast cancers are due to an inherited familial predisposition; a number of predisposing genes such as *BRCA1*, *BRCA2* and *TP53* have been identified. The remainder are sporadic, and risk factors include a positive family history, early menarche, late menopause, no pregnancy or late first pregnancy, exogenous oestrogens (e.g. contraceptive pill and hormone replacement therapy) and benign proliferative breast disease, especially atypical hyperplasia.

Pathology

As in this case, many patients present with a lump. With the mammographic screening programme in place, some women will be diagnosed earlier due to the presence of microcalcification or a soft tissue mass. This lady had a screening mammogram 2 years previously, hence she had an 'interval cancer'. The normal interval between mammograms is 3 years at present. The history of 4 months is short and this is sometimes the case with 'interval' cancers, possibly due to rapid growth of the tumour. She had a positive family history, which is a risk factor for breast cancer. Her clinical findings and radiological examination of a hard mass fixed to the skin, which was spiculated in appearance, indicate a malignant rather than benign tumour. The tethering to the skin is due to infiltration of tongues of tumour cells into adjacent tissues. Benign tumours, by contrast, have a smooth pushing edge. The 'erythema' around the nipple is a classical sign of Paget disease and is due to spread of tumour cells up the ductal system and into the epidermis of the nipple (Fig. B9). This then induces

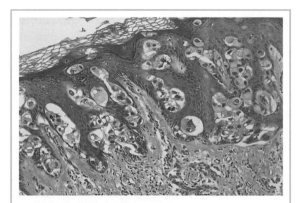

Fig. B9 Nipple showing invasion by tumour cells: pale areas within the epidermis. This is classical of Paget disease of the nipple.

an inflammatory reaction. FNA is used to suck out cells from the mass and examination of the cells indicated that it was malignant, i.e. showed features such as pleomorphism, increased nuclear:cytoplasmic ratio, increased mitotic activity and disorganization of cellular arrangement: C5 indicates definite malignancy. C4 is suspicious malignancy, C3 suspicious but probably benign, C2 benign and C1 inadequate for diagnosis. Her routine blood tests

were normal, suggesting that she was unlikely to have disseminated metastatic disease.

With the diagnosis established using the 'triple' approach (clinical examination, radiology, cytology), the mass was excised. Four important pieces of information were then provided by the histopathological examination:

- the type of tumour: she had an *in-situ* and invasive ductal carcinoma. There are many different types within the breast, the ductal type being the commonest (approx. 70%). Other types include lobular, tubular, mucinous and medullary to name just a few.
- the grade: she had a grade III tumour. Grading refers to degree of differentiation and, within the breast, is based on the assessment of tubule formation, pleomorphism and mitotic activity.
- stage: the pathological staging is provided by the size of the tumour (2.2 cm is T2, 2.0 and 5.0 cm are cut-off points for T1 and T3) and the lymph node status, which in her case was positive.
- the excision margins: her tumour was completely excised and this reduces the chances of local recurrence.

The information provided by type, grade and stage determine the prognosis: the higher the grade and stage, the worse the prognosis. Type is also important; tubular carcinoma has a better prognosis than ordinary ductal type. Other prognostic features include vascular permeation and hormone receptor status (ER+ and PR+ in her case means a good prognosis as well as predicting response to endocrine therapy).

Management

The management is dependent on the overall stage, which includes the pathological stage combined with the clinical staging. The clinical staging involves blood tests to determine whether organs such as bone marrow or liver are likely to be involved (her blood tests were normal) as well as radiological investigations such as chest radiograph, bone scan, liver ultrasound and CT scans. This will determine if the patient needs radiotherapy, chemotherapy, endocrine therapy or a combination of these.

BRITTLE BONE DISEASE: A disorder of collagen synthesis which leads to changes in the sclera, ligaments, joints, teeth, and skin. Also known as osteogenesis imperfecta.

BRODIE ABSCESS: The result of localized acute osteomyelitis, which becomes walled off to create a small bone abscess.

B

BRONCHIAL CARCINOMA: See Lung carcinoma.

BRONCHIECTASIS: An abnormal dilatation of the bronchial airways as a result of chronic necrotizing infections.

Aetiology and risk factors
The causes include congenital conditions such as congenital bronchiectasis and cystic fibrosis. It may also result from bronchial obstruction by either foreign bodies, mucus or tumour, or from chronic and severe pneumonia, e.g. tuberculous or staphylococcal.

Pathology
Patients with bronchiectasis usually present with a chronic cough, fever and expectoration of foul-smelling sputum. The major underlying pathogenesis is that of obstruction of the bronchial airways and infection. Obstruction of the airways secondary to either tumour or mucus impaction leads to absorption of the air distal to obstruction and collapse (atelectasis). There is also usually secondary infection of the lung parenchyma. The combination of obstruction, infection and inflammation leads to damage of the bronchial walls and subsequent dilatation (Fig. B10). Bronchiectasis usually affects the lower lobes bilaterally.

Complications of bronchiectasis include cor pulmonale (pulmonary hypertension and right ventricular hypertrophy), amyloidosis, and metastatic abscess in the brain.

Management
Management comprises adequate treatment of underlying infection and relieving any obstruction by impacted mucus, as in cystic fibrosis or by

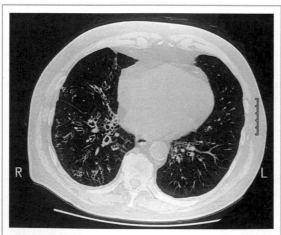

Fig. B10 CT scan showing dilated bronchi in lung. (Reproduced with permission from Curtis J, Whitehouse G. *Radiology for the MRCP*. London: Arnold, 1998)

tumours. Antibiotic or antituberculous treatment may be necessary as appropriate.

 Bronchopneumonia; Cystic fibrosis; Lung carcinoma

BRONCHIOLITIS: Acute pulmonary infection occurring early in life caused by viruses, principally, respiratory syncytial virus (RSV).

BRONCHOPNEUMONIA: Disseminated infection in the lungs caused by a variety of different bacteria leading to acute inflammation.

BRUCELLOSIS: Infection with *Brucella* spp.

Case
A 34-year-old vet was admitted to hospital for investigation of a pyrexia of several weeks' duration. She gave a history of visits to Africa and South America some weeks prior to the onset of her illness. She complained of intermittent fevers accompanied by a feeling of malaise and generalized myalgia, and she also complained of night sweats. Her only localizing complaint was of a persistent backache. On examination, an enlarged liver and spleen were noted. The patient was investigated as a case of pyrexia of unknown origin (PUO).

Haematology: The patient had a haemoglobin of 10 g/dl, a white cell count of 4000×10^6/l and a platelet count of 150×10^9/l. Thick and thin films for malaria were repeatedly negative.
Histopathology: Bone marrow aspirates showed pancytopenia with granulomatous lesions evident. Ziehl–Neelsen stain was negative.
Microbiology: Blood and bone marrow cultures grew *Brucella melitensis* after 4 weeks of incubation. *Brucella* serology was positive at a serum dilution of 2560.

Aetiology and risk factors
Brucella is a fastidious Gram-negative bacterium that causes infection in many animals. It is acquired by consuming unpasteurized dairy products or by occupational exposure to infected animals where the organism can cause infection by inhalation or through minor abrasion of the skin. The organisms are disseminated to various organs of the body and thus may produce a variety of signs and symptoms.

Pathology
Organs particularly affected are the liver, spleen, brain and bones. The histopathological appearance in the liver depends to some extent on the infecting

species (*Brucella abortus*, *Brucella melitensis*, *Brucella suis*, *Brucella canis*, etc.), but may include hepatocellular necrosis surrounded by mononuclear cells or well-defined granuloma. Pulmonary and genitourinary involvement can also occur with pleural effusion and orchitis. The patient may present with meningitis or endocarditis. The organisms are taken up by cells of the monocyte/ macrophage system but are not killed by them, instead replicating in the phagosome or endoplasmic reticulum. *Brucella* is able to inhibit phagolysosome fusion and also myeloperoxidase-generated halides. In addition, *Brucella* evades the host defences by inhibiting TNF synthesis. *Brucella* spp. upregulate IL-12 production, stimulating a Th1 response with the production of IFN-γ. The synthesis of IL-1, and endogenous pyrogen, are also increased following infection. By stimulating PGE synthesis in the hypothalamus, IL-1 resets the temperature-regulating mechanism to produce a pyrexia. Fever is a favourable host response to infection and causes a reduction in iron concentrations (thus depriving the organism, in this case *Brucella*, of a vital growth factor) by releasing lactoferrin and decreasing iron absorption through the gastrointestinal tract. Fever also causes a catabolic response with a negative nitrogen balance and loss of muscle mass. Investigation of a PUO follows the scheme shown in Table B1.

Table B1 Investigation of a PUO

Clinical history/ physical examination	Geographical, occupational, sexual and drug history important
Routine laboratory investigations	
Haematology	Full blood count, film for malarial parasites
Chemistry	Liver function tests
Radiology	Chest x-ray
Microbiology	Blood culture, faeces, MSU, throat swab
Special laboratory investigations	
Haematology	Bone marrow and trephine
Histology	Biopsy, e.g. liver
Microbiology	Serology, e.g. *Brucella*, EMU
Chemistry	Protein electrophoresis
Radiology	Sinus x-ray, ultrasound, CT scan, MRI scan, radioactive scans
Immunology	Autoantibody screen
Clinical	Laparotomy, therapeutic trial

The diagnosis of brucellosis is usually serological or by isolation of the organism from a blood or bone marrow culture.

Management
Management is with tetracycline and an aminoglycoside.

BRUTON DISEASE: A form of hypogammaglobulinaemia* due to absence of functioning B-lymphocytes. It is X-linked and therefore inherited by boys from their normal 'carrier' mothers. The incidence in the UK is about 1 in 100 000. Symptoms of repeated pyogenic infections typically begin at about 6 months of age with the disappearance of maternally transferred IgG antibodies. Treatment is by regular injections of pooled normal human immunoglobulin.

 Antibody deficiency

BUDD–CHIARI SYNDROME: Enlarged liver, ascites and abdominal pain due to thrombosis* of the hepatic vein.

BULLOUS SKIN DISEASES: A group of skin diseases characterized by blisters (bullae), many of which are immune-mediated.

Case
A 65-year-old man presented with several large tense blisters (diameter 1–2 cm) on his back and lower limbs which he said had appeared about 2 weeks earlier (Fig. B11). He also complained of

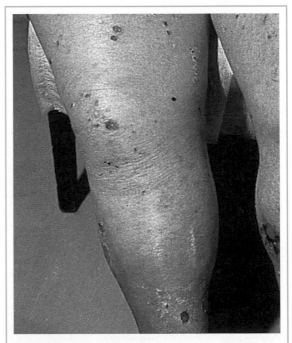

Fig. B11 Blisters seen on the lower limbs of a patient with bullous pemphigoid.

B

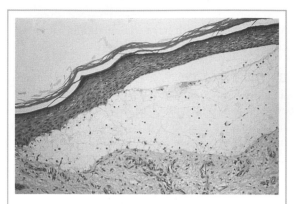

Fig. B12 Subepidermal blister containing eosinophils, characteristic of bullous pemphigoid.

(especially antibiotics) in the aetiology. There are four types of pemphigus: vulgaris, vegetans, foliaceus and erythematosus. A variant of foliaceus, fogo selvagem, affects children and adults in Brazil and it is probably the result of an infectious agent carried by an arthropod vector. The characteristics of the major bullous diseases are shown in Table B2. Note that there are some HLA haplotype associations with most of the diseases but the significance of this is presently unknown. Dermatitis herpetiformis is often accompanied by mild coeliac disease* and is thought to be a manifestation of gluten sensitivity.

Pathology

The pathogenesis of bullous pemphigoid is mediated through a type II hypersensitivity* reaction. IgG autoantibodies bind to the bullous pemphigoid protein antigens BP180 (180 kDa, type XVII collagen) and BP230 (230 kDa) and probably others in the hemidesmosome basement membrane complex of the basal keratinocytes. Similarly, in pemphigus, autoantibodies bind to the pemphigus antigen desmoglein 3 (160 kDa) on epidermal keratinocytes and probably keratinocyte cholinergic receptors. Complement is activated when the autoantibodies bind to their antigen and C3a and C5a are responsible for attraction of eosinophils, their products and those of mast cells contributing to the split occurring in the basement membrane, leading to blister formation and to the immunohistological picture used in diagnosis. There does not appear to be any correlation of titre of IgG autoantibodies in the serum and disease severity. IgE is raised in 50% of cases of pemphigoid but the relevance of this is unknown. The autoimmune nature of the pathogenesis of the pemphigus/pemphigoid diseases has been shown by transfer of the disease to experimental animals through IgG autoantibodies.

discomfort in his mouth. On examination, he had mild gingivitis and erythema in his oral cavity. His GP sent him to the local hospital for a blister biopsy and a blood test. He was given topical steroids and asked to return a week later. The biopsy revealed that his blisters were subepithelial and the blister cavities and adjacent epidermis contained eosinophils (Fig. B12). Immunoglobulin and complement were deposited at the dermoepidermal junction in the basement membrane region.

IgG antibodies to a 180 kDa glycoprotein were present in his serum. Bullous pemphigoid was diagnosed.

Aetiology and risk factors

Bullous pemphigoid is one of the commonest bullous diseases, most of which are immunologically mediated. There is some evidence in some cases of a role for drug treatment or UV/x-irradiation in the aetiology. It can be life-threatening in old people. The more serious disease pemphigus is rarer in the UK, but commoner in tropical countries. Again there is evidence for drug treatment

Table B2 Characteristics of the major bullous diseases

	Pemphigoid	Pemphigus	Herpes gestationis (pemphigoid gestationis)	Dermatitis herpetiformis
Group affected	Mainly elderly	Most ages	During pregnancy or the puerperium	Mostly young to middle age
Presentation	Tense large blisters	Often with oral ulceration	Similar to pemphigoid	Itchy vesicles
Site of blisters	Subepidermal	Intraepidermal	Subepidermal	Subepidermal
Pattern of immuno-fluorescence	Linear deposits IgG, C3 at dermoepidermal junction	Intercellular deposits IgG and C3	Similar to pemphigoid	Granular IgA deposits in dermal papillae
HLA associations	HLA-DQ7 (men only)	A10, B13, DR4	DR3,4	B8, DR3

Management

The mainstay treatment for these diseases is topical and parenteral administration of steroids. The exception to this is dermatitis herpetiformis which is associated with coeliac disease* and is treated by a gluten-free diet.

 Autoimmunity; Hypersensitivity

BURKITT LYMPHOMA: A B-cell lymphoma mainly affecting young children and found most commonly, but not exclusively, in tropical countries (especially East Africa).

Case

An 8-year-old boy visited his doctor in a village outside Kampala complaining of recent headaches, nausea and vomiting. He also had a swelling on the left side of his face (Fig. B13). On examination the mass appeared to be associated with his maxilla but his cervical nodes were not enlarged. A blood test was taken and from the blood film he was diagnosed as having malaria. A fine-needle aspirate of the swelling showed cells of Burkitt lymphoma. He was immediately started on primaquine for his malaria and cyclophosphamide treatment for his

lymphoma. Being young, he has a good prognosis for complete remission.

Aetiology and risk factors

In tropical countries, Burkitt lymphoma is commoner in young males than females, with an average age of onset of 7 years. It is mainly seen in malaria endemic regions. The vast majority of cases are associated with the Epstein–Barr virus, the EBV genome and EBV-associated antigens being detectable in the tumour cells. The exact role of EBV (and of malaria) in the development of Burkitt lymphoma is unclear. EBV is probably responsible for the activation of oncogenes which result in the B-cell proliferation, whereas malaria has been postulated as a cofactor for tumorigenesis by suppressing T-cell responses, which allows the development of transformed B-cell clones. EBV is associated with a number of other tumours, notably nasopharyngeal carcinoma*. Burkitt lymphoma can occur without any association with EBV, usually in non-tropical areas and in older children, and also in immunosuppressed patients.

Pathology

Burkitt is a high-grade non-Hodgkin B-cell lymphoma. In general, there is less involvement of peripheral nodes and the tumour rarely becomes leukaemic. In males, the jaw is commonly the site of primary involvement, whereas in females, the ovaries are usually affected first. The rapid growth of the tumour is reflected in the high mitotic rates and the presence of many macrophages (histiocytes) containing nuclear debris of apoptotic cells. This gives rise to a diagnostic 'starry-sky' histological picture (Fig. B14). In common with most B-cell

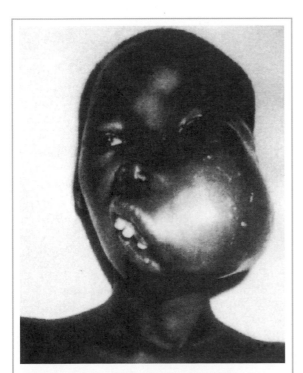

Fig. B13 Young child with a large maxillary tumour distorting the face. This is a classical presentation of Burkitt lymphoma. (Reproduced with permission from Lakhani SR, Dilly SA, Finlayson CJ. *Basic Pathology*, 2nd edn. London: Arnold, 1998)

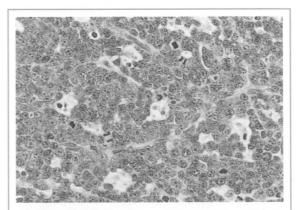

Fig. B14 Photomicrograph showing classical 'starry sky' appearance of Burkitt lymphoma. (Reproduced with permission from Lakhani SR, Dilly SA, Finlayson CJ. *Basic Pathology*, 2nd edn. London: Arnold, 1998)

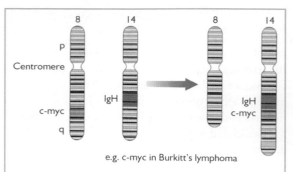

e.g. c-myc in Burkitt's lymphoma

Fig. B15 Translocation. (Reproduced with permission from Lakhani SR, Dilly SA, Finlayson CJ. *Basic Pathology*, 2nd edn. London: Arnold, 1998)

lymphomas, there is a chromosomal translocation. In Burkitt lymphoma, the translocation is usually between chromosome (chr) 8 and 14 – t(8;14). The breakpoint on chr 8 is near to the c-*myc* oncogene which is involved in control of cell proliferation. This joins adjacent to the immunoglobulin heavy chain joining or constant region on chr 14, bringing together the c-*myc* oncogene with the heavy chain region of immunoglobulin (Fig. B15). Translocations can also occur between chr 8 and the lambda light chain constant region of chr 2 or the kappa light chain region on chr 22.

Management

Directed x-irradiation treatment is appropriate but wide field irradiation should be avoided to avoid skeletal deformities later in life. As for all high-grade lymphomas, cytotoxic drugs are given (e.g. cyclophosphamide) and, where possible, combination therapy with CNS prophylaxis (see Acute lymphoblastic leukaemia) is used.

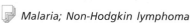 *Malaria; Non-Hodgkin lymphoma*

BURULI ULCER: Skin ulceration caused by *Mycobacterium ulcerans*.

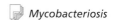 *Mycobacteriosis*

C

CACHEXIA: This refers to a generalized state of ill health in which there is loss of body mass and wasting. It is often associated with malignant disease.

 Paraneoplastic syndromes

CAISSON DISEASE: See Decompression sickness.

CALCULUS: The presence of stones within the urogenital tract. The vast majority occur in the renal pelvis or bladder.

Aetiology
This is a fairly common problem occurring in about 0.5–2% of the population. The commonest calculus is a calcium oxalate, which is seen in about 70% of patients. Patients usually present with acute obstruction or haematuria.

Pathology
Table C1 provides a list of causes associated with hypercalcaemia and the mechanisms involved where known.

Table C1 Causes associated with hypercalcaemia and mechanisms involved

Stone	Predisposing factor

Calcium oxalate (70%)	Hypercalcaemia
	  Primary hyperparathyroidism
	  Metastatic bone disease
	Idiopathic hypercalciuria
	Hyperoxaluria
	  Inherited
	  Intestinal disease
	  High intake of green vegetables
	  High vitamin C intake
	  Ethylene glycol intake

Phosphate calculi (calcium phosphate, and magnesium ammonium phosphate) (15%)	Urinary tract infection by urea splitting bacteria
Uric acid (10%)	Gout, but dose occurs in patients with normal serum acid levels
Cystine and xanthine stones	Cystinuria, xanthinuria

Investigations

Blood: bone profile (calcium, albumin, phosphate, alkaline phosphatase); electrolytes and urea; parathyroid hormone (PTH); thyroid hormones (T4, T3 and TSH); angiotensin-converting enzyme (ACE); protein electrophoresis; vitamin D metabolites [1,25(OH)$_2$D, 25(OH)$_2$D]; parathyroid hormone related protein (PTHrP); uric acid; cystine; oxalate; bone marrow examination
Urine: calcium (24 hour), cystine, oxalate, microscopy/culture/sensitivity
Radiological: bone scan, chest radiograph, plain abdominal radiograph, intravenous or retrograde pyelography.

Management
Management consists of treating the cause of hypercalcaemia. The treatment of small stones is by observation and allowing the stone to be passed naturally, whilst controlling pain with analgesics. Treatment of large and complicated stones usually requires lithotripsy, ultrasonic breaking or surgery.

CANDIDIASIS: Diseases caused by *Candida* species, notably *Candida albicans*.

Aetiology and risk factors
Candida albicans is a yeast that is part of the normal flora of many individuals (Fig. C1). Disease can be mucocutaneous or systemic. There is usually a predisposing factor in developing candidal infection such as a side-effect of antibiotic usage, diabetes, or immunosuppression. Occasionally, other *Candida* species such as *Candida krusei* and *Candida tropicalis* may cause disease. These also occur in immunocompromised individuals.

C

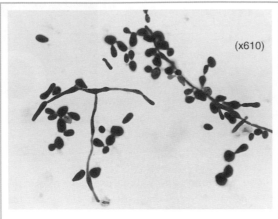

(x610)

Fig. C1 Photograph showing a Gram stain of *Candida*. (X 610)

Pathology

Disturbance of the normal flora allows the opportunity for *Candida* to proliferate and cause mucosal disease. This may present as oral or vaginal 'thrush' which is seen as white plaques, consisting of superficial epithelial cells, necrotic debris, polymorphs and the yeast, on the mucosa. *Candida* may also penetrate the keratinized epithelium giving rise to nodular skin lesions and can also cause paronychia when the *Candida* invades the nail fold, usually following trauma. Disease is caused by invasion of the tissue and consequent damage to the mucosa, skin or solid organ. Defects in T-cells are linked to tissue invasion as may occur in oesophagitis in patients with HIV or patients with chronic mucocutaneous candidiasis. In the latter condition there is cutaneous anergy to *Candida* antigens and the condition presents as severe infiltration and proliferation of the yeast on the mucosa and mucocutaneous junctions. In *Candida* oesophagitis the whole of the oesophagus may be covered by the yeast, which also invades into the wall of the oesophagus, giving rise to dysphagia. Disseminated infection may also occur in the compromised and abscesses may form in any organ, e.g. liver, spleen, or the patient may develop endocarditis. A particularly characteristic complication of disseminated disease is endophthalmitis where the *Candida* grows in the vitreous humour of the eye, giving rise to blurred vision. *Candida* can bind to many cell types as well as to plastic and thus infections are associated with those receiving total parenteral nutrition or chronic ambulatory peritoneal dialysis (CAPD).

Management

Management includes the azole group of antifungal agents (fluconazole, clotrimazole), flucytosine or amphotericin. Often the non-albicans *Candida* species are resistant to the azoles.

CAPLAN SYNDROME: The combination of rheumatoid arthritis and progressive massive lung fibrosis due to inhalation of dust, silica, etc.

CARCINOID TUMOUR: A tumour arising from neural crest tissue and enterochromaffin cells, of low-grade malignancy and frequently invading local tissue, distant metastases being a rarity (Fig. C2). Ninety per cent of these tumours are found in the appendix and ileocaecal region. Clinically, most are asymptomatic until metastases are present, the frequent site of carcinoid metastases being the liver.

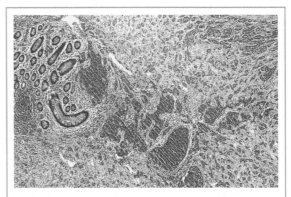

Fig. C2 Section of appendix involved with carcinoid tumour. Normal appendix mucosa is seen to the left. The tumour, composed of small cells forming sheets or trabeculae, is seen on the right half of the section.

Location of tumour by site of embryonic origin

- Foregut: oesophagus, stomach, duodenum, pancreas, gallbladder and bile duct, ampulla of Vater, larynx, bronchus and thymus
- Midgut: jejunum, ileum, appendix, colon, liver, ovary, testes and cervix
- Hindgut: rectum

Pathology

Carcinoid cells produce adrenocorticotropic hormone (ACTH), calcitonin, gastrin, glucagon, growth hormone, insulin, motilin, neuropeptide K, neurotensin, somatostatin, serotonin, pancreatic polypeptide, substance K, substance P and vasoactive intestinal peptide. Serotonin (5-hydroxytryptamine) is synthesized from the amino acid tryptophan and is the major byproduct secreted by the midgut tumours, whilst the main product secreted by the foregut tumours is 5-hydroxytryptophan.

The **carcinoid syndrome** occurs as a consequence of the release of these peptides into the circulation. Many of these peptides are vasoactive and cause vasodilatation, resulting in flushing. Other symptoms include diarrhoea, hyperperistalsis, nausea, vomiting, colicky pain, wheezing, increased salivation and lacrimation. There are also chronic complications such as fibrosis of the pulmonary and tricuspid heart valves, mesenteric fibrosis and hyperkeratosis of the skin. The symptoms are usually seen in patients with bronchial tumours, which spill their peptides into the systemic circulation directly or in patients with tumours from the gut with metastases to the liver. The presence of 5-HIAA in the urine is diagnostic.

Management of this condition is quite difficult. Medical management with serotonin antagonists is not very effective in controlling the symptoms. Inhibitors of tryptophan 5-hydroxylase are also used. Surgical removal of the tumour is also performed, unless metastases are present. Chemotherapy and destruction of blood supply to hepatic metastases by embolization of the hepatic arteries have been helpful.

CARCINOMA: A malignant tumour of epithelial tissues such as squamous and glandular epithelium.

CARCINOMA *IN SITU*: Refers to cytologically malignant cells, which have not yet broken through the basement membrane and hence do not have metastatic potential.

 Dysplasia

CARDIAC FAILURE: See Heart failure.

CARDIAC TAMPONADE: Compression of the heart due to fluid or blood within the pericardial space, obstructing the normal functioning and contractions of the myocardium.

CARDIOGENIC SHOCK: A state of severe failure of tissue perfusion as a result of severe reduction in cardiac output due to primary cardiac disease, e.g. myocardial infarction, acute myocarditis and arrhythmias.

CARDIOMYOPATHY: This term refers to a variety of non-inflammatory disorders of the heart muscle.

Aetiology and risk factors

The aetiology of the cardiomyopathies is unknown. Some of these disorders may have a genetic predisposition. Where the aetiological agent or risk factor is understood, these are referred to as secondary cardiomyopathies. Causes of secondary cardiomyopathy include infections, haemochromatosis*, amyloidosis*, fibrosis, x-irradiation, sarcoidosis* and drug toxicity (e.g. adriamycin).

Pathology

The cardiomyopathies of unknown aetiology can be divided into three main groups, as follows:
- dilated or congestive cardiomyopathy
- hypertrophic or obstructive cardiomyopathy
- restrictive cardiomyopathy.

Dilated cardiomyopathy In this type of cardiomyopathy all four chambers of the heart are dilated (Fig. C3) and patients usually have severe cardiac failure. Idiopathic dilated cardiomyopathy has a familial incidence of approximately 20%. Secondary dilated cardiomyopathy is usually due to an infective myocarditis or secondary to disorders such as haemochromatosis and sarcoidosis. Chronic alcohol abuse also leads to this type of cardiomyopathy Adriamycin treatment, which is used for chemotherapy of neoplastic lesions, is also a recognized cause of dilated cardiomyopathy.

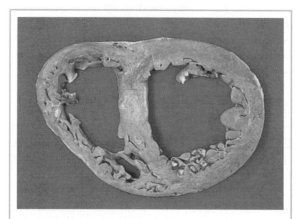

Fig. C3 Dilated cardiomyopathy as a result of untreated hypertension. Note the dilated right and left ventricles. (Reproduced with permission from Lakhani SR, Dilly SA, Finlayson CJ. *Basic Pathology*, 2nd edn. London: Arnold, 1998)

Hypertrophic cardiomyopathy In this disorder there is marked hypertrophy (increase in cell size) of the myocytes. The hypertrophy is usually asymmetrical and leads to outflow obstruction of the blood from the ventricular chamber. Approximately half the patients with hypertrophic cardiomyopathy have a positive family history and the disease is thought to be transmitted in an autosomal dominant fashion. The clinical course is variable and many patients present with atrial

C

fibrillation and subsequent thrombosis and embolism. These patients are also at risk of sudden death from cardiac arrhythmia.

Restrictive cardiomyopathy In this type of cardiomyopathy there is a restriction to ventricular filling as a result of deposition of material within the ventricular wall. The commonest causes of secondary restrictive cardiomyopathy are amyloid deposition, radiation-induced fibrosis and endomyocardial fibrosis of unknown aetiology. The decreased compliance of the ventricular wall as a result of such depositions leads to cardiac failure.

Management

The management of dilated cardiomyopathy relates to treatment of cardiac failure. Cardiac failure and cardiac arrhythmia are the commonest causes of death. Because of the dilated chambers these patients are at risk of thrombosis and embolism. In selected cases, cardiac transplantation may be an option. The management of hypertrophic cardiomyopathy is usually by medical therapy to cause ventricular relaxation. Although the asymmetrical ventricular hypertrophy is a cause of outflow obstruction, this does not always lead to symptoms. However, resection of the hypertrophic muscle is sometimes recommended in these patients. Restrictive cardiomyopathy is extremely difficult to treat, as the deposition (e.g. by amyloid) is diffuse and therefore not surgically removable.

 Amyloidosis; Haemochromatosis; Hypertension; Sarcoidosis

CARPAL TUNNEL SYNDROME: Results from compression of the medium nerve within the carpal tunnel. It may be due to amyloid deposition.

CATARACT: An opacity of the lens of the eye. The most common cause is ageing, but cataracts may also be congenital or associated with trauma, diabetes, congenital rubella syndrome, hypoparathyroidism, dystrophia myotonica or drugs (e.g. steroids). The lens becomes oedematous and necrotic and there is disruption of continuity of lens fibres.

CAT-SCRATCH DISEASE: A self-limiting disease caused by *Bartonella henselae*, transmitted from cats and dogs, usually through a scratch or bite. It presents with a papule at the site of inoculation, tender regional lymphadenopathy and fever. Rarely, a systemic illness may follow, with a rash, hepatic granuloma, splenomegaly or encephalitis. Histopathologically the enlarged lymph nodes show granulomata and stellate microabscesses infil-

trated with polymorphs. Diagnosis is by serology, isolation of the organism or the polymerase chain reaction. As the condition is self-limiting, treatment is not usually required.

 Bartonellosis

CELLULITIS: A general term for infection of the skin and subcutaneous tissues that can be caused by a wide range of organisms, most commonly *Streptococcus pyogenes* and *Staphylococcus aureus*.

 Gas gangrene; Necrotizing fasciitis

CEREBROVASCULAR DISEASE: Injury to cerebral tissue as a result of impairment of the circulation to the brain.

Case

A 50-year-old man was seen in the clinic following an episode of 'paralysis' in the night. He was woken from his sleep by a strange dream. When he tried to get up to go to the bathroom, he almost fell to the ground. He managed to get himself back into bed and discovered that he had difficulty moving the left side of his body. After the initial panic had settled, he managed to alert his wife but the weakness began to disappear within a few minutes and they decided to wait till the morning to see the doctor.

This was the first such episode. He had been diagnosed as having hypertension 3 years previously and he was on regular medication. His father had died of a 'stroke' at the age of 63 years.

On examination, his pulse was 80 beats/min and blood pressure 130/90 mmHg. His apex beat was displaced to the left. Auscultation revealed normal heart sounds but a carotid bruit was heard on the right side.

An urgent referral was made to the cardiologist, but 2 days later he was admitted to A&E with a left-sided hemiplegia. Examination revealed complete loss of movement with extensor plantar response. He continued to deteriorate over the next 2 days and died. A postmortem examination was requested.

Postmortem findings The main findings were in the cardiovascular system. He had extensive atheroma throughout the vascular tree, in particular the aorta and carotid arteries (Fig. C4). There was plaque fissuring in the left carotid artery with thrombus formation. The heart was enlarged with left ventricular hypertrophy but no evidence of myocardial infarction. Examination of the brain showed atheroma in the cerebral vessels

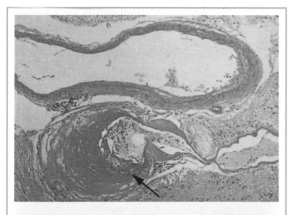
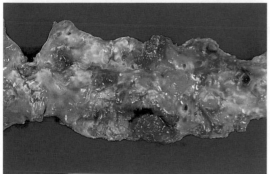

Fig. C4 Section of cerebral microaneurysm (top, arrowed); descending aorta showing severe atherosclerosis (bottom).

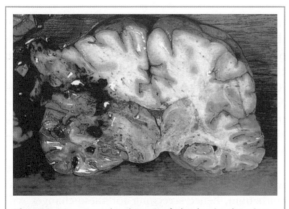

Fig. C5 Macroscopic picture of the brain showing cerebral infarction. (Reproduced with permission from Lakhani SR, Dilly SA, Finlayson CJ. *Basic Pathology*, 2nd edn. London: Arnold, 1998)

and mild atrophy. The right parietal cortex showed softening (Fig. C5) over the motor cortex and histology confirmed infarction. Cause of death:

- 1a: cerebrovascular accident (CVA) due to
- 1b: embolus from carotid thrombus
- 1c: atherosclerosis.

Aetiology and risk factors

Cerebrovascular disease is usually a result of atherosclerosis; hence, risk factors include those of atherosclerosis. These are hypertension, hyperlipidaemia, obesity, diabetes and smoking. CVA, due to haemorrhage, may occur in about 20% of cases.

Pathology

The initial presentation here was with a transient ischaemic attack (TIA). This is usually due to an embolus causing a transient obstruction and ischaemia of the cerebral circulation. Since it passes without leaving a permanent deficit, its importance is as a sign of potentially fatal CVA. This man had a known history of hypertension and his clinical examination suggested left ventricular hypertrophy. Hypertension is a risk factor for atherosclerosis and hence for myocardial infarction and CVA. Hypertension, if uncontrolled, can also lead to a cerebral bleed, which may also manifest as a CVA. This man, however, had an embolic episode and examination suggested that the site was the right carotid artery. He had an audible bruit indicating turbulent flow as a result of atherosclerosis. Unfortunately, he suffered a fatal CVA soon afterwards.

The postmortem examination confirmed widespread atherosclerotic disease and also a complicated atheromatous plaque in the carotid. Plaque fissuring results in thrombus formation due to exposure of the lipid and collagen, which excites the coagulation pathway. A potential complication of thrombus formation is embolism, which is the most likely scenario in this man.

Management

Treatment of patients with widespread atherosclerotic disease is difficult and comprises changes in lifestyle (stop smoking), antihypertensive or antilipidaemia therapy if appropriate, and surgical intervention. Carotid narrowing can be relieved by an endarterectomy but this 're-boring' is not without risk and the surgery itself can induce a CVA.

 Atheroma; Hypertension; Myocardial infarction

CERVICAL CARCINOMA: A malignant neoplasm arising from the squamous or glandular epithelium of the cervix.

Case

A 42-year-old lady presented to the clinic for a routine smear test. The smear was reported as suspicious but inadequate for assessment and a repeat smear was suggested. The clinic tried to contact the patient without success. She represented a year later for her smear.

C

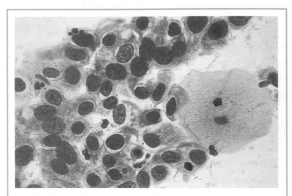

Fig. C6 Cervical smear showing one normal keratinocyte together with large number of cells exhibiting severe dyskaryosis.

Cytology: The smear showed marked wart virus change and severe dyskaryosis (Fig. C6).

She was referred for colposcopic examination of her cervix. Further questioning by the gynaecologist revealed that she was a single mother living with her boyfriend. She had divorced 1 year previously and gave a history of multiple sexual partners prior to her marriage, her first sexual contact being at the age of 16. There was no family history of note and she was not on any medication.

At colposcopy an abnormal aceto-white area was identified which was biopsied. Histological examination confirmed CIN III (cervical intraepithelial neoplasia stage III) and she underwent a cone biopsy.

Cone biopsy: Sections showed extensive koilocytic change together with CIN III extending into the crypts. A focus of invasive squamous cell carcinoma invading to a depth of 2 mm was also seen. CIN extended to the excision margin (Fig. C7).

The surgeon recommended that she should have a hysterectomy. The decision was a difficult one for her but she eventually agreed. No further treatment was required.

Aetiology and risk factors
Risk factors include multiple sexual partners, early age of first sexual contact, and infection with human papilloma virus (HPV) especially HPV 16.

Pathology
Within the UK and many other countries, a cervical screening programme has been established to try and reduce the morbidity and mortality from this disease. Cervical carcinoma is effectively a sexually

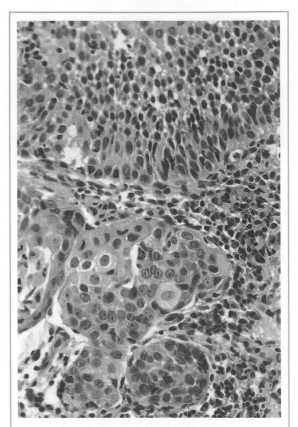

Fig. C7 Histological section showing severe dysplasia and foci of invasive carcinoma.

transmitted disease and it is important to realize that early onset of sexual contact and multiple partners are strong risk factors as they increase the chances of contracting infection with HPV. Reducing promiscuity and the use of barrier contraceptives such as condoms are therefore effective preventive measures. The screening programme is also a type of preventive strategy and relies on the knowledge of the 'multistep model of carcinogenesis'. This model suggests that invasive carcinoma will arise via dysplastic changes in the cervical epithelium, hence screening for these changes will allow detection of the tumour at an earlier stage of the process. This screening procedure is carried out using the cervical smear test. Cells from the transformation zone of the cervix are scraped off with a spatula and examined microscopically. The term dyskaryosis (used in cervical cytology reporting) is synonymous with dysplasia. Dyskaryosis is graded as mild, moderate and severe and is the smear equivalent to CIN (cervical intraepithelial neoplasia) I, II and III. These represent increasingly worse dysplastic changes so that in CIN III, the full thickness of the cervical epithelium is affected, amounting in essence to carcinoma *in situ*. It is impossible on smear test to make a definite diagnosis of invasive cancer since the cells are scraped from the surface. If significant abnormalities (i.e. dyskaryosis) are seen on the smear, the patient is referred for colposcopic examination. Here the cervix is viewed using a special microscope and biopsies are taken of any suspicious areas. In this patient, not only did she have CIN III (severe dysplasia) but also a focus of invasive cancer. It is impossible to rule out further invasive disease on biopsy of this sort and formal staging (extent of disease) requires that the uterus is removed. This is a difficult decision for a woman of 42 as she may still want to have children in the future. However, she has little choice since untreated carcinoma of the cervix carries a significant mortality.

Management

The management is initially surgical but patients may also need local radiotherapy. In the event of systemic disease, chemotherapy would also be considered.

 Dysplasia

CHAGAS DISEASE: Also called South American trypanosomiasis, an infection with *Trypanosoma cruzi*.

Aetiology and risk factors

Trypanosoma cruzi is a flagellate protozoon. The disease is a zoonosis* and the organism is transmitted to humans by a reduviid bug which, whilst feeding, also defecates on the skin, the organism then being inadvertently inoculated into the host's blood following scratching of the bite.

Pathology

The infection may remain entirely asymptomatic or cause disease of the heart or gastrointestinal tract. Primary infection presents as a soft tissue swelling called a chagoma characteristically adjacent to the eye. Thereafter, a small proportion of people will ultimately develop disease with cardiomyopathy, megacolon or mega-oesophagus. The amastigote penetrates and replicates in the cytoplasm of host cells, usually muscle cells. The precise mechanisms of pathogenesis are unclear but the parasite may directly induce damage to the heart muscle cells and/or may induce antibodies cross-reacting with cardiac cells. Histopathologically, the heart is infiltrated by mononuclear cells. The muscle cells are degenerate and there is dense fibrosis. This eventually leads to biventricular thinning, aneurysm formation, valvular incompetence and congestive cardiac failure. Intraventricular thrombi may form. Inflammation and fibrosis of thoracic or mesenteric parasympathetic ganglia lead to disorders of peristalsis in the gut with either mega-oesophagus, difficulty in swallowing, aspiration and lung abscesses or constipation, megacolon and volvulus. Diagnosis is by serology and histology and treatment of acute infection is with benznidazole.

CHANCROID: A venereal disease, usually occurring in tropical countries, caused by *Haemophilus ducreyi*. The organism enters via damaged epithelium on the genitals and produces a papule, which then ulcerates. There is a mononuclear cell infiltrate with granuloma formation and a polymorph infiltrate. Regional lymphadenopathy occurs in about half the patients and the enlarged nodes may suppurate. The ulcer has a sharply demarcated edge and is painful. Frequently, several ulcers merge into a single ulcer. The mainstay of laboratory diagnosis is by culture of the organism. Treatment is with co-trimoxazole, ceftriaxone or ciprofloxacin.

CHEDIAK–HIGASHI SYNDROME: A genetic (autosomal recessive) form of immunodeficiency associated with defects in the cytoplasmic granules of neutrophils. These are visible as giant granules, and expressed as a failure to kill Gram-positive bacteria, e.g. *Streptococcus pneumococcus*. Oxidative killing, however, is normal. There are also defects in neutrophil chemotaxis and NK cell function.

CHICKENPOX: An exanthema occurring predominantly in children, caused by varicella-zoster virus (a herpes virus).

Aetiology and risk factors

Chickenpox is transmitted by the respiratory route. The primary infection is chickenpox (varicella). After resolution of the primary infection, the virus is not eliminated from the body but becomes latent in the dorsal root ganglia. The virus may reactivate, induced by a number of factors (e.g. immunosuppression) and clinically present as shingles (zoster), usually in adults. Both forms of the disease are highly infectious but non-immune contacts of cases of shingles present with the primary infection – chickenpox, not shingles. Shingles is thus a manifestation of the carrier state and not a primary infection.

Pathology

At primary infection the virus replicates in cells in the nasopharynx producing typical intranuclear eosinophilic inclusions with multinucleate giant cells. The virus spreads locally from cell to cell and may also infect white cells and be spread around the body. The disease presents clinically with fever, malaise and the characteristic rash, which goes

Table C2 *Chlamydia* species and associated illnesses

Species	Disease	Source	Route
Ch. trachomatis serovar A–C	Trachoma – eye	Human	Direct contact or via flies
Ch. trachomatis serovar D–K	Non-gonococcal urethritis – urethra Inclusion conjunctivitis – eye Ophthalmia neonatorum – eye	Human	Sexual contact Infected mother at birth
Ch. trachomatis L1–3	Lymphogranuloma venereum – genitals	Human	Sexual contact
Ch. psittaci	Psittacosis – lungs	Birds	Respiratory
Ch. pneumoniae	Pneumonia – lungs	Human	Respiratory

through the stages: maculopapular, vesicular, pustular, scab formation. The rash first appears centrally, spreading to the limbs, and occurs in successive crops with all stages of development present at any one time. Eventually all the ruptured pustules scab over and the patient is then non-infectious.

Complications may occur, such as Reye syndrome, systemic disease with pneumonia or encephalitis, an extensive haemorrhagic rash or secondary bacterial infection, particularly with *Streptococcus pyogenes*. Complications are more common in the immunocompromised. Infection in pregnancy can lead to congenital malformations in the fetus and perinatal disease carries a high mortality for the neonate. Reactivation of virus replication to produce shingles presents as localized unilateral pain followed by a vesicular eruption with a dermatome distribution. Involvement of the fifth cranial nerve can lead to ophthalmic complications and the seventh cranial nerve to lesions in the mouth. Severe post-herpetic pain may occur in some patients. Encephalitis and myelitis are rare complications of shingles. Laboratory diagnosis includes culture, serology and PCR.

Management
Treatment, if required, is with aciclovir. Prophylaxis of immunocompromised contacts is with zoster immunoglobulin (ZIG). An attenuated vaccine is available, but its use is still controversial.

CHLAMYDIAL DISEASE: Infection caused by the obligate intracellular pathogen *Chlamydia*.

Aetiology and risk factors
There are three different *Chlamydia* species associated with different illnesses (see Table C2).

Pathology
The life cycle is shown in Fig. C8.

The characteristic histopathological feature of chlamydial disease is the lymphoid follicle composed of B-cells and macrophages surrounded by T-cells. In the tissue between follicles there is a neutrophil infiltrate accompanied at a later stage by macrophages and lymphocytes. An important inflammatory stimulus to the host is chronic exposure to the 60 kDa heat shock protein of the micro-organism which may be responsible for the scarring found in trachoma and salpingitis.

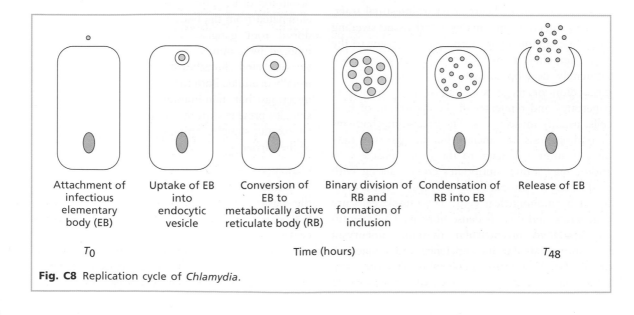

| Attachment of infectious elementary body (EB) | Uptake of EB into endocytic vesicle | Conversion of EB to metabolically active reticulate body (RB) | Binary division of RB and formation of inclusion | Condensation of RB into EB | Release of EB |

T_0 Time (hours) T_{48}

Fig. C8 Replication cycle of *Chlamydia*.

The clinical conditions are:

- trachoma: a follicular keratoconjunctivitis which heals by fibrosis and vascularization, leading to scarring and opacity of the cornea and blindness.
- inclusion conjunctivitis: similar to trachoma, presenting as a follicular conjunctivitis with a purulent discharge but not usually leading to blindness.
- ophthalmia neonatorum: does not usually show follicles, presenting as a mucopurulent discharge with swollen eyelids, but may cause blindness if untreated. Some neonates may also develop pneumonia.
- genital infections: inflammation of the urethra, cervix and rectum can occur and the patient presents with a purulent discharge and may complain of pain. In females, infection of the cervix is often asymptomatic and they are an important source of infection in the community. Infection can spread, causing salpingitis or endometritis and eventual sterility due to tubal adhesions caused by the scarring that occurs (see Pelvic inflammatory disease).
- lymphogranuloma venereum: the infection causes an ulcer on the penis or fourchette with acute onset painful regional lymphadenopathy. There is associated fever, malaise and arthralgia. Proctitis may also occur. Complications include strictures in the genitourinary system and scrotal lymphodema.
- psittacosis and *Ch. pneumoniae*: see Atypical pneumonia.

Laboratory diagnosis is usually by serology, rapid antigen detection methods or for genital infections with serovars D–K, the ligase chain reaction (LCR).

Management

Management is with erythromycin or tetracycline and for sexually transmitted disease, contact tracing. Ophthalmia neonatorum is a notifiable disease.

CHOLANGIOCARCINOMA: A primary malignant tumour of the liver arising from the bile duct epithelium. It is an uncommon tumour. By definition it is an adenocarcinoma. It is associated with exposure to Thorotrast (used in the past for radiological examination) and infection with liver flukes. It tends to present late in its natural history and death usually occurs within 6 months of diagnosis.

Hepatocellular carcinoma

CHOLANGITIS: Inflammation of the bile duct and intrahepatic biliary system which can be caused by many different bacteria and associated with cholecystitis. Obstruction of biliary drainage by, for example, an extrinsic mass or a gallstone, leads to damage to the mucosa, necrosis of the endothelium, proliferation of bacteria (frequently *Enterobacteriaceae* (*Escherichia*) and anaerobes (*Bacteroides*) and an acute inflammatory reaction, often with periportal abscesses. Clinically it is indistinguishable from cholecystitis and presents with right upper quadrant pain and tenderness with fever, rigors and jaundice (Charcot's triad). There is an elevated peripheral white count with neutrophilia, an elevated serum conjugated bilirubin, alkaline phosphatase and moderately elevated aspartate aminotransferase levels. Complications include septic shock and liver abscess. Treatment is by antibiotics and surgical relief of any obstruction.

CHOLECYSTITIS: Inflammation of the gallbladder, typically associated with obstruction by gallstones. The pathology of inflammation is the same as with cholangitis – obstruction causing an increased pressure in the viscus with mucosal necrosis, bile stasis and bacterial proliferation. Frequently there is evidence of previous episodes of inflammation, characterized by chronic inflammatory cells, mucosal herniation and fibrosis in the gallbladder wall , as a background to the acute inflammatory reaction. Clinically it presents in the same way as cholangitis, with an elevated white count, although the biochemical abnormalities are frequently not as marked. Complications include septic shock, ascending cholangitis, liver abscess, gangrene or rupture of the gallbladder and peritonitis. Treatment is with antibiotics, cholecystectomy or surgical relief of any obstruction.

CHOLERA: A disease caused by the Gram-negative bacillus *Vibrio cholerae*.

Aetiology and risk factors

The disease is acquired by drinking contaminated water.

Pathology

The organism attaches to the enterocytes of the small intestine and produces a toxin which causes the disease cholera. The toxin leads to elevated levels of cAMP which in turn opens the cystic fibrosis transmembrane conductance channel leading to loss of NaCl and water (Fig. C9). The net effect is the loss of isotonic fluid from the intestine leading to dehydration.

The patient complains of passing large volumes of 'rice water' stools. The patient is acidotic with a pH of about 7.0, and low serum bicarbonate, but

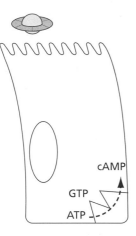

Binding of cholera toxin to luminal surface

Synthesis of cAMP from ATP with binding of GTP by the G protein of the adenyl cyclase complex

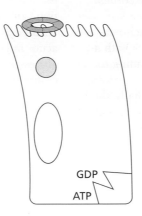

Membrane transport of the active subunit of cholera toxin across the cell membrane

Hydrolysis of GTP to GDP by G protein (a GTPase) and inactivity of adenyl cyclase complex

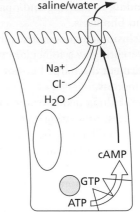

cAMP opens cystic fibrosis transmembrane conductance channel with loss of isotonic saline/water

Modification of G subunit by active subunit of cholera toxin, resulting in lack of GTPase activity, leading to continuous production of cAMP

Fig. C9 Diagram showing the action of cholera toxin.

paradoxically normal serum sodium and slightly elevated potassium and chloride brought about by loss of fluid and dehydration. The serum protein and specific gravity of the blood is elevated. This metabolic imbalance leads to hyperventilation, altered consciousness and cardiac irregularities. Laboratory diagnosis depends upon isolating the organism from the faeces.

Management
Treatment is by rehydration given parenterally and antibiotics – tetracycline. In some situations only oral rehydration is possible in which case glucose should be added to the sodium chloride, sodium bicarbonate and potassium chloride mixture as the cholera toxin does not affect the glucose-facilitated sodium absorption pathway. There is a killed vaccine, but its value is debatable, and vaccines based on toxin-attenuated strains or the toxin itself are under trial. The disease is notifiable.

CHOLESTASIS: Accumulation of bile constituents in the body due to failure in bile excretion from the liver.

Aetiology and risk factors
A number of factors involving the bile secretion mechanism of the hepatocytes or the obstructing of the biliary tree can cause cholestasis. Some of these are shown in Table C3.

Table C3 Common causes of cholestasis

Hepatocytic cholestasis
Alcohol
Drugs (chlorpromazine, isoniazid, contraceptive pill)
Viral hepatitis*
Severe bacterial infections
Pregnancy
Obstructive cholestasis
Choledocholithiasis
Tumours (pancreas, ampulla, bile ducts)
Primary biliary cirrhosis*
Primary sclerosing cholangitis
Cystic fibrosis*
Pancreatitis*

Pathology
In cholestasis the pathology predominantly reflects the underlying cause. However, there are some characteristic features, which are often observed irrespective of the underlying aetiology. Serum alkaline phosphatase activity is increased several-fold. This enzyme is produced mainly in the liver and the bone. In the liver it is located in the canalicular and sinusoidal membranes of the hepatocytes and when the hepatocytes are damaged only a mild increase in blood levels is observed. However, in cholestasis the serum alkaline phosphatase activity is increased as a result of enzyme induction of the cells lining the biliary canaliculi. Detection of

increased blood alkaline phosphatase is not specific for liver disease, as it can be seen in other conditions such as pregnancy (from the placenta), increased osteoblastic activity in adolescence, Paget disease of bone*, rickets*, hyperparathyroidism and metastatic bone disease. In situations where it is not clear whether the increase in blood alkaline phosphatase is due to liver disease or not, the measurement of γ-glutamyltransferase levels may be helpful. This is a microsomal enzyme present in the hepatocytes that is also increased as a result of enzyme induction. The highest activity is seen in biliary obstruction but significant increases can also be present in parenchymal liver disease, e.g. viral hepatitis. A reduction in serum alkaline phosphatase activity indicates a resolution in the cholestasis.

In some instances, there is secondary hepatocellular damage as a result of cholestasis, resulting in an increase in the serum transaminase (AST and ALT) levels (though very high levels are a marker of hepatitis).

In cholestasis, blood levels of main bile constituents such as bile salts, bilirubin and cholesterol are also increased.

The main histological feature of cholestasis is accumulation of bile pigment in the liver parenchyma. Plugs of bile are usually seen in the bile ducts and small droplets of bile are visible in the hepatocyte cytoplasm. If bile canaliculi are ruptured, the bile is extravasated and phagocytosed by Kupffer cells. The other histological features depend on the underlying pathology. In obstructive cholestasis, distal obstruction leads to proliferation of small distal bile ducts. This feature may be helpful in the diagnosis of obstructive cholestasis.

The common presenting symptoms of cholestasis, pruritus and jaundice, are the result of accumulation of bile constituents such as bile salts and bilirubin. The stools are pale in colour as bilirubin cannot be excreted into the intestinal lumen, and the urine is usually dark in colour due to excretion of excess bilirubin through the kidneys. Another accompanying biochemical feature is that of increased blood cholesterol levels, leading to the formation of xanthelasma and xanthomas* late in the disease. Lack of bile salts in the intestinal lumen may occasionally lead to malabsorption, steatorrhoea and weight loss.

Alcoholic liver disease; Hepatitis B infection; Jaundice; Primary biliary cirrhosis

CHORIOCARCINOMA: A malignant epithelial tumour of trophoblastic tissue. It may occur secondary to either normal or abnormal pregnancy.

Aetiology and risk factors
Choriocarcinoma is associated with a history of hydatidiform mole, previous abortion and teratoma. Occasionally it arises following a normal pregnancy.

Pathology
Macroscopically, it is a soft yellow-white tumour with large areas of softening and cystic degeneration, composed of trophoblastic proliferation without evidence of chorionic villi. The trophoblastic proliferation is composed of both cytotrophoblast and syncytiotrophoblast. It tends to invade the underlying myometrial muscle and lymphatic and vascular permeation is commonly seen. Because of its very rapid growth it tends to become ischaemic and necrotic. Metastasis from choriocarcinoma may be seen within the lung, liver, brain, bone marrow and many other systemic sites.

Patients present with irregular bleeding and discharge following either normal or abnormal pregnancy.

Management
Beta-hCG is valuable in diagnosis as the amount of the hormone produced by the tumour correlates with the amount of trophoblast tissue. Management comprises evacuation of the contents of the uterus followed by surgery and chemotherapy. Although it is a very rapidly progressive disease, it is sensitive to chemotherapy and many patients achieve complete remissions and cures.

CHRISTMAS DISEASE: See Haemophilia.

CHROMOSOMAL ABNORMALITIES: Aberrations of chromosomal material due to mutation.

Aetiology and risk factors
Chromosomal abnormalities may be due to changes in the number or the structure of chromosomes, their importance being due to the fact that they result in abnormalities at the genetic (DNA) level. Abnormal chromosome number tends to occur because of errors at the anaphase stage of meiosis, which leads to unequal sharing of the chromosomes. In non-disjunction, the pairs of chromosomes fail to separate while in anaphase lag, and there is delay of movement of the chromosomes so that the extra chromosomes are left on the wrong side of the dividing wall. The cause of this is unknown. Abnormalities of chromosome structure occur when breaks within the chromosomes are not repaired appropriately. This may occur randomly, although certain regions of the chromosomes appear to be more liable to damage.

C

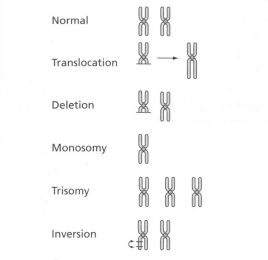

Fig. C10 Specific types of structural abnormalities.

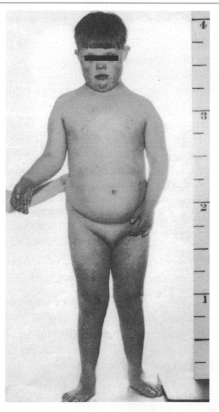

Fig. C11 Patient with Down syndrome. Note short stature, floppiness and typical facial features. (Reproduced from Browse NL. *An Introduction to the Symptoms and Signs of Surgical Disease*, 3rd edn. London: Arnold, 1997)

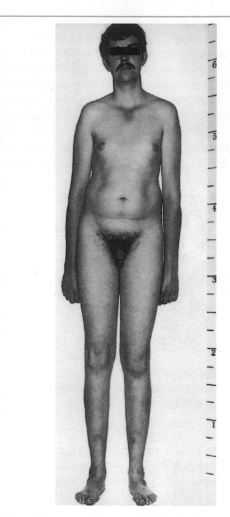

Fig. C12 A young man with Klinefelter syndrome – a tall male with a female distribution of body fat. (Reproduced from Browse NL. *An Introduction to the Symptoms and Signs of Surgical Disease*, 3rd edn. London: Arnold, 1997)

Specific types of structural abnormalities include translocations, deletions, amplifications and inversions (Fig. C10).

Pathology

The pathology of chromosomal abnormalities depends on the disorder produced by the alteration either in number on in structure. A classic example of abnormal chromosome number is Down syndrome in which there is trisomy 21. Other examples include Edward syndrome (trisomy 18) and Patau syndrome (trisomy 13). In Klinefelter syndrome, patients have an extra X chromosome (XXY). These patients are tall, but have hypogonadism and infertility. In Turner syndrome there is a loss of one X chromosome (X0). Many of the fetuses with Turner syndrome undergo spontaneous abortion. Those who survive show evidence of short stature, webbing of the neck, infertility, aortic coarctation, and an increased carrying angle of the arm (cubitus valgus) (Figs C11, C12, C13).

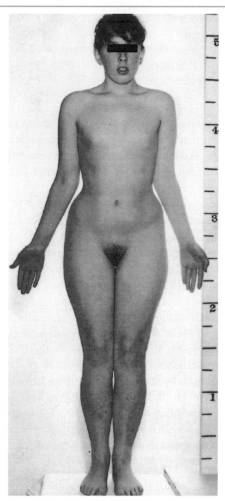

Fig. C13 A young woman with Turner syndrome – a short female with a masculine shape and amenorrhoea. (Reproduced from Browse NL. *An Introduction to the Symptoms and Signs of Surgical Disease*, 3rd edn. London: Arnold, 1997)

Abnormalities of chromosome structure, i.e. translocation, deletion or inversion, tend to occur in malignancy. Translocations are a common feature of chronic myeloid leukaemia* (translocation of chromosome 9 and 22) and Burkitt lymphoma* (translocation of chromosome 8 to 14). Translocations are rarer in solid tumours although they do occur, e.g. deletions of various chromosome arms including chromosomes 13q (retinoblastoma) and 11p (Wilms tumour). Amplifications of chromosome regions are classically seen in neuroblastoma where there is amplification of the N-*myc* gene.

Management
Management of inherited chromosomal disorders is difficult and essentially relies on genetic counselling of families. Prenatal testing is available for some of the disorders. The detection of characteristic chromosome abnormalities in haematological malignancies is useful in diagnosis, prognosis, and treatment (e.g. see Acute myeloid leukaemia*).

 Down syndrome

CHRONIC BRONCHITIS: Excess mucus production associated with, e.g. smoking. Exacerbations are caused by infection with *Streptococcus pneumoniae* or *Haemophilus influenzae*.

 Chronic obstructive airways disease

CHRONIC GRANULOMATOUS DISEASE: A group of rare congenital immunodeficiency diseases in which phagocytes fail to produce reactive oxygen intermediates on activation, resulting in failure to control certain infectious organisms.

Case
A 6-month-old boy, underweight for his age, presented with discharging abscesses in the inguinal and axillary regions. He had a healthy sister but an elder brother had died from osteomyelitis. On examination he was febrile and his spleen, liver and several lymph nodes were enlarged. He was admitted to hospital, where his abscesses were drained and microbiological culture revealed *Staphylococcus aureus*. His blood count showed slight anaemia (11.0 g/dl) and a marked neutrophil leucocytosis (total white cells, $25 \times 10^9/l$: 80% neutrophils). His immunoglobulin levels were raised, particularly IgA (2.8 g/l) and IgG (19.5 g/l). Further investigation of neutrophils by the NBT test showed that his neutrophils were incapable of giving a respiratory burst, and in an *in vitro* assay using *Staph. aureus*, intracellular killing was markedly impaired.

He was treated with systemic flucloxacillin. Two months later he was readmitted with a further abscess in the leg, again staphylococcal. Subsequently, he developed repeated infections with bacteria and fungi (*Candida albicans*). Now aged 5, he receives prophylactic antibiotic therapy, but continues to suffer from repeated infections.

Aetiology and risk factors
A primary immunodeficiency due to several abnormalities in the respiratory burst of phagocytes. In the commonest variant (70% of cases), the defect is in cytochrome b_{558}, a molecule required for the generation of superoxide, hydrogen peroxide and other 'oxygen radicals'.

There is frequently a family history of similarly affected male relatives, inheritance being through the female line. However, in about 30% of cases (autosomal inheritance) females can be affected.

Table C4 Common infections in CGD

Staphylococcus aureus
Escherichia coli
Klebsiella spp.
Pseudomonas spp.
Proteus spp.
Salmonella spp.
Candida albicans
Aspergillus spp.

Symptoms may start within weeks of birth and survival beyond the second decade is uncommon. The incidence is estimated to be about 1 per million births.

Pathology

The infections characteristic of CGD are those normally killed by the respiratory burst in neutrophils (see Table C4). The raised neutrophil count and raised levels of immunoglobulins, especially IgG, reflect the presence of chronic infection. Note that phagocytosis itself proceeds normally. The failure of neutrophils to eliminate phagocytosed organisms leads to the attraction and activation of macrophages which also cannot kill the organisms. This leads to the development of granulomas in which giant cells may be prominent but caseation does not occur (see Tuberculosis).

Management

Treatment depends on antibiotics, but is not always effective, since many organisms are inside cells which antibiotics cannot penetrate. Interferon-γ has shown promise in some cases.

Genetic analysis has revealed several mutations of the b_{558} gene. The X-linked disease is a potential candidate for gene replacement therapy.

Abscess; Candidiasis; Granuloma; Immunodeficiency

CHRONIC LYMPHOCYTIC LEUKAEMIA: A clonal proliferation of small lymphocytes resulting in a blood lymphocytosis.

Case

An 81-year-old man suffered a bout of bronchitis which was successfully treated with oral antibiotics. He was noted to be pale and a blood count was performed:

WBC 87.3 × 10⁹/l
RBC 3.24 × 10¹²/l; Hb 9.2 g/dl; Hct (ratio) 0.272
MCV 83.8 fl; MCH 34.6 pg

MCHC 34.1 g/dl; RDW 15.2 %
Plt 121 × 10⁹/l
Differential white cell count: neutrophils 28% = 0.36 × 10⁹/l; lymphocytes 70% = 0.91 × 10⁹/l; monocytes 2% = 0.02 × 10⁹/l.

On examination he was found to have a generalized lymphadenopathy and his spleen was just palpable on deep inspiration. He was referred to the local haematology clinic where further investigations were performed.

Immunophenotyping of his peripheral blood lymphocytes showed that they expressed both CD19 (a B-cell marker) and CD5 (a T-cell marker). The lymphocytes also expressed surface immunoglobulin, all cells showing kappa light chain type (monoclonal). These results are typical of B-cell chronic lymphocytic leukaemia.

Direct antiglobulin (Coombs) test was weakly positive. Protein electrophoresis showed reduced gammaglobulin levels, confirmed by the finding of low immunoglobulin levels.

No treatment was given for his leukaemia for 2 years when he complained that the enlarged lymph nodes in his neck were visible and he was treated with oral chlorambucil, which shrank the nodes in his neck and reduced the blood lymphocytosis.

Aetiology and risk factors

Little is known of the aetiology of chronic lymphocytic leukaemia (CLL). CLL is rare in the Far East and common in Western countries. Two-thirds of cases are males. Cytogenetic abnormalities are found in half of all cases studied. Because the lymphocytes divide infrequently, it is necessary to culture them with a mitogen in the laboratory to stimulate cell division so that the chromosomes can be examined. One of the most common abnormalities is an extra chromosome 12, thought to be a secondary phenomenon rather than a direct cause of leukaemogenesis. Another common cytogenetic abnormality is a deletion or translocation involving chromosome 13 at band 14 on the short arm. How this is related to the development of CLL is not known but might be related to inactivation of tumour-suppressor genes in this region.

Pathology

CLL accounts for 60% of all lymphoproliferative diseases and is predominantly a disease of the elderly, more than 60% of cases being over 60 years old at presentation. As in this case it is often discovered incidentally when a blood count is done for other reasons. More than 95% of cases are of B-cell lineage. A blood lymphocytosis is found, the

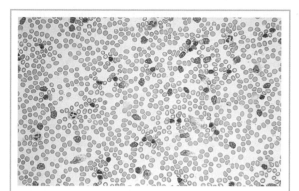

Fig. C14 Blood film in chronic lymphocytic leukaemia. The predominant white cell is the mature-looking small lymphocyte, many of which have been crushed during the spreading of the film – smear or smudge cells.

lymphocytes are fragile and often crushed during the spreading of the film (Fig. C14).

As the disease advances, increasing enlargement of lymph nodes, liver and spleen are found. Bone marrow infiltration eventually results in marrow failure with anaemia, neutropenia and thrombocytopenia.

B-cells are responsible for antibody-mediated immunity and in CLL there is defective antibody production with low immunoglobulin levels resulting in an increased susceptibility to infection. There is also an increased incidence of warm autoimmune haemolytic anaemia and autoimmune thrombocytopenia in patients with CLL. Haemolysis may be precipitated by treatment with fludarabine, a cytotoxic agent that not only kills CLL lymphocytes but also affects the balance of T-lymphocytes controlling autoimmunity.

Management

Many cases of CLL require no treatment, as the disease progresses very slowly in many cases and elderly patients may die of another condition. Supportive treatment includes red cell transfusion for the correction of anaemia, and prompt antibiotic treatment for intercurrent infection. Some CLL patients with low immunoglobulin levels and recurrent infections may benefit from immunoglobulin administration, particularly in the winter months. When chemotherapy is required, single-agent oral alkylating agent treatment is usual. Younger patients, or those with more aggressive disease, may benefit from combination chemotherapy similar to that employed in lymphomas.

CHRONIC MYELOID LEUKAEMIA: One of the myeloproliferative disorders* associated with increased production of relatively mature myeloid cells, particularly granulocytes.

Case

A 42-year-old woman attended her local women's health clinic with a 3-month history of tiredness and intermittent fever. She had lost approximately a stone in weight over this time, though her appetite had been normal. On examination her spleen was found to be enlarged 4 cm below the costal margin.

A blood count was performed:

WBC 456.0 × 10⁹/l
RBC 3.58 × 10¹²/l; Hb 9.4 g/dl; Hct (ratio) 0.294
MCV 82 fl; MCH 26.3 pg
MCHC 32.0 g/dl; RDW 12.9 %
Plt 88 × 10⁹/l.

The blood film showed a massive neutrophilia with occasional myelocytes, metamyelocytes and 1% blast cells. A bone marrow aspirate was grossly hypercellular, with granulocytic hyperplasia and left shift, but no excess of blasts. The features were typical of chronic myeloid leukaemia (CML).

Cytogenetic examination of bone marrow showed all cells to possess the Philadelphia chromosome (Fig. C15).

Aetiology and risk

Philadelphia chromosome (Ph) in CML More than 90% of cases of CML have Philadelphia

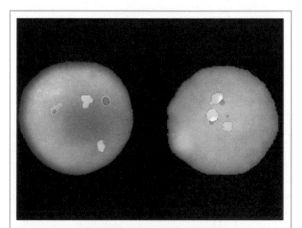

Fig. C15 Fluorescent *in-situ* hybridization of a normal nucleus and one containing the genetic rearrangement *bcr/abl*. Probes to *bcr* on chromosome 9 fluoresce green, that to *abl* on chromosome 22 red. Where the red and green signals overlap in the abnormal new gene *bcr/abl* found on the Philadelphia chromosome the fluorescence is yellow ('traffic lights' appearance).

chromosome and this is an important marker of the disease. Although the truncated chromosome 22 appears to lose an important piece of DNA in the translocation 9;22, the *ABL* gene from chromosome 9 ends up on chromosome 22. Here it is juxtaposed to the BCR (breakpoint cluster region) of DNA, forming a new hybrid gene termed *BCR-ABL*. The protein products of this fusion gene are related to the development and progression of CML in ways that are as yet poorly understood.

Although some cases of apparently typical CML may lack the Philadelphia chromosome, analysis at DNA level will usually show that they have the *BCR-ABL* rearrangement of DNA, even though large enough amounts of chromosome have not been translocated to be detected microscopically.

The Philadelphia chromosome may also be found in a small number of cases of acute lymphoblastic leukaemia* and acute myeloid (myeloblastic) leukaemia*. Although the abnormal chromosome found in these diseases cannot be distinguished from that found in CML by microscopic appearances, analysis of the site of DNA breakage on chromosome 22 shows different areas of cleavage. In CML the breakpoint is termed p210, and in acute lymphoblastic leukaemia p190. These different hybrid genes produce different proteins in the different types of leukaemia in which Ph is found. When Ph is found in a leukaemia other than CML it generally confers a bad prognosis.

Pathology

The presenting symptoms of CML are usually of a non-specific type, as in the case described above. Some cases of CML are found incidentally on blood counts done for other reasons. Rarely, presentation may be with acute symptoms associated with leucostasis. In this situation the blood viscosity is grossly elevated because of a very high white cell count leading to stagnant flow and thrombosis. The circulation of the spleen or penis can be affected, leading to splenic infarction or priapism. In the lungs, transient pulmonary infiltrates and hypoxaemia can be found. Because red cells also contribute to whole blood viscosity, it is best not to transfuse red cells to patients with very high leukaemic white cell counts unless they are very anaemic, because of the danger of precipitating leucostasis. Leucopheresis on a cell separator provides a quick way of reducing the white cell count, allowing transfusion. The harvested white cells can be cryopreserved for later use (see Management, below).

All the common features of myeloproliferative disorders* may be present in a case of CML in chronic phase. Control of the disease during chronic phase is usually a fairly simple matter using single-agent oral cytotoxics such as hydroxyurea. However, almost all cases eventually enter an accelerated phase of their disease, when control is much more difficult. This transformation occurs an average of 3 years after diagnosis but may be seen at any stage from 1 to 11 years after first presentation. This phase is usually heralded by increasing numbers of blast cells in bone marrow and blood, weight loss, anorexia, bone pains, fever and cytopenias. Sometimes large numbers of blast cells may simulate an acute leukaemia (blast crisis). These blast cells may be lymphoid, myeloid, or of mixed lymphoid-myeloid lineage.

Management

In chronic phase CML, oral hydroxyurea tablets usually return the blood count to normal levels, shrink the enlarged spleen and abolish constitutional symptoms. However, such treatment does not change the underlying cytogenetic abnormality or prevent disease transformation, and patients with transformed disease have a poor prognosis. If an HLA matched sibling donor is available, bone marrow transplantation* provides a good chance of curing the disease, with harvested peripheral blood stem cells collected at diagnosis providing the option of autologous chronic phase reconstitution in the event of graft failure. Regular self-administered injections of the antiviral cytokine interferon can provide good blood count control and restore Ph-negative haemopoiesis in a small number of cases. Overall, the use of interferon adds about another 2 years to the length of chronic phase in most patients.

CHRONIC OBSTRUCTIVE AIRWAYS DISEASE (COAD): A group of disorders in which there is obstruction to airflow resulting in shortness of breath, comprising chronic bronchitis, asthma, emphysema and bronchiectasis.

Case

A 67-year-old man presented to his doctor complaining of increasing shortness of breath (SOB) over the previous 2 months. His exercise tolerance had dropped to walking 50 m. He did not have a cough and did not produce excessive sputum. There was no family history of cardiac or respiratory disease and he was not on any medication. He admitted to smoking 30 cigarettes per day since the age of 18 years.

On examination, he was breathing through pursed lips and was tachycardic, tachypnoeic and mildly cyanosed. His blood pressure was normal.

Examination of his chest revealed a resonant percussion note with decreased air sounds.

He was admitted to hospital for further investigations:

> Chest radiograph: hyperinflated chest with decreased vascular markings. Heart mildly enlarged. No evidence of pleural or pericardial effusions.
> Blood gases: Po_2 7 kPa, Pco_2 8 kPa, pH 7.2, HCO_3^- 30 mmol/l.
> Respiratory function test: decreased vital capacity (VC) and forced expiratory volume (FEV) with reduced FEV/VC ratio.

A diagnosis of chronic obstructive airway disease was made.

Aetiology and risk factors

Smoking, air pollutants, infections and inflammatory conditions leading to lung tissue destruction are the commonest causes of COAD.

Pathology

Four different conditions fall under the heading of COAD: asthma, bronchiectasis, chronic bronchitis and emphysema. In asthma, there is reversible obstruction due to bronchoconstriction that may have an immunological mechanism. In bronchiectasis, there is destruction of lung parenchyma due to recurrent infections. Chronic bronchitis is defined as productive cough with sputum, occurring for at least 3 months for 2 consecutive years. The patient described above does not fit into any of these three categories. He fits into the fourth category, emphysema, which is defined as permanent dilatation of airspaces distal to the terminal bronchioles, due to destruction of the walls but without fibrosis. Unlike chronic bronchitis, this is a histopathological definition and strictly speaking can only be diagnosed at autopsy; however, it is the most likely diagnosis given the history and findings on investigations.

Emphysema is divided into four types depending on which part of the acinus is involved (the acinus is composed of the terminal bronchiole, alveolar duct and cluster of alveolar acini). In **centrilobular emphysema**, the proximal part (terminal bronchiole) is affected. In **panacinar**, the entire acinus is involved. **Paraseptal emphysema**, also known as **distal emphysema**, involves the alveolar duct and acini. In **irregular emphysema**, the acinus is affected in an irregular fashion. Centrilobular emphysema is the most common type seen in smokers.

The exact mechanism by which emphysema develops is unclear. The most likely explanation for the tissue destruction is referred to as the 'protease-antiprotease hypothesis'. According to this hypothesis, the destruction of tissue is a result of an imbalance between proteases (elastase) secreted by neutrophils, macrophages, mast cells and bacteria, and antiproteases (α1-antitrypsin, secretory leucoprotease inhibitor) found in serum and the lung. Smoking has been shown to increase elastase activity as well as decrease anti-elastase activity, leading to tissue destruction and emphysema.

Management

The best form of treatment is preventive, i.e. giving up smoking and reducing the risk of recurrent infections by adequate antibiotic treatment. Once emphysema is established, the management is symptomatic with antibiotics, if needed, and oxygen therapy to reduce the hypoxia.

 Asthma; Bronchiectasis; Chronic bronchitis

CHURG–STRAUSS DISEASE: A form of vasculitis involving the lung, in which there is an allergic granulomatosis. It is associated with asthma and eosinophilia.

CIRRHOSIS: Irreversible destruction of the liver architecture by fibrosis and nodular regeneration.

Case

A 48-year-old man visited his general practitioner with increasing pruritus. The doctor noticed that he was mildly jaundiced. On further enquiry, he said that the pruritus had got worse over the last few months. He had no other symptoms. He stated that he drank 'socially' but on direct questioning admitted to drinking 8 pints of beer in addition to half a bottle of whisky a day, since he was a businessman and had to entertain customers regularly. He denied taking any medication and had been using a topical moisturizer for the pruritus.

On examination, he was jaundiced and had pallor of his conjunctiva. A number of 'spider naevi' were seen on his neck and upper trunk. Examination of the heart and lung did not reveal any abnormalities. His abdomen was distended and it was difficult to palpate his liver. The doctor felt that he had chronic liver damage and referred him to a gastroenterologist.

Blood tests at the hospital showed a haemoglobin of 10 g/l and platelet count of 300 × 10⁹/l. Coagulation studies revealed a mild increase in clotting time. His urea and creatinine were mildly raised. Liver function tests revealed raised levels of alkaline phosphatase, AST and ALT.

A chest radiograph was unremarkable. A liver biopsy was performed and showed distortion of the

C

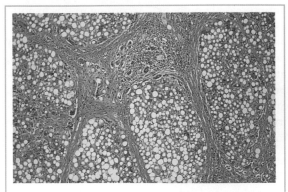

Fig. C16 Histological section of the liver showing severe fatty change (vacuolation) and thick bands of fibrous tissue dividing up the nodules.

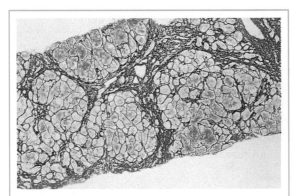

Fig. C17 Histological section of the liver stained with reticulin to highlight the dense fibrous bands and the regenerating nodules.

normal architecture by dense fibrosis and nodular regeneration. There was bridging fibrosis between portal tracts and between portal tracts and central veins. The liver parenchyma showed individual cell necrosis and an inflammatory infiltrate. There was also fatty change and Mallory hyaline was seen in some cells. Iron was seen within Kupffer cells. The features are of alcoholic cirrhosis (Figs C16 and C17).

The patient was advised to abstain from alcohol and given medication to relieve his pruritus. Follow-up care was arranged.

Aetiology and risk factors

Risk factors for cirrhosis include alcohol abuse, biliary disease, hepatitis B and C and, more rarely, haemochromatosis*, Wilson disease* and α1-antitrypsin deficiency.

Pathology

Cirrhosis is one of the major killers in Western countries as a result of alcohol abuse, biliary disease and viral hepatitis.

There are two main features of cirrhosis: fibrosis and nodular regeneration of the liver parenchyma. The end result is a generalized distortion of the liver parenchyma. The fibrosis, once established, is irreversible and the resultant distortion to architecture leads to a change in the blood flow through the liver.

Fibrosis occurs either as delicate bands or as large scars and connects portal tracts to portal tracts, portal tracts to central veins, or central veins to central veins. Liver cells are able to secrete collagen but the main source of collagen deposition in cirrhosis is the Ito cells found in the space of Disse. Deposition of collagen in the space of Disse is responsible for loss of fenestration in the sinusoidal endothelium.

The distortion of the parenchymal and vascular architecture is responsible for the raised serum bilirubin (jaundice and pruritus), portal hypertension and ascites and varices. Other features include anaemia, spider naevi, loss of body hair and testicular atrophy as a result of abnormal hormonal metabolism. In the late stages of the disease, patients may develop encephalopathy.

Management

Patients are advised to refrain from alcohol and drugs that may further damage the liver. Patients with the rare disorders, such as haemochromatosis, can be given chelation therapy to help excrete the excess iron. Once cirrhosis is established, it is not possible to reverse the fibrosis and management is of symptoms and complications (e.g. bleeding varices).

 Haemochromatosis; Hepatitis; Wilson disease

COARCTATION: A narrowing or stricture of the aorta.

 Congenital heart disease

COCCIDIOMYCOSIS: A systemic infection with the dimorphic fungus *Coccidioides immitis*.

Aetiology and risk factors

The infection is endemic in the arid south-western half of North America (California) and Northern Mexico. The infection is acquired by inhalation of spores.

Pathology

There is a peripheral and tissue eosinophilia and serum IgE levels are elevated. In established infection there is granuloma formation in the tissue and caseation may occur. Clinically the patient may remain asymptomatic, or develop a flu-like illness, chronic pulmonary disease with cavities, or disseminated disease to skin, bone, joints, or meninges. The chronic pulmonary disease, like the other systemic mycoses (blastomycosis, histoplasmosis) clinically resembles tuberculosis, with fever, weight loss and haemoptysis. Erythema nodosum* may also occur. Diagnosis is by histology, isolation of the fungus and serology. Treatment is with amphotericin or an azole, e.g. fluconazole. Surgery may be required for cavitating disease with severe haemoptysis.

COELIAC DISEASE: A chronic disease of intestinal mucosa resulting in malabsorption, which improves on removal of gliadin from the diet. The disease is also known as gluten-sensitive enteropathy and non-tropical sprue.

Case

A 4-year-old boy presented to his GP with failure to thrive. He had been well until 6 months previously. Since that time, he had begun to lose weight, was lethargic and had episodes of diarrhoea. There was no significant past history and he was not on any medication. He had a brother, 2 years older than him, who was well.

On examination, he looked tired and thin for his age but no specific abnormalities were identified. He was referred to a paediatrician for further assessment.

At the hospital, a full dietary history was obtained and haematological and biochemical investigations were ordered. He was mildly anaemic but the rest of the investigations were normal. Stool samples were sent for microbiological analysis but did not reveal an infective cause for his diarrhoea. The paediatrician suspected coeliac disease and an upper gastrointestinal endoscopy was carried out. Biopsies from the stomach and proximal duodenum were sent for histology:

> Gastric biopsies: mild non-specific chronic inflammation.
> Duodenal biopsies: sections show almost complete villous atrophy with an increase in intraepithelial lymphocytes. There is also elongation of the crypts with hyperplasia. An increase in chronic inflammatory cells is also seen in the lamina propria. Features are consistent with coeliac disease (Figs C18, C19).

The family was seen by a dietitian who gave advice on a gluten-free diet. It was initially difficult for the family to exclude all wheat, oats and rye from the diet of a 4-year-old who was about to start school. However, persistence with the diet was soon rewarded by a dramatic improvement in the boy's symptoms. He began to gain weight and his diarrhoea settled.

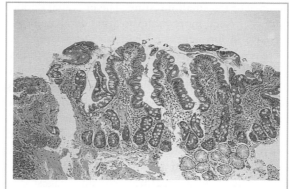

Fig. C18 Histological section of normal duodenal mucosa.

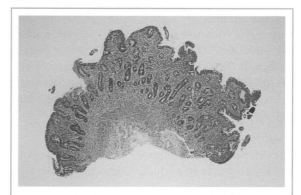

Fig. C19 Histological section of the duodenum showing blunting of the villi and chronic inflammation suggesting coeliac disease.

Biopsy after 3 months on the diet showed a marked improvement of the villous atrophy although a mild chronic inflammatory infiltrate was still present.

Aetiology and risk factors

The disorder is a result of sensitivity to gliadin protein found in oats, barley and rye, antigliadin antibodies being present during active disease. The actual damage to the intestinal mucosa, however, is probably T-cell mediated. A cross-reactivity with E1b protein of adenovirus has been suggested, implicating an environmental aetiology. A genetic susceptibility and familial clustering is also known to be present and there is an association with HLA-B8, DR3 and 7, and Dqw2.

Coeliac disease occurring with bullous skin lesions is known as dermatitis herpetiformis*.

Pathology

The essential pathology is of enteritis (inflammation) with loss of the villous architecture and hence the absorptive capacity due to the immune-mediated damage of the small intestine. The proximal duodenum is affected more than the distal duodenum. An increase in intraepithelial lymphocytes is seen and there is reactive hyperplasia of the underlying crypts. The clinical features of weight loss and lethargy are all related to the malabsorption that occurs secondary to villous damage. Occasionally, coeliac disease does not present until adulthood.

Although the histological features described above are strongly suggestive of coeliac disease, the diagnosis is made on a clinicopathological correlation. The clinical features should suggest the diagnosis and the pathology should lend weight to this. But further, it must be shown that withdrawal of the offending agent (gliadin) from the diet leads to clinical and histopathological improvement.

Most patients who stick to the gluten-free diet remain free of symptoms. There is, however, a small risk of malignancy. Patients with coeliac disease have a small increase in risk of intestinal T-cell lymphoma. Epithelial cancers of the gastrointestinal tract and breast have also been described with slightly increased frequency.

Management
The management comprises good dietary advice and support to help exclude all gluten from the diet.

 Dermatitis herpetiformis; Malabsorption

COLD ABSCESS: A chronic abscess caused by *Mycobacterium tuberculosis*.

COLD AGGLUTININS: Cold-acting antibodies directed against the I/i red cell antigen system which cause clumping and haemolysis of red cells.

Cold agglutinins are most frequently discovered by the haematology laboratory when a blood count is attempted on a sample which has been allowed to cool to room temperature. Because clumps of cells rather than individual red cells are counted, nonsense results are produced. These clumps of red cells may also be seen on the blood film (Fig. C20).

Aetiology and risk factors
- Idiopathic cold autoimmune haemolytic anaemia – usually monoclonal antibody.
- In low-grade B-cell lymphoproliferative disorders – usually monoclonal antibody.
- Associated with mycoplasma pneumonia* infection – usually polyclonal antibody.
- Associated with glandular fever* – usually polyclonal antibody.

The antibody associated with cold agglutination is directed against the I/i antigen system. All red cells bear this antigen but at birth mostly as i antigen,

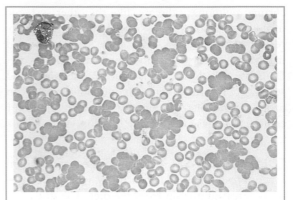

Fig. C20 Cold agglutinates on the blood film in a case of autoimmune anaemia.

which changes to I with increasing age. In glandular fever, the cold agglutinin is usually anti-i and in other causes of cold agglutination usually anti-I. The specificity can be established by titration against adult and cord red cells.

The blood count and blood film abnormalities may be abolished by warming the blood sample to 37°C before processing.

Pathology
In the patient, agglutination of red cells in cold peripheries may obstruct small blood vessels. This results in peripheral cyanosis that disappears on warming and symptoms similar to Raynaud disease*. Agglutinated red cells are filtered from the circulation by the reticuloendothelial system, resulting in predominantly extravascular haemolysis. All the general features of haemolytic anaemia* may be present. The direct antiglobulin test, performed at 37°C, will be negative as the IgM elutes off the red cells, but complement components may be detected.

Management
The most important feature of management is keeping the patient warm. Transfusion, through an in-line blood warmer, may be required for the treatment of severe anaemia. In contrast to warm autoimmune haemolytic anaemia*, steroids are relatively ineffective, but immunosuppression with chlorambucil may used. As in other causes of haemolytic anaemia, folic acid supplements should be given.

COLITIS: Inflammation of the colon.

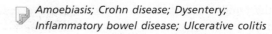 *Amoebiasis; Crohn disease; Dysentery; Inflammatory bowel disease; Ulcerative colitis*

COLORECTAL CARCINOMA: A malignant tumour arising from the mucin-secreting epithelium of the large bowel.

Case

A 56-year-old lady presented to surgical outpatients with a 3-month history of rectal bleeding. She had noticed fresh blood in her stools on a number of occasions but there was no pain associated with opening her bowels. She was otherwise well and had no other symptoms. Her husband and children were all alive and well and there was no family history of note.

On systemic examination, the surgeon could not find any abnormalities and rectal examination did not reveal any masses. A sigmoidoscopy was carried out which revealed a 2 cm ulcerated lesion within the proximal sigmoid colon and a biopsy was taken from the edge of the lesion. She was sent for blood tests and radiography.

Routine blood tests showed an Hb of 11.1 g/l. Other haematological tests were normal. Biochemistry, including tests for liver and renal function, was normal. Chest and abdominal radiographs were unremarkable. Abdominal ultrasound was also normal.

Histopathology: Sections of the sigmoid biopsy showed a moderately differentiated adenocarcinoma. She underwent a left hemicolectomy. Gross examination of the specimen revealed a 2.5 cm ulcerated mass in the sigmoid that appeared to penetrate the full thickness of the bowel wall. The rest of the bowel was normal without evidence of polyps. Lymph nodes from the mesentery were sampled. Microscopical examination showed a moderately differentiated adenocarcinoma (Fig. C21), which penetrated the full thickness of the bowel wall and involved 4/10 lymph nodes (Duke C).

She remained well for 6 months at which stage she began to complain of weight loss and lethargy. She was found to have an enlarged liver on palpation.

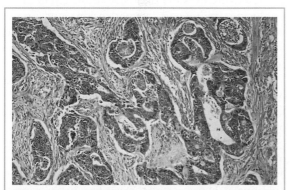

Fig. C21 Histological section showing a moderately differentiated adenocarcinoma of colon.

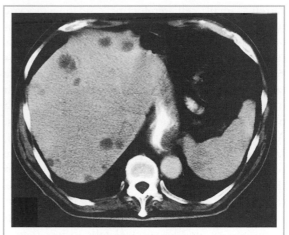

Fig. C22 CT scan showing metastatic nodules in liver. (Reproduced with permission from Curtis J, Whitehouse G. *Radiology for the MRCP*. London: Arnold, 1998)

CT scan of the liver showed multiple lesions in the parenchyma consistent with metastases (Fig. C22).

Liver biopsy revealed metastatic adenocarcinoma consistent with origin from a colonic primary.

She died 3 months later.

Aetiology and risk factors

Colorectal carcinoma may be familial, as part of the FAP (familial adenomatous polyposis) syndrome, Gardner syndrome or HNPCC (hereditary non-polyposis colorectal carcinoma), or it may be sporadic. Suspected risk factors include dietary factors, chronic constipation and long-standing inflammatory bowel disease.

Pathology

Colorectal carcinoma usually presents with a change in bowel habit and bleeding *per rectum*. Although some patients may put the bleeding down to 'piles', it should always be taken seriously and investigated thoroughly. Other presenting symptoms may relate to metastatic disease if present, or due to non-metastatic effects of tumours such as lethargy, weight loss and tiredness.

Tumours are more common in the left side, although in HNPCC they are commoner in the right colon. In FAP, hundreds or thousands of adenomatous polyps are present and these are precursors of the invasive carcinoma. These patients have a 100% risk of developing a carcinoma in their lifetime. The tumours tend to ulcerate and erosion of blood vessels leads to the bleeding, a common presenting complaint.

As these tumours arise from the glandular mucin-secreting epithelium, they are adenocarcinomas.

Rarely, small cell, endocrine and melanocytic tumours can arise. The staging system for colorectal carcinoma is the Duke classification. Duke's A is tumour that invades lamina propria and muscularis propria but not all the way through the muscle layer. Duke's B is tumour that invades through muscularis propria but does not involve lymph nodes. Duke's C is involvement of lymph nodes. Although not part of the original Duke's system, Duke's D is sometimes used to denote the presence of distant metastases. The prognosis is related to the staging, Duke's A having a very good prognosis (85% 5-year survival) whilst Duke's C has a poor prognosis (35% 5-year survival). Once distant metastases occur, the survival falls to less than a year.

Management

The primary management is surgical excision, which allows pathological diagnosis and staging as well as treating symptoms, especially if the tumour is obstructing the bowel. If tumours are left *in situ*, there is a risk of bleeding and perforation with peritonitis, which could be fatal. Chemotherapy and radiotherapy are given to prevent recurrence and metastases but the outcome for advanced disease is poor.

 Adenomatous polyposis coli; Dysplasia

COMPLEMENT DEFICIENCIES: A group of genetic deficiencies in the complement system.

Genetic deficiencies of virtually all of the complement components (proteins) involved in both the classical and alternative pathways of complement activation have been found. In most cases they show phenotypically autosomal recessive patterns of inheritance. The complement deficiencies are most usefully grouped according to the outcome of the deficiency (Table C5). The most common form of complement deficiency is hereditary angio-edema*.

CONGENITAL HEART DISEASE: A term used to describe abnormalities of the heart or large vessels, present from birth.

Aetiology and risk factors

These disorders arise because of problems during embryogenesis and hence the aetiology is generally unknown. It is probably a combination of genetic and environmental factors. Although there appears to be familial predisposition to such disorders, the concordance in monozygotic twins is only about 10% for abnormalities such as ventricular septal defect. This suggests that environmental factors

Table C5 Complement deficiencies

Group	Type	Deficiency
1	Immune complex deficiency, e.g. SLE (classical pathway components involved in IC dissolution)	C1q, C1s, C1r and C1s, C2, C4
2	Angioedema	C1 inhibitor
3	Recurrent pyogenic infections (C3 important in opsonization)	C3, factor H, factor I
4	Recurrent neisserial infections (role of alternative pathway and membrane attack complex in lysis of these organisms)	C5, C6, C7, C8, properdin, factor D
5	Asymptomatic	C9

must play a major role. Some genetic disorders such as Turner syndrome (X0) are associated with cardiac malformation.

Pathology

There is a vast number of different cardiac malformations that may occur. The commonest are ventricular septal defect (VSD), patent ductal arteriosus (PDA), Fallot tetralogy*, aortic stenosis, pulmonary stenosis, coarctation of the aorta, atrial septal defect (ASD) and transposition of the great arteries. These abnormalities can be divided into two groups: shunts or obstructions. When there is a communication either between the chambers of the heart, between the heart and a blood vessel, or between different blood vessels, this is referred to as a shunt. In a right-to-left shunt, deoxygenated blood from the right side of the heart enters the left side, producing cyanosis. Examples of such cyanotic congenital heart diseases include Fallot tetralogy and transposition of the great arteries. With a left-to-right shunt, blood from the left side of the heart enters the right side of the circulation, producing pulmonary hypertension and right ventricular hypertrophy. This may occur if the foramen ovale or the ductus arteriosus remain patent after birth.

Occasionally congenital abnormalities produce obstruction rather than shunting of blood. Examples of such abnormalities include coarctation of the aorta and valvular stenosis.

Whether congenital abnormalities cause shunting or obstruction, the long-term consequences to the myocardial function are related to either pulmonary hypertension or cardiac hypertrophy. The turbulence of blood flow caused by these anomalies also predisposes to cardiac infections.

Children with cardiac abnormalities may also show failure to thrive and retarded development.

Management
Some forms of cardiac anomalies are amenable to surgical repair.

 Pulmonary hypertension

CONGESTIVE HEART FAILURE: See Heart failure.

CONJUNCTIVITIS: Acute inflammation of the conjunctiva caused by a number of different infectious and toxic agents.

Aetiology and risk factors
Some common infective causes of conjunctivitis are given in Table C6. In addition, a wide variety of chemicals, drugs and allergic reactions can cause conjunctivitis.

Pathology
Conjunctivitis presents with pain, swelling, erythema and a discharge. There is regional lymphadenopathy and follicular hyperplasia in the conjunctiva. Pharyngoconjunctival fever and keratoconjunctivitis present with pharyngitis, fever and conjunctivitis, the latter developing subepithelial cellular infiltration. Haemorrhagic conjunctivitis presents with sudden onset of bilateral conjunctivitis and conjunctival haemorrhages. All have systemic symptoms and occur as epidemics.

Laboratory diagnosis is by isolation of the pathogen. Conjunctivitis is usually self-limiting although topical antibiotics may be required.

Gonococcal or chlamydial conjunctivitis requires referral to an STD clinic and contact tracing or if in a neonate, appropriate specimens and counselling of the mother.

CONN SYNDROME: A rare condition resulting from excessive aldosterone production (hyperaldosteronism).

Aetiology and risk factors
Primary hyperaldosteronism is usually a result of an aldosterone-secreting adrenal adenoma (60–80% of cases). It also occurs less commonly in bilateral hyperplasia of the cells of the zona glomerulosa. Very rarely do adrenal carcinomas cause primary hyperaldosteronism. Secondary hyperaldosteronism is more commonly observed and occurs as a complication of congestive cardiac failure, cirrhosis of the liver with ascites, nephrotic syndrome, renal artery stenosis, malignant hypertension, Bartter syndrome and renin-secreting tumours.

Pathology
In most patients with primary hyperaldosteronism the microscopic and macroscopic features are those of an adenoma, whereas in secondary hyperaldosteronism the adrenals appear normal. In secondary hyperaldosteronism, there is a high renin output, as a result of the response of the juxtaglomerular cells of the kidney to renal ischaemia, reduced effective plasma volume, and hyperplasia of the juxtaglomerular cells.

Biochemically, the excess aldosterone secreted causes sodium retention in the kidney in exchange for potassium and hydrogen. Thus serum potas-

Table C6 Some common infective causes of conjunctivitis

Organism	Comments
Viral	
Adenovirus	Commonest cause and may be part of pharyngoconjunctival fever (serotypes 3,7), keratoconjunctivitis (serotype 8), haemorrhagic conjunctivitis (serotype 11)
Herpes virus	HSV and VZV may both cause conjunctivitis, the latter as part of chickenpox or shingles
Influenza virus, measles	Common symptom during influenza. Conjunctivitis may develop as part of the exanthema. Koplik spots may be found on the conjunctiva as well as the oral mucosa
Enterovirus	Serotype 70 causes haemorrhagic conjunctivitis
Coxsackievirus	Serotype A24 causes haemorrhagic conjunctivitis
Bacterial	
Staphylococcus aureus	
Streptococcus pneumoniae	
Haemophilus influenzae	
Neisseria gonorrhoeae	A cause of ophthalmia neonatorum which is a notifiable disease
Chlamydia trachomatis	A cause of ophthalmia neonatorum which is a notifiable disease
Pseudomonas aeruginosa	Common in association with contact lenses. May progress to severe corneal ulceration
Mycobacterium tuberculosis	Causes a conjunctival granulomatous nodule rather than the clinical presentation of acute inflammation

C

sium is low and usually associated with metabolic alkalosis. The clinical features are hypertension, muscle weakness, fatigue, paralysis, paraesthesia, tetany, polydipsia and polyuria. Oedema is rare in patients with primary hyperaldosteronism.

The diagnosis must be suspected in any patient with hypertension. In primary hyperaldosteronism, there is an elevated serum aldosterone level with low serum renin. This is confirmed by demonstrating a failure of suppression of aldosterone secretion following salt loading. In secondary hyperaldosteronism, both aldosterone and renin levels are elevated.

Management

Primary hyperaldosteronism is treated by surgically removing the adrenal adenoma. In patients with bilateral adrenal hyperplasia, treatment with spironolactone (antagonizes action of aldosterone) may be helpful.

CONTACT DERMATITIS: A skin disease resulting from contact with a specific inducing agent, which may or may not be mediated by allergic mechanisms (see also Eczema).

Irritant contact dermatitis can result from contact with a variety of detergents, alkalis, mineral oils and organic solvents. Atopic individuals are particularly susceptible and housewives, together with persons in a number of occupations, e.g. hairdressers, are at risk. The condition is due to direct skin damage by the agent.

Allergic contact dermatitis (also called eczematous contact allergy) is a disease which occurs world wide and can affect males and females at all ages. It is mediated by T-cells (type IV hypersensitivity), both sensitization and elicitation of the hypersensitivity reaction involving skin contact with allergens which include both natural and synthetic chemicals (see Eczema for a list of these). One common allergen, penta-decylcatechol, found in poison ivy and poison oak affects more than 50% of the US population! Another is nickel, e.g. from underwear. Diagnosis is confirmed by a 'patch' test where test allergens in concentrations eliciting allergic but not irritant reactions are applied to the skin. Reactions are read at 48 hours and are positive when localized eczema is seen. Photoallergic contact dermatitis, like allergic contact dermatitis, is caused by type IV hypersensitivity but the allergens require sunlight activation, e.g. some soaps, perfumes. Some drugs taken systemically can also cause photodermatitis reactions, e.g. sulphonamides, phenothiazines.

Dermatitis; Eczema; Hypersensitivity

COT DEATH: Death of a baby that remains unexplained even after postmortem examination. Also known as sudden infant death syndrome (SIDS)*.

CREUTZFELDT–JAKOB DISEASE: A disease of the brain caused by infection with prion protein and characterized by rapidly progressive dementia.

Case

A 40-year-old man went to his family doctor complaining of feeling unwell. He did not give any specific symptoms but said that over the previous few months, his memory was not as good as it was and he had found himself being irritable with close family members. Looking through his records, the doctor noticed that he had been on growth hormone replacement therapy as a child, as treatment for short stature, but there was nothing else of note. There was nothing to find on examination and blood tests for haematology and biochemistry were all normal. The doctor reassured him and asked him to return if he did not feel better within a month.

The patient did not return, but 3 months later his wife asked for a home visit for her husband. At this stage, the patient showed profound memory impairment and was exhibiting signs of ataxia. He was referred to the hospital where the neurologist confirmed that he had signs of dementia. Further, while on the ward, he exhibited startle myoclonus. The neurologist felt that the most likely cause of his dementia was infection with the prion protein as a result of contaminated growth hormone replacement in his childhood. Six months later, the man died of bronchopneumonia.

Postmortem findings The brain did not exhibit atrophy and the principal findings were of spongiform (vacuolar) changes in the cerebral cortex. The features were consistent with spongiform encephalopathy (CJD) (Fig. C23).

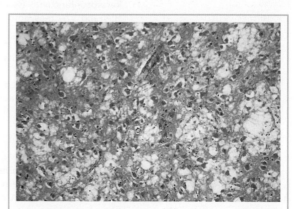

Fig. C23 Histological section of the brain showing spongiform change.

Aetiology and risk factors

The aetiology is infection with prion protein. The infection may be sporadic (majority of cases), familial, or iatrogenic (growth hormone replacement, corneal transplant, implantation of electrodes in the brain). Recently a new variant of CJD has been described which is thought to have a dietary aetiology – eating beef contaminated with the bovine spongiform encephalopathy (BSE) prion.

Pathology

CJD is part of a group of disorders collectively known as the spongiform encephalopathies. They also include kuru in humans (due to cannibal practices of eating brain), scrapie in sheep and goats, transmissible encephalopathy in minks and bovine spongiform encephalopathy (BSE). In the past, growth hormone was prepared from human pituitaries and contamination of infected brain tissue in these extracts is thought to be responsible for some cases of CJD, as in the case above. Growth hormone is no longer produced in this way, a recombinant product having been available since 1985. There is a long latent period before the appearance of symptoms but once it manifests, the progress is rapid and fatal. Few survive beyond a year. The hallmark of the disease is spongiform change in the cerebral cortex. Due to the rapid progression, atrophy of the brain as seen in senile dementia is not a common finding.

Recently, a new variant CJD has been described which occurs in younger patients and a link with eating contaminated beef has been suggested. The transmission of disease across species and especially by a protein molecule is both intriguing and worrying.

Management

There is no known cure. Prevention by avoiding contaminated materials is the best approach but since our knowledge is still scanty, this is problematic. Further, the latent period appears to be very long, making a realistic assessment of potential risk factors difficult.

 Spongiform encephalopathy

CROHN DISEASE: A chronic granulomatous inflammatory disorder resulting in transmural inflammation of the bowel, mucosal damage and systemic manifestations.

Case

A 24-year-old lady presented to the gastroenterologist with a 6-month history of intermittent diarrhoea. The first episode was mild with some abdominal pain and this settled in a couple of days. The second episode did not occur until 6 weeks later when she had further diarrhoea, fever and abdominal pain. She did not see her own doctor as she thought it was 'food poisoning' following a meal at a restaurant. Over the last week, she had developed diarrhoea again but this time she had noticed blood in her stools. On questioning, she did not have any other history of note. She had not travelled abroad in the previous 2 years.

On examination, she was thin but otherwise well. She had pallor of the conjunctiva and abdominal examination revealed generalized tenderness without guarding. A sigmoidoscopy was carried out and apart from mild erythema, no abnormalities were seen. A biopsy was taken for histology. She also had blood samples taken and stools were sent for microbiology.

Histology of the rectal biopsy was normal. Blood tests confirmed that she was anaemic with a haemoglobin of 10 g/l. The ESR was raised at 23. Microbiological analysis did not reveal an infective cause for her diarrhoea.

A colonoscopy was arranged and biopsies were obtained from the caecum and terminal ileum, which appeared to be inflamed:

> Caecum: mild chronic inflammation
> Terminal ileum: acute and chronic inflammation with extension of the inflammation through the bowel wall to involve the serosa. Occasional crypt abscesses were also seen. A single non-caseating granuloma was present. Features are suggestive of Crohn disease.

She was started on a course of steroids and her diarrhoea and abdominal pain settled. Six months later, she presented to casualty in the middle of the night as an emergency with severe abdominal pain and signs of peritoneal irritation. An emergency laparotomy was carried out at which a segment of inflamed terminal ileum and the appendix was removed.

Histology of the bowel showed severe ulceration of the mucosa with fissuring ulcers, transmural inflammation and granulomata in keeping with Crohn disease. There was also oedema in the lamina propria and hypertrophy of the muscularis was noted. The inflamed mucosa was separated by relatively normal mucosa (skip lesions). The appendix was normal (Figs C24 and C25).

A year later, she again presented to the clinic with symptoms of a colovesicular fistula, which was confirmed on a barium follow-through. This was repaired surgically.

Aetiology and risk factors

Crohn disease is a granulomatous disorder of

C

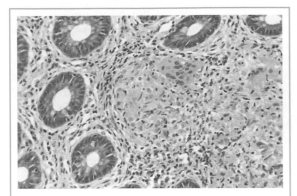

Fig. C24 Histological section of bowel showing a granuloma with giant cells in Crohn disease.

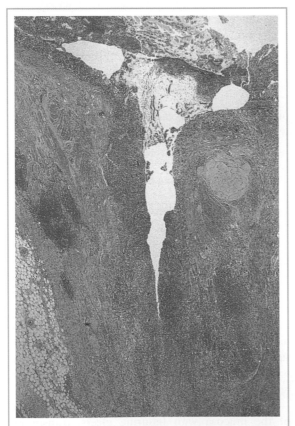

Fig. C25 Histological section showing a fissuring ulcer involving bowel mucosa in Crohn disease.

unknown aetiology. Some form of immune over-reactivity to food antigens has been suspected but not proved.

Pathology

The insidious onset and history of intermittent mild diarrhoea in a young patient are typical of the disease. It is slightly more common in women than men. There may be long periods when the disease is quiescent. It is a granulomatous disorder but the

antigen producing the immune response has not been identified. There is some evidence for the role of slow-growing micro-organisms, including mycobacteria. Unlike tuberculosis (which is a differential diagnosis), the granulomata are non-caseating.

The classical histopathological features are oedema, inflammation (infiltrate of activated T-cells and macrophages), ulceration (fissuring and linear) and granulomata. Crohn disease shows transmural inflammation and 'skip lesions' which help to differentiate it from ulcerative colitis. The presence of transmural inflammation means that the serosa also becomes inflamed and patients may therefore have signs of peritonitis. This also accounts for fistula formation between different segments of the bowel and between the bowel and other viscera such as bladder and vagina.

In the past, Crohn disease was also known as terminal ileitis as it was believed to be confined to that area; however, it is now known that it can affect any part of the gastrointestinal tract from mouth to anus. Approximately a third of the patients have involvement of the mouth, oesophagus, stomach or duodenum. The involvement of the small bowel, especially the ileum, leads to malabsorption and anaemia.

Crohn disease may also present with extracolonic manifestations, which include erythema nodosum, clubbing of the fingers and migratory polyarthritis. Patients also have a risk of colonic carcinoma, but less so than in ulcerative colitis.

Management

This relies mainly on steroids to reduce the inflammation. Surgery is avoided, if possible, as this increases the likelihood of fistula formation; however, it is not an absolute contraindication. The chronic intermittent relapses and the risk of fistula mean that patients may have to endure many years of hardship.

 Erythema nodosum; Granuloma; Inflammatory bowel disease; Ulcerative colitis

CRYOGLOBULINAEMIA: Precipitation of serum when cooled, due to an immunoglobulin molecule (cryoglobulin) that precipitates in the cold.

Symptoms are those of peripheral microvascular occlusion on exposure to cold, including Raynaud phenomenon. Cryoglobulins should be distinguished from cold agglutinins* which have antibody activity directed against red cell antigens, whereas the antibody specificity of cryoglobulins is usually not known. Cryoglobulinaemia may be an incidental finding (idiopathic) but is also found in paraproteinaemia and in autoimmune diseases.

CRYPTOCOCCOSIS: Infection with *Cryptococcus neoformans*.

Aetiology and risk factors

The infection typically affects AIDS patients and is acquired from the environment presumably by inhalation. The yeast is found in pigeon droppings, soil and on fruit.

Pathology

Once present in the body, the yeast develops an abundant capsule which is protective. The yeast produces disease primarily in the central nervous system (meningoencephalitis) as this has relatively poor cellular and humoral defences against crypto-cocci. It can also localize to other organs such as the lungs, liver, or skin, where granulomata may be formed (Fig. C26). Clinically the patient presents

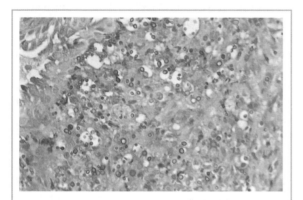

Fig. C26 Cryptococcus in tissue stained in PAS.

with a low-grade temperature, headache, and mental changes. The presentation is usually of slow onset – more like tuberculous meningitis rather than meningococcal meningitis. The cell count in the cerebrospinal fluid is elevated with a monocyte response, decreased glucose, and elevated protein. Occasionally the patient may present with pulmonary disease: either pneumonia or an isolated focus of infection called a cryptococcoma. Cryptococcomas may also be found in the central nervous system, in which case the patient may present with focal neurological signs. Diagnosis is by microscopy, histology, detection of capsular antigen in blood or cerebrospinal fluid, or isolation of the yeast. Treatment is with amphotericin or fluconazole.

CRYPTOSPORIDIOSIS: Infection with the proto-zoon *Cryptosporidium parvum*, which is found widely distributed in the animal kingdom. In humans this causes a gastrointestinal infection.

Aetiology and risk factors

The disease is acquired by drinking contaminated water or by contact with infected animals, e.g. puppies and farm animals.

Pathology

The organism can infect the whole gastrointestinal tract but usually localizes to the brush border of the enterocytes in the ileum. Occasionally it can infect the biliary or respiratory tract. Histologically there is stunting of the microvilli, lengthening of the crypts and a neutrophilic infiltrate in the lamina propria. The mechanism of production of the secre-tory-type diarrhoea associated with infection is currently unknown. In immunocompetent individ-uals the presentation is with offensive, watery diarrhoea, abdominal pain and distension. In some patients there may be mild flu-like symptoms. The infection lasts about 7–10 days, slowly resolving. In immunocompromised (e.g. AIDS) patients, the diarrhoea becomes chronic, and the infection may be ultimately fatal. Extraintestinal infections are more common, particularly of the biliary tract where the infection causes a sclerosing cholangitis with elevated serum levels of alkaline phosphatase and normal bilirubin levels. Laboratory diagnosis is by demonstration of the parasite in the faeces.

Management

In immunocompetent patients the infection is self-limiting. No single agent has been found to be universally effective although improvement has been reported with bovine colostrum, azithromycin and paromomycin, amongst others. Management of immunocompromised individuals relies on symptomatic control.

CUSHING SYNDROME: A group of disorders in which the affected individuals present with signs and symptoms resulting from an excessive amount of cortisol in the blood.

Case

A 45-year-old shop assistant presented at the clinic with complaints of progressive muscle weakness and headaches. He also noticed that he was drinking a lot of fluids and urinating more frequently. On examination, he was obese, with a flushed face (Fig. C27). He had proximal muscle wasting and abdom-inal striae. His blood pressure was 190/110 mmHg.

Laboratory investigations revealed the following:

Serum sodium 150 mmol/l; potassium 3.4 mmol/l; bicarbonate 34 mmol/l
Glucose 8.0 mmol/l (fasting)

C

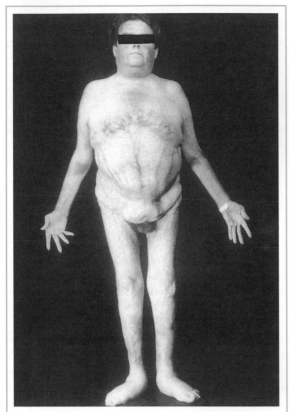

Fig. C27 Patient with Cushing syndrome. The characteristic features are the truncal obesity, striae, round moon face, thin limbs and foot oedema. (Reproduced with permission from Toghill, PJ (ed.) *Examining Patients. An Introduction to Clinical Medicine*. London: Edward Arnold, 1995)

Cortisol (9 a.m.) 1200 nmol/l; (midnight) 1256 nmol/l
Urine: cortisol 600 nmol/24 hours.

He had a low-dose dexamethasone suppression test which showed a 9 a.m. serum cortisol of 960 nmol/l. This was followed by a high-dose dexamethasone suppression test in which his 9 a.m. serum cortisol was 96 nmol/l. A CT scan performed revealed the presence of a 3 mm mass in the pituitary fossa.

Aetiology and risk factors

Excessive amounts of glucocorticoids are produced in conditions that increase adrenal cortical cell function, from ectopic or excessive ACTH production or from excessive administration of glucocorticoids. The various causes of Cushing syndrome can be divided into three main categories: ACTH-dependent, ACTH-independent and others (Table C7).

Table C7 The principal causes of Cushing syndrome

Pituitary origin	Adrenal origin	Others
Adenoma (Cushing disease); 70–80%; usually < 10 mm	Adenoma 5–10%	Ectopic ACTH production
	Carcinoma	Iatrogenic
		Alcoholic pseudo-Cushing syndrome Severe depression

Pathology

The symptoms, signs and laboratory findings in this patient are the result of exposure to excessive amounts of cortisol. Cortisol breaks down protein, thus resulting in tissue destruction. This produces skin atrophy, causing a weakening of the elastic lamina, resulting in disruption of the dermis along lines of stretch. This causes the striae seen on the breast, abdomen and thighs. Reduction in the tensile strength of the capillaries results in purpura and easy bruising. Muscle wasting and weakness also occur. The facial plethora is a result of an increase in platelets and red blood cells produced by cortisol excess.

The biochemical manifestations of excessive cortisol are increased gluconeogenesis and increased mineralocorticoid activity, which result in a raised blood sugar (hyperglycaemia), salt retention and potassium depletion giving rise to the oedema, hypernatraemia, hypokalaemia and alkalosis all seen in this patient. Marked electrolyte disturbances are most common in ectopic Cushing's. The salt retention also results in a raised blood pressure as observed in this patient. The excess of cortisol is demonstrated by the increased amount in the free cortisol in the urine.

Urinary free cortisol (24 hour) This test involves measuring the free cortisol in the urine that has filtered from the blood. The reason free cortisol is measured rather than total cortisol is because total cortisol is affected by steroid hormones and a host of other factors that affect cortisol-binding globulin. In this patient the free cortisol in his urine is 600 nmol/l per 24 hours, which is far in excess of the normal (180 nmol/l). This test also confirms Cushing syndrome. In the blood, there is no suppression of cortisol at midnight, indicating a loss of the diurnal variation in the cortisol secretion.

Diurnal plasma cortisol This test involves measuring a morning and midnight plasma cortisol. In normal individuals, cortisol is secreted in a diurnal fashion – high in the morning and low at night. However, in this patient this diurnal rhythm is disrupted and the midnight cortisol is greater than 280 nmol/l. This test establishes the existence of Cushing syndrome.

Low-dose dexamethasone suppression test When a low-dose dexamethasone suppression test was performed there was no significant reduction in the blood cortisol. This test confirms that the patient does have Cushing syndrome, but does not establish the cause.

High-dose dexamethasone suppression test This dynamic function test is used to ascertain whether the elevated plasma cortisol will respond to a course of dexamethasone. Physiologically, there should be a feedback reduction in the elevated levels of cortisol. In patients with Cushing syndrome, there is no suppression using a low dose of dexamethasone as seen in this patient. However, the cortisol is reduced when a high dose is used. This response is seen in patients with Cushing disease (pituitary-dependent Cushing syndrome). Patients with an adrenal carcinoma or ectopic ACTH production will not suppress their cortisol even in the presence of a high dose. The high-dose dexamethasone suppression test therefore helps to identify the aetiology of the Cushing disease. In this case Cushing disease was confirmed on CT scan which revealed a mass in the pituitary fossa. This was subsequently removed and histologically diagnosed as a pituitary adenoma.

Management
Functional adrenal and pituitary neoplasms are surgically removed. The management of ectopic ACTH-producing tumours is directed at the responsible tumour.

CUTANEOUS LARVA MIGRANS: An infection with animal hookworms leading to inflammatory and pruritic lesions in the skin that migrate as the nematodes move through the skin.

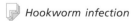 *Hookworm infection*

CYCLOSPORIASIS: Infection with *Cyclospora cayetanensis* causing a self-limiting gastrointestinal infection presenting with watery diarrhoea.

CYSTICERCOSIS: Infection with the cyst stage of the tapeworms *Taenia solium* or *Hymenolepis nana*.

Pathology
The clinical presentation depends upon the localization of the cysts. Disease is caused by the space-

occupying nature of the cysts and the inflammatory reaction against them. The tissues surrounding the cysts are infiltrated with neutrophils and eosinophils and fibrosis encapsulates the cyst. Subsequently, there is infiltration by macrophages and a granuloma develops. The patient expresses delayed hypersensitivity to the cyst antigens. Neurologically, the patient may present with epilepsy, hydrocephalus or dementia. If in the eye, blindness may develop and if in the muscle the cysts may be apparent on palpation. There is a peripheral eosinophilia. If the cyst ruptures there may be a severe anaphylactic reaction, though not so commonly as in hydatid disease*. Radiology can demonstrate the presence of the cysts and laboratory confirmation is by histology and serology. Treatment is with praziquantel or albendazole.

 Hydatid disease; Tapeworm infection

CYSTIC FIBROSIS: An autosomal recessive multisystem disease affecting chloride transport across membranes.

Case
A 10-month-old child was noted to have recurrent chest infections and was not thriving, having lower than normal size and weight for his age. The child had episodes of fever accompanied by coughing. The mother also complained that the faeces were abnormally offensive. Two older brothers were healthy. A clinical suspicion of cystic fibrosis was raised.

> Chemistry: A sweat test on two occasions showed levels of 80 and 110 mmol of sodium per litre.
> Faecal immunoreactive lipase level: < 1 μm per gram faeces.
> Cytogenetics: Genotyping positive (see below)

The diagnosis of cystic fibrosis was confirmed and the patient started on appropriate management.

Aetiology and risk factors
Cystic fibrosis affects about 1 in 2000 live births. Mutations occur in the gene coding for the cystic fibrosis transmembrane conductance regulator (CFTR). The commonest mutation is a deletion of the nucleotides coding for phenylalanine on chromosome 7, and the defective protein does not transport chloride ions across epithelial membranes. This leads to lack of sodium reabsorption from sweat and mucus (hence the positive sweat test) and deficient transport of water into the secretions. This in turn leads to viscid secretions such as mucus, which explains the varied pathological effects.

C

Pathology

In the gastrointestinal tract there is blocking of the pancreatic ducts, fibrosis of the glandular epithelium and a resultant deficient secretion of pancreatic enzymes which leads to malabsorption and steatorrhoea. Infants may present with meconium ileus. In older patients diabetes may occur. As the child ages, the bronchi become blocked with secretions leading to atelectasis, damage to the bronchial walls and eventually bronchiectasis. Recurrent chest infections are common, particularly with *Staphylococcus aureus*, *Pseudomonas aeruginosa* and *Burkholderia*. These organisms exacerbate the tissue damage by secreting proteases; damage also occurs from immune-complex-mediated degranulation of the patient's own polymorphs which are recruited into the lung by the presence of the bacteria. Amyloidosis may occur as a complication of prolonged suppurative lung disease. Blockage of the intrahepatic bile ducts leads to focal fibrosis and eventually cirrhosis. Portal hypertension follows, which can lead to oesophageal varices and bleeding. Hepatic encephalopathy may occur. Males may be infertile owing to azoospermia.

Diagnosis is by the pilocarpine-induced sweat test (normal sodium 70 mmol/l), combined with tests for malabsorption, or by genotyping. Antenatal screening is available.

Management

Management may include antibiotics, physiotherapy, pancreatic enzyme replacement, α1-antitrypsin therapy, heart–lung transplant or possibly in the future, replacement of the faulty gene.

CYSTITIS: Acute inflammation of the bladder, caused principally by bacteria.

Aetiology and risk factors

The source of the organisms causing cystitis is predominantly the bowel flora and the route of infection is principally ascending via the urethra. The commonest infective cause is *Escherichia coli* although in females *Staphylococcus saprophyticus* is an important cause. Cystitis is more common in females than males because potential pathogens that contaminate the introitus can more easily enter the bladder due to the short urethra. Residual urine in the bladder is also a predisposing factor for developing cystitis. Cystitis in females frequently occurs following coitus – so-called 'honeymoon cystitis'.

Pathology

The infection presents with frequency, dysuria, suprapubic pain and haematuria. The patient has a temperature and there is a peripheral neutrophilia

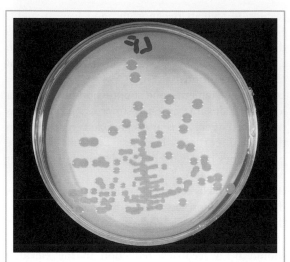

Fig. C28 Growth of *E. coli* (lactose-fermenting and therefore yellow on this medium) from the urine.

with elevated serum levels of acute phase proteins. When bacteria gain entry to the bladder they attach to the uroepithelium, often by means of fimbriae. These adhesins bind to receptors on the uroepithelium, the amount of which may be genetically determined, and thus predispose to urinary tract infections. Some adhesins, such as the P-fimbria which has binding specificity for the P blood group antigen expressed on uroepithelial cells, are commonly found on uropathogenic *E. coli*.

The presence of bacteria adherent to the bladder epithelium starts an acute inflammatory response and leads to the symptoms of cystitis. The organisms may pass up into the kidney, particularly if vesicoureteric reflux or some congenital abnormality is present, causing pyelonephritis. In some patients bacteria may colonize the bladder but the patient remains asymptomatic. This is only important in children and pregnant women as asymptomatic bacteriuria may predispose to pyelonephritis in these groups. Alternatively, some women may have symptoms of cystitis but bacteria are not found in the urine. This is the 'urethral syndrome' and may be caused by common uropathogenic bacteria present in low numbers or by organisms that are not detected by routine investigations, or it may have a non-infectious cause (chemical, allergic). Haemorrhagic cystitis is caused by viruses (adenovirus type II and BK virus) but the condition is uncommon. Laboratory diagnosis of cystitis is by semiquantitative culture of a midstream specimen of urine (MSU) (Fig. C28) when >10^5 organisms per millilitre of urine is considered as a significant bacteriuria. Treatment is with the appropriate antibiotics.

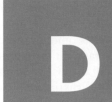

DECOMPRESSION SICKNESS: A form of gas embolism (nitrogen) which occurs in caisson workers and deep-sea divers when they come to the surface too rapidly after long periods of submersion. Also known as caisson disease.

Aetiology

In caisson workers and deep-sea divers when air is breathed under high underwater pressure, an equilibrium exists between the oxygen and nitrogen in the blood and the tissues. On rapid ascent to the surface of the water, the dissolved gases come out of solution; whilst oxygen is rapidly reabsorbed, nitrogen is not, and forms bubbles in the blood and tissues which act as emboli. Decompression sickness can also occur in rapid unpressurized ascent, e.g. in mountaineers climbing too rapidly to high altitude.

Pathology

If nitrogen emboli occur in the pulmonary vessels, divers experience retrosternal discomfort, dyspnoea and cough. Involvement of the brain may cause cortical blindness, hemiparesis and sensory disturbances; in severe cases, extensive necrosis results and ultimately death. In less severe cases, nerve and muscle involvement results in muscle contraction, giving rise to muscle pain ('the bends'). In addition, platelets adhere to nitrogen bubbles and activate the coagulation cascade, which results in disseminated intravascular coagulation*. A long-term complication seen in deep-sea divers is aseptic necrosis of the femoral head as a result of infarction of the nutrient artery by nitrogen bubbles.

Management

Management is with oxygen and decompression chambers.

DEMENTIA: This refers to loss of intellectual functions due to cerebral damage.

 Alzheimer disease

DEMYELINATING DISEASES: Disorders in which there is a loss of myelin sheath around the axon.

Aetiology and risk factors

Demyelination occurs as a result of damage to either oligodendrocytes or the myelin sheath. There are two main groups of disorders included in this category: multiple sclerosis and perivenous encephalomyelitis. Multiple sclerosis is thought to have a genetic predisposition, which may be triggered by viral infection (see below). Perivenous encephalomyelitis is essentially a postinfectious encephalomyelitis and is usually preceded by viral infection, e.g. measles, mumps, chickenpox, whooping cough or rubella.

Multiple sclerosis is usually seen in temperate higher latitude climates of both northern and southern hemispheres. It is rare amongst Africans, American Indians and Orientals. Females are affected more than males and there is an association with B7 and DR2. It has been suggested that the canine distemper virus is aetiologically related to multiple sclerosis; however, direct evidence is lacking.

Pathology

The histological hallmark of multiple sclerosis is areas of demyelination which are referred to as plaques. These tend to occur around the cerebral ventricles, although they may be found anywhere within the central nervous system. The earliest loss of the myelin occurs around small venules. Because of the presence of mononuclear cells and lymphocytes around these vessels and at the edge of plaques, cell-mediated immunity has been implicated in the pathogenesis. There is often an increase of IgG in the CSF, but this is not specific to multiple sclerosis.

Multiple sclerosis usually presents between the ages of 20 and 40 years and patients have a relapsing course of many years. Common manifestations include sensory and motor loss, retrobulbar neuritis and cerebellar problems. In the worst cases, the patient becomes disabled over a long period of time with incontinence, paraplegia, ataxia and mental dysfunction.

There are two main types of perivenous encephalomyelitis. Acute disseminated encephalomyelitis usually occurs, secondary to viral infection, as mentioned above. Acute necrotizing haemorrhage leucoencephalitis is very rare and is preceded by a non-specific viral respiratory infection. Histologically there are focal areas of perivenous demyelination. Both these entities are probably a reaction to the immune-mediated damage following viral infection.

Management

This is symptomatic and no specific treatment is available for either disorder at present.

 Multiple sclerosis

DE QUERVAIN THYROIDITIS: A subacute self-limiting form of thyroiditis, characterized by thyroid swelling with areas of inflammation, giant cells and granuloma formation. There may be transient symptoms of hyperthyroidism. The cause of the disease is unknown, but it frequently follows a virus infection, e.g mumps, Coxsackie, ECHO, EBV, and probably represents a viral thyroiditis. Full recovery usually occurs in weeks or months.

DERMATITIS: Acute or chronic inflammation of the skin, usually due to contact with exogenous irritants, and further subdivided according to cause. The term is essentially synonymous with eczema.

DERMATITIS HERPETIFORMIS: A chronic skin disease characterized by extremely itchy, small vesicles on extensor surfaces including knees, elbows, buttocks, neck and shoulders (see Bullous skin diseases). Often patients have an enteropathy, indistinguishable from gluten-sensitive coeliac disease, which is usually mild and asymptomatic; however, as in coeliac disease*, there is an increased risk of lymphoma. Treatment of the skin disease is with dapsone.

DERMATOMYOSITIS: An inflammatory muscle disease (polymyositis*) with skin involvement, typically a photosensitive facial rash accompanied by oedema. In adults, there is an association with malignancy, particularly carcinoma.

DERMATOPHYTOSIS: Infection of the skin caused by one of the keratinophilic fungi called dermatophytes.

 Ringworm

DERMOID CYST: A cyst lined by skin and filled with keratin material. It may occur as a benign cyst within the skin (sebaceous cyst). When found within the ovary, it is a form of benign teratoma

DIABETES INSIPIDUS (DI): A condition caused by a lack of antidiuretic hormone (ADH) produced, or a failure to respond to ADH by the renal tubules, resulting in polydipsia and polyuria.

Aetiology
Cranial DI is caused by any condition that results in an impaired or absent release of ADH from the pituitary. Nephrogenic DI is caused by any condition that results in a lack of sensitivity of the kidney to ADH (see Table D1).

Table D1 Causes of diabetes insipidus

Cranial DI	Nephrogenic DI
Unknown (50%)	Low potassium
Head injury	High calcium
Hypophysectomy	Drugs (lithium, demeclocycline)
Metastases	Pyelonephritis
Pituitary tumour	Hydronephrosis
Sarcoidosis	
Meningitis	

Pathology
A lack of ADH production or its effect on the renal tubules results in deficient water reabsorption from the tubules. The patient then produces large amounts (polyuria) of dilute (low specific gravity) urine. This results in an increase in serum osmolality (high sodium), which in turn induces thirst and excessive fluid intake (polydipsia). Therefore, the clinical features of diabetes insipidus are similar to that of diabetes mellitus, with the absence of glucose in the urine.

The diagnosis is based on the clinical signs and symptoms and confirmed by performing a water deprivation test. In cranial DI, the low specific gravity of the urine fails to increase but this is reversed following intranasal desmopressin. On the other hand, patients with nephrogenic DI, who also fail to increase their urine concentration after deprivation, do not respond even when give desmopressin.

Management
Treatment of cranial DI is with intranasal desmopressin. Nephrogenic DI may be treated with carbamazepine, chlorpropamide and thiazide diuretics.

DIABETES MELLITUS: A metabolic disorder in which there is an impairment of glucose metabolism. This may be due to lack of insulin (type I) or to insulin insensitivity (type II).

Case
A 45-year-old man attended the medical clinic complaining of deteriorating vision. He was a known insulin-dependent diabetic (IDDM) and had been using insulin injection since the age of 6 years. He had been well recently and did not complain of any other symptoms. On direct questioning, however, he did admit to mild numbness of his feet (sensory neuropathy) and to being tired. He also admitted that over the last 12 months, he had not paid enough attention to monitoring his blood sugar and on one occasion, had to be admitted to hospital with hyperglycaemic ketoacidosis.

On examination, he was overweight and his weight had gone up by 6 kg in 12 months. His pulse was 100 beats/min and his blood pressure 145/100

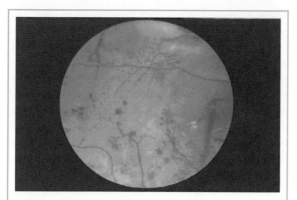

Fig. D1 Photograph showing proliferative retinopathy with haemorrhages. (Reproduced with permission from Toghill, PJ (ed.) *Examining Patients. An Introduction to Clinical Medicine*. London: Edward Arnold, 1995)

mmHg. His apex beat was displaced laterally. Auscultation of his chest was normal but he had mild pitting oedema of his legs. Formal neurological examination confirmed a mild sensory deficit in his hands and legs. Ophthalmoscopy revealed that he had an early cataract in his right eye but in addition, there was evidence of oedema (soft exudates) and neovascularization in both eyes (Fig. D1).

Blood tests showed normal haematological indices but a raised urea and creatinine. Blood sugar was raised at 16 mmol/l. Urine testing revealed proteinuria and glycosuria. His chest radiograph confirmed left ventricular hypertrophy.

A renal biopsy was carried out and showed nodular glomerulosclerosis in keeping with diabetes (Fig. D2). He was advised to lose weight and monitor his sugar more carefully, and laser treatment of his retinal abnormalities was arranged.

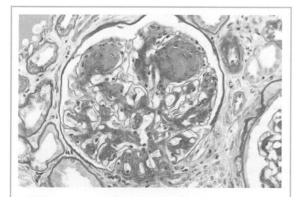

Fig. D2 Histological section of the kidney showing nodular glomerulosclerosis in diabetes.

Aetiology and risk factors

Insulin-dependent diabetes (type I) is thought to arise as the result of a genetic susceptibility combined with an autoimmune reaction against the insulin-secreting cells, possibly triggered by an environmental agent such as a viral infection. HLA-DR3 and DR4 are commoner, and DR-2 rarer, in diabetics than in the general population, and antibodies are found against insulin, pancreatic islet cells (islet cell antibodies, ICA), the enzyme glutamic acid decarboxylase (GAD) and heat shock protein 65 (hsp65). The damage to the insulin-producing β-islet cells, however, is thought to be T-cell mediated.

Type II diabetes (maturity onset; non-insulin-dependent) is about four times commoner than type I, and is associated with obesity, but the reasons for insulin insensitivity at target tissues is unclear.

Diabetes may also occur secondary to pancreatitis, pancreatic tumours, drugs (e.g. steroids), haemochromatosis (bronze diabetes) and in some genetic disorders such as the lipodystrophies.

Pathology

Diabetes is a multisystem disorder resulting from glucose intolerance. The symptoms are related to abnormalities in glucose metabolism. A low insulin level generally leads to hyperglycaemia, which causes glycosuria (glucose in urine), and this in turn causes polyuria and polydipsia (increased frequency of passing urine and increased thirst). The patient may eventually go into coma if uncontrolled. This is further exacerbated by the increased free fatty acid oxidation and hence ketoacidosis that results in hyperglycaemic states. Hypoglycaemia, which may occur due to excessive exercise, inadequate diet, or insulin overdosage, can also lead to coma.

Patients with long-standing diabetes, especially if uncontrolled, tend to have problems with four major systems: microangiopathy, retinopathy, neuropathy and nephropathy.

Diabetic patients have a risk of cardiac disease as a result of atherosclerosis and hypertension. Atheroma of the coronary vessels leads to cardiac ischaemia and myocardial infarction and this risk is further exacerbated by hypertensive heart disease, the hypertension often being secondary to renal disease. The patients are also at risk of cerebrovascular disease due to atheroma in the carotids and within the intracerebral vessels. Peripheral vascular disease leads to distal ischaemia and gangrene.

Small-vessel disease is responsible for the retinopathy, which leads to exudates (soft exudates), and infarcts (hard exudates). A proliferation of small new vessels occurs (neovascularization) and these may bleed, leading to retinal haemorrhages. In the long run, visual impairment of varying degrees is a significant problem.

Diabetic patients are also at risk of both peripheral and autonomic neuropathy. The neuropathy is sometimes responsible for traumatic injury as a result of decreased sensory perception and this, combined with decreased peripheral circulation, leads to chronic non-healing ulcers and gangrene, which may ultimately necessitate amputation.

Renal damage occurs due to ischaemia and patients with diabetes may develop either diffuse or nodular glomerulosclerosis. Diabetics are also prone to infection and hence chronic pyelonephritis may contribute to chronic renal damage.

In summary, abnormalities in glucose metabolism result in multisystem damage with cardiovascular events as the principal cause of death.

Management

For type I diabetes, insulin replacement, regular diet and close monitoring of blood glucose is required. Type II diabetics are advised to lose weight and in some cases this suffices. Alternatively, oral hypoglycaemic agents can be used. The rest of the management is symptomatic. Hypertension is treated with medication and retinopathy can be treated with laser ablation of neovascularized tissue. Little can be done about the neuropathy apart from educating the patients to take care not to injure themselves due to the sensory deficit.

 Atheroma; Hypertension; Myocardial infarction; Neuropathy

DI GEORGE SYNDROME: A rare and severe form of T-cell immunodeficiency caused by failure of the thymus to develop in fetal life, associated with other developmental defects involving the eyes, ears, mouth, parathyroids, and the heart and great vessels. Tetany is an early symptom, due to hypocalcaemia. Functional T-cells are absent, which leads to recurrent infections with viruses, bacteria, fungi, or protozoa. B-cells are normal. Treatment by fetal thymus transplantation has shown some success.

DIPHTHERIA: A systemic disease caused by the Gram-positive toxigenic bacillus *Corynebacterium diphtheriae*. The organism is transmitted by droplet infection and colonizes the nasopharynx.

Pathology

As the organism multiplies in the nasopharynx it produces a thick membrane composed of fibrin, bacteria and sloughed respiratory epithelial cells.

There is frequently regional lymphadenopathy. The presence of the membrane causes symptoms of a sore throat or, if the membrane is extensive (e.g. extending into the trachea and bronchi), respiratory obstruction. The toxin inhibits protein synthesis in many cell types. In addition to the local effects of the organism, the patient may complain of diplopia, dysphonia, lack of accommodation or difficulty in swallowing, due to the effect of the toxin on the cranial nerves. Peripheral neuritis may also develop, affecting mainly the motor fibres. Histologically, there is degeneration of the axons and segmental demyelination. In addition, the toxin affects the autonomic supply to the heart and causes a myocarditis. Therefore, the patient may present with cardiac arrhythmias such as bundle branch block, cardiac enlargement, congestive heart failure, or even sudden death due to ventricular fibrillation or complete heart block.

Rarely, cutaneous infection may be seen with *C. diphtheriae*. This is a tropical infection and the patient presents with a sharply demarcated punched-out cutaneous ulcer. Toxic manifestations may accompany the cutaneous form of diphtheria. Laboratory diagnosis is by isolation of the organism and demonstrating the toxigenicity of the isolate.

Management

Treatment is with antitoxin and erythromycin to eradicate the organism. Close contacts of patients are also given erythromycin as prophylaxis. The disease can be prevented by administration of a vaccine consisting of inactivated toxin ('toxoid'), which is given together with tetanus toxoid and pertussis as a triple vaccine. The disease is notifiable.

DISCOID LUPUS ERYTHEMATOSUS: A chronic skin disease which is usually benign but may progress to systemic lupus erythematosus.

Discoid lupus erythematosus (DLE) shares some features with systemic lupus erythematosus (SLE) but without systemic involvement, and is therefore considered to be at one end of the clinical spectrum of lupus erythematosus, SLE representing the other. Skin lesions usually arise in sun-exposed areas and are round or irregular scaly erythematous patches on the face, ears and scalp which tend to heal with scarring. Systemic involvement should be eliminated at presentation. Patients characteristically have antinuclear antibodies (25%) with <5% having anti-Ro antibodies. Most patients with DLE and SLE have a lupus band (i.e. granular deposition of antibodies and complement in the dermis of lesions). Discoid lupus patients, however, unlike 75% of SLE patients, do not have a lupus band in non-lesional sun-exposed skin. About 10% of DLE patients progress to SLE. There is an intermediate condition (subacute cutaneous lupus erythematosus) in which the skin features are more widespread but non-scarring, with mild systemic illness, especially fever. Treatment of DLE is mainly with topical steroids and antimalarials.

DISSEMINATED INTRAVASCULAR COAGULATION (DIC):
A bleeding disorder, often severe, due to consumption of all coagulation factors by release into the circulation of a procoagulant.

Case
A 50-year-old man was running from police when he was hit by a bus. He was admitted to the hospital A&E department and was not able to give a history. On examination blood pressure was 90/40 mmHg, pulse 110 beats/min and regular. Auscultation of his chest revealed absent breath sounds on the left side. The abdomen was distended and silent, with an uncoordinated pain response on palpation. There was a clear closed fracture of the left humerus. An intravenous infusion of saline was set up, followed by hydroxyethylstarch. He was transferred to the radiology department but suffered a cardiac arrest in the lift. The cardiac arrest team was called and he was resuscitated with further intravenous fluids, external cardiac massage and a direct current shock for ventricular fibrillation. He was transferred to the intensive care unit where a chest drain was inserted and 2 litres of blood drained. Grouped-but-unmatched red cell transfusion was set up. The results of his investigations now became available. The blood count showed an elevated white cell count with neutrophilia and occasional nucleated red cells, a low haemoglobin of 6 g/dl and a low platelet count of 13 × 10⁹/l. The blood film showed fragmented red cells and helmet cells, and reduced platelets (Fig. D3).

Coagulation screen: prothrombin time, 34 seconds (control 13 seconds); INR 4.1
APTT: 94 seconds (control 37 seconds)
APTT on 50/50 mixture with normal plasma: 41 seconds
Thrombin time: 23 seconds (control 14 seconds)
Fibrin degradation products (D-dimers): 4.0 (normal <0.25 mg/l)

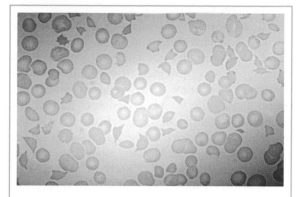

Fig. D3 Blood film from a case of disseminated intravascular coagulation showing fragmented cells and helmet cells with very few platelets.

Aetiology and risk factors
Disseminated intravascular coagulation usually follows the release into the circulation of a procoagulant. This may be tissue thromboplastin released from damaged cells, as in the case described above, or bacterial toxins in a case of septicaemia, or other causes as detailed in Table D2.

Table D2 Causes of DIC

Obstetric causes	Non-obstetric causes
Retained dead fetus	Crush injury
Amniotic fluid embolus	Haemolytic transfusion reaction
Retroplacental haemorrhage	Septicaemia

Pathology
The procoagulant released into the circulation triggers the coagulation mechanism, resulting in the deposition of fibrin strands in small blood vessels. These fibrin strands damage passing red blood cells. When a red cell membrane is damaged, it can often reseal itself, resulting in a half red cell or helmet cell. If damaged in several places, a fragmented cell results. Some cells are so badly damaged that they are destroyed, causing intravascular haemolysis.

This process consumes all coagulation factors and platelets. This results in a severe bleeding tendency and prolongation of all coagulation times. In order to prevent obstruction of small blood vessels, the fibrinolytic system is also activated, dissolving the fibrin rapidly. This prevents ischaemic damage to major organs but worsens the clinical bleeding tendency. The fibrin is split into fibrin degradation products (FDPs) by plasmin. Elevated levels of FDPs may be measured in the plasma, confirming the diagnosis of DIC.

D

Management

The first priority in management is to correct the cause, if possible – for example, treat septicaemia, deliver a dead fetus, etc. Then appropriate treatment with blood products is given. In this case transfusion of fresh frozen plasma was used, containing all the plasma coagulation factors and platelet concentrate. Red cell transfusion will also be required to correct the anaemia, as severe anaemia prolongs the bleeding time. The coagulation screening tests and blood count should be repeated after a few hours and further appropriate blood products given if required.

A controversial method for controlling difficult cases of DIC is the administration of low doses of heparin. This may damp down the consumption of coagulation factors but runs the risk of increasing bleeding by its anticoagulant action.

DIVERTICULITIS: Diverticula are flask-shaped outpouchings of the mucosa into the bowel wall and peri-intestinal tissues, most commonly in the colon. Diverticulitis is inflammation of one or more diverticula in diverticular disease of the colon.

Case

A 67-year-old woman was admitted to the hospital complaining of severe abdominal pain, vomiting, fever and chills. On examination her temperature was 38.5°C, pulse 110 beats/min and blood pressure 90/50 mmHg. The abdomen showed muscle rigidity, reflex guarding and sensitivity in the left lower quadrant. She had been well until 2 years ago when her bowel habits started to change, with increasing constipation, intermittent cramps and failure to feel empty after defecation. A month ago she had a bout of rectal bleeding for a day which was not investigated.

> **Haematology**
> Blood count: Hb 11 g/dl, WBC 14 000 ×10⁶/l, ESR 60 mm/h

Emergency surgery revealed perforation of the sigmoid colon and peritonitis associated with diverticulosis. Twelve centimetres of the sigmoid colon was resected and end-to-end anastomosis performed.

> **Histopathology:** Macroscopically the serosal surface of the resected segment of sigmoid colon was covered with fibrinous exudate. When opened, the mucosa contained multiple diverticula where the colonic mucosa was seen herniating through the

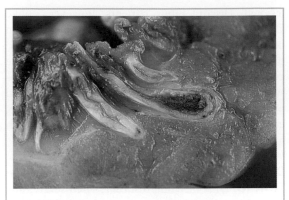

Fig. D4 Macroscopic picture showing resected colon in which there is herniation of mucosa into pericolic fat.

muscle layer and forming small pouches in the serosal fat tissue (Fig. D4). One of the diverticula was enlarged and contained pus and was connected to the peritoneal surface. Microscopical examination confirmed diverticulosis. The perforated diverticulum showed inflammatory exudate in the lumen, extensive ulceration of the mucosa and active chronic inflammation with fibrosis in the surrounding pericolonic soft tissue.

Aetiology and risk factors

The cause of diverticulosis of colon is not known. However, both increase in the intraluminal pressure and weakness in the colonic wall may contribute. The lower incidence observed in societies with a high fibre intake indicates an association with dietary factors and constipation.

Pathology

Diverticulosis is a common disease affecting 5–10% of the population in the West, although only a small number of cases are symptomatic. The most common segment of the colon involved is the sigmoid; however, all of the colon can be affected. Symptoms relate to slow bowel movement and retention of faeces within the diverticula and include changing bowel habits in the form of increasing constipation or periods of intermittent constipation alternating with diarrhoea, lower abdominal discomfort and pain, and abdominal distension. Obstruction of the neck of the diverticula and retention of the faeces within the lumen may lead to diverticulitis with mucosal ulceration and a severe acute inflammatory response to the faecal contents. There is often associated focal peritonitis and acute abdominal symptoms as described in this case. Usually the diverticulitis can be controlled by medical treatment; however, occasionally, as in this case, it can lead to perforation of the bowel wall with more extensive peritonitis and sometimes development of septic shock. Perforation usually requires urgent surgical intervention. If the area of perforation is sealed by adjacent soft tissues, pericolic abscesses can develop. If the inflammation extends into other hollow organs of the pelvic region, colovaginal, colovesical or coloenteric fistulous tracts can form. Repeated attacks of diverticulitis can produce extensive fibrosis and obstruction and mimic colonic carcinoma. Inflammation can also damage mucosal or submucosal blood vessels and cause chronic or intermittent rectal bleeding and anaemia.

Management
In uncomplicated diverticulosis, measures to relieve the constipation, such as high fibre diet or laxatives, are usually sufficient. Diverticulitis is usually managed by antibacterial agents. Other complications such as perforation and bleeding may require urgent or elective surgical intervention.

DIVERTICULOSIS: Diverticula are blind-ended pouches found within the gastrointestinal tract. They may result from developmental defects, such as in Meckel diverticulum, or may be acquired within the colon due to weakness of the bowel wall.

DOWN SYNDROME: A cytogenetic disorder in which there is trisomy of chromosome 21.

Aetiology and risk factors
The most common cause of trisomy of 21 is meiotic non-disjunction. There is an association of Down syndrome with increasing maternal age.

Pathology
Patients with Down syndrome have a flat face, oblique palpebral fissures and prominent epicanthic folds, and are usually mentally retarded. Pathological manifestations include congenital heart disease, the most common being septal defects. They also have a high risk of developing leukaemia, especially acute lymphoblastic leukaemia. Children with Down syndrome are also prone to respiratory tract infections. If they survive beyond the age of 30–35 years, they have a high incidence of Alzheimer disease.

Antenatal screening involves use of the biochemical 'triple test' at week 16. This is an assay of maternal serum alpha-fetoprotein, unconjugated oestriol and beta human chorionic gonadotrophin. In combination with maternal age and weight, this provides a risk score of the fetus having Down syndrome. Diagnosis is by chromosomal examination of fetal tissue.

Management
Since Down syndrome is a chromosomal disorder, genetic counselling can be offered to the families. Specific management is only required when the children develop recurrent respiratory tract infections or leukaemia.

 Acute lymphoblastic leukaemia; Acute myeloid leukaemia; Alzheimer disease; Bronchopneumonia; Congenital heart disease

DRACUNCULIASIS: Infection with the Guinea worm, *Dracunculus medinensis*. The infection is acquired by drinking water containing crustacea infected with the *Dracunculus* larvae. These migrate from the gastrointestinal tract into the peritoneum where they mate. The gravid female migrates to the subcutaneous tissues and the overlying skin ulcerates, releasing the larval stage on contact with water. The larvae then infect crustacea to complete the life cycle. The infection is endemic in Africa, India and the Middle East. Clinically, the first indication of infection is the appearance of the worm in a subcutaneous papule, which ulcerates, to expose the worm. Diagnosis is by demonstration of the worm in the skin and treatment is by mechanical removal of the worm, as there is no specific antihelminth available. Better is prevention by provision of safe potable water supply.

DRESSELER SYNDROME: Pericarditis and sometimes pleurisy associated with myocardial infarction. It occurs 1–6 weeks following myocardial infarction, and may be due to an autoimmune reaction of unknown aetiology.

DUCHENNE MUSCULAR DYSTROPHY: A rare, inherited, X-linked recessive muscular dystrophy seen in childhood, the earliest in onset and most serious of the muscular dystrophies.

Pathology
The condition is caused by the absence of a membrane-associated structure protein, dystrophin, which maintains muscle fibre integrity during contraction. This protein is absent because the gene is absent from the short arm of the X chromosome at the Xp21 site. Female genetic carriers (abnormal gene) give birth to males who are normal at birth but subsequently manifest the disease in childhood. The disease progresses rapidly and death occurs at the end of the second decade. The muscles involved are mainly those of the pelvic girdle and weakness is usually symmetrical. In the early stages of the disease the muscles appear larger as a result of fatty infiltration (pseudohypertrophy). Walking becomes

D

very difficult with the individual finally having a typical waddling gait. Female carriers usually have high creatine kinase levels and fetal creatine kinase estimation may help in prenatal diagnosis of this disease.

DUPUYTREN CONTRACTURE: Palmar fibromatosis. It consists of a nodule and poorly defined deposition of mature collagen, resulting in contracture of the hand.

 Fibromatosis

DWARFISM (ACHONDROPLASIA): A genetic (autosomal dominant) disease that results in abnormal synthesis of cartilage matrix protein.

Due to this, there is a failure of cartilage cell proliferation at the epiphyseal plates, resulting in failure of longitudinal bone growth and subsequent short stature. This affects mainly long bones and not membranous bones, so that the retardation in growth is only restricted to the long bones. The typical achondroplastic dwarf has short limbs and a large head with a prominent forehead and deep indented nose. Intelligence, life expectancy and general health are normal. In homozygotes, however, death may occur in early infancy.

DYSENTERY: Frequent mucopurulent blood-stained faeces.

Case

A 39-year-old woman went to her GP complaining of colicky abdominal pain and sudden onset of watery blood-stained diarrhoea. She felt generally unwell and the GP noted she had a fever. She gave a history of having returned from a holiday in Africa 2 days previously. The GP sent a specimen of faeces to the laboratory for culture and ova, cysts and parasites.

> Microbiology: *Entamoeba histolytica* was not demonstrated in the faeces. Culture for *Salmonella*, *Campylobacter* and *E. coli* O157 were negative. *Shigella flexneri* was isolated from the faeces.

Aetiology and risk factors

Dysentery can be caused by *Entamoeba histolytica* (amoebic dysentery), enteroinvasive *E. coli* (EIEC) and *Shigella* (bacillary dysentery).

Shigella is a Gram-negative bacterium that is transmitted by person-to-person faeco-oral spread associated with poor hygienic standards. Spread can also occur by contaminated food or water and in some cases flies may spread the organism. There are four species of *Shigella*: *Shigella dysenteriae*, *Shigella flexneri*, *Shigella boydii* and *Shigella*

sonnei. *Sh. sonnei* is the common organism present in the UK; the other three species are more usually found in tropical countries. The organism is highly infectious, 100–200 organisms being able to cause the disease (compared with *Salmonella* or *Vibrio cholerae* where 10^6–10^7 organisms are needed to cause disease).

Pathology

After a short period of multiplication in the small intestine, the organism is found in the colon. *Shigella* are initially taken up by macrophages or polymorphs in the colonic epithelium and transported to the lamina propria, where the host cell is killed either by a *Shigella* toxin or by induction of apoptosis. The bacteria then invade the colonic epithelial cells via their basolateral surface, polymerizing the actin of the colonic cell and inducing bacteria-directed phagocytosis. The proteins necessary for the adhesion and invasion of *Shigella* are coded for by a large plasmid carried by the organism. The organism escapes from the phagosome and penetrates adjacent cells. Within the colonic epithelial cell the bacterium is able to precipitate actin in a polarized manner and thus move through the cytoplasm (Fig. D5).

Infected cells are ultimately killed as the organism spreads from cell to cell to produce a superficial ulcer. This gives rise to the symptoms of abdominal colic and blood-stained diarrhoea. *Shigella* also produce a potent toxin (particularly *Sh. dysenteriae*), which is virtually identical to the Vero-toxin of *E. coli* O157 in both structure and mode of action. The haemolytic uraemic syndrome can follow infection with *Shigella* as it can with *E. coli* O157. Diagnosis is by isolation of the organism from the faeces.

Management

Treatment is usually not required, especially for the mild disease caused by *Sh. sonnei*. If symptoms are severe, antibiotics (e.g. ciprofloxacin) can be given and fluid replacement may be required. Dysentery is a notifiable disease.

 Amoebiasis; Gastroenteritis; Haemolytic uraemic syndrome

DYSGERMINOMA: A germ cell tumour of the ovary, the ovarian counterpart of seminoma of the testis*.

DYSPLASIA: When applied to epithelial or mesenchymal tissues, this refers to cytological and architectural atypia signifying a precancerous state. 'Dysplastic' changes may also be seen in tissues after chemotherapy treatment.

D

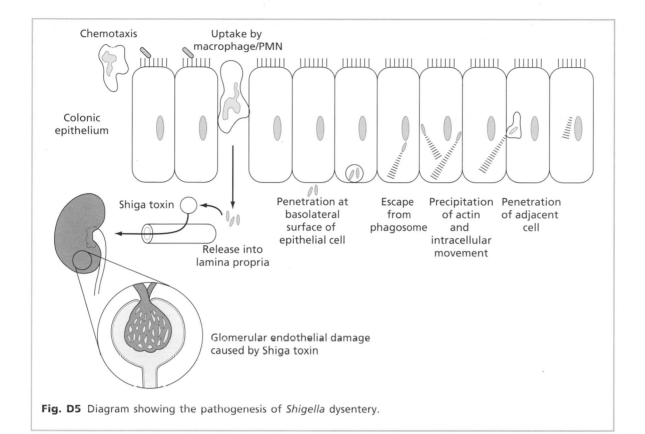

Fig. D5 Diagram showing the pathogenesis of *Shigella* dysentery.

(labels within figure)

Chemotaxis

Uptake by macrophage/PMN

Colonic epithelium

Shiga toxin

Release into lamina propria

Penetration at basolateral surface of epithelial cell

Escape from phagosome

Precipitation of actin and intracellular movement

Penetration of adjacent cell

Glomerular endothelial damage caused by Shiga toxin

Aetiology and risk factors

The risk factors are varied and range from inherited susceptibility, as in dysplastic adenomas arising with familial adenomatous polyposis, to viral infections, as in human papilloma virus-related cervical dysplasia.

Pathology

Dysplasia, which occurs principally in epithelial tissues, describes a set of cytological and architectural characteristics, which signify a precancerous state. There is a loss of normal polarity of cell arrangement together with alterations in nuclear

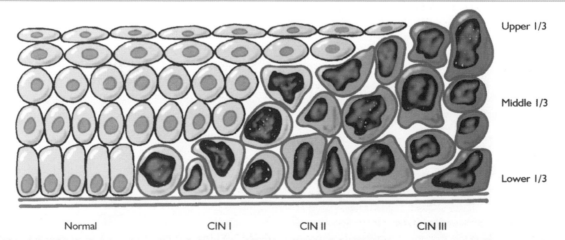

(labels within figure)

Upper 1/3

Middle 1/3

Lower 1/3

Normal   CIN I   CIN II   CIN III

Fig. D6 Schematic representation of dysplasia affecting the transformation zone in cervix. Different grades of dysplasia are shown from left to right. Left is normal, extreme right high-grade dysplasia (CIN3). (Reproduced with permission from Lakhani SR, Dilly SA, Finlayson CJ. *Basic Pathology*, 2nd edn. London: Arnold, 1998)

size and shape (pleomorphism) (Fig. D6). The cells also show increased mitotic activity and there may be abnormal mitotic figures. Such epithelial changes may also be identified adjacent to frankly invasive carcinoma.

Although dysplasia in this context signifies a precancerous lesion, it is not inevitable that the dysplastic foci will progress to frankly invasive carcinoma. It is clear from studies on the cervix and other tissues that lower grades of dysplasia may regress. The concept of dysplasia is important because it signifies an intermediate stage in the transition from normal to frankly invasive carcinoma. It is the recognition of these intermediate stages that has led to the institution of screening programmes such as those for the cervix and breast, with a view to identifying early dysplastic lesions so that patients can be managed before they develop an invasive carcinoma.

Management

Low grades of dysplasia such as CIN1 in the cervix may not require any treatment and many of these lesions regress spontaneously. Higher grades of dysplasia are treated with surgical resection and a close follow-up is instituted to check for progression.

 Adenoma; Adenomatous polyposis; Cervical carcinoma; Myelodysplasia

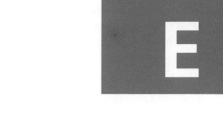

ECTHYMA GANGRENOSUM: Necrotic infection of the skin usually caused by *Pseudomonas* sp., occurring in neutropenic patients.

ECTHYMA INFECTIOSUM: Also called Fifth disease or 'slapped cheek disease', caused by Parvovirus B19. Associated with aplastic crises in patients with sickle cell disease and abortion if infected in the second trimester of pregnancy.

 Exanthema

ECTOPIC HORMONE PRODUCTION: The production of a hormone in malignant neoplasms from cells that do not secrete that particular hormone under normal circumstances.

Aetiology and risk factors
This condition may result as a derepression of genes associated with the neoplastic process, as there is some evidence to show that mRNA coding for the particular hormone may be found in the tumour tissue.

Pathology
The hormone is produced at a site that does not normally secrete it and is demonstrable in the veins draining the tumour; its production exceeds physiological concentrations, does not appear to be controlled by the normal physiological stimulatory mechanisms, and does not respond to feedback suppression. The malignant cells may secrete more than one hormone. Treatment of the malignancy resolves the condition.

Table E1 gives some examples of various malignancies and the hormone they produce.

ECTOPIC PREGNANCY: Implantation of the embryo at sites other than the uterine cavity.

Aetiology and risk factors
The most important underlying predisposing condition is pelvic inflammatory disease, especially gonococcal endosalpingitis. Other predisposing factors include previous surgery, for instance for appendicitis or endometriosis. The use of intrauterine contraceptive devices (IUCDs) is also thought to increase the risk of ectopic pregnancy.

Pathology
The commonest site for ectopic pregnancy is within the fallopian tubes. Other sites include the ovary and the abdominal cavity. Whatever the site of the ectopic implantation, the embryo begins its usual development with formation of the amniotic sac, placental tissue, placental implantation site and decidua. Serum pregnancy tests are positive in only about 50% of cases. However, the β-subunit hCG assay is positive in about 95%. Urine pregnancy test results are variable. A decrease in serum β-hCG after curettage indicates completed abortion, whereas a rise implies ectopic pregnancy or incomplete abortion.

Table E1 Examples of malignancies and hormones produced

Hormone or hormones secreted	Malignancies
Human chorionic gonadotrophin	Carcinoma of lung, breast, stomach, colon, prostate and pancreas
Parathyroid hormone related peptide (PTHrP)	Squamous carcinoma of lung, head and neck, oesophagus, cervix, renal adenocarcinoma, multiple myeloma and large cell carcinoma of lung
Adrenocorticotropic hormone (ACTH)	Small cell carcinoma of lung, pancreatic islet cells neoplasms, phaechromocytoma, medullary thyroid carcinoma, and bronchial carcinoid tumour
Antidiuretic hormone (ADH)	Small cell carcinoma of the lung
Insulin	Hepatocellular carcinoma and retroperitoneal sarcomas
Erythropoietin	Renal adenocarcinoma, cerebellar haemangioblastoma, hepatocellular carcinoma and uterine fibroids
Growth hormone	Lung and gastric carcinoma
Glucagon	Renal carcinoma and anaplastic lung carcinoma and non-β-islet cell tumour
Calcitonin	Small cell carcinoma of the lung, pulmonary carcinoid tumour

E

If the ectopic pregnancy occurs within the fallopian tubes, the implantation into the wall leads to intratubal haemorrhage and possible tubal rupture with intraperitoneal haemorrhage. The patient presents with severe abdominal pains and shock.

Management

Management consists of early diagnosis and, if necessary, surgical intervention either through laparoscopy or laparotomy. The predisposing causes such as endosalpingitis are worth investigation as it may be possible to avoid future ectopic pregnancies.

 Inflammation; Shock

ECZEMA: This is a pattern of inflammation in the skin, rather than a disease and has several causes. The term is often used synonymously with dermatitis.

Aetiology and risk factors

Patients usually present with itchy red skin and have oedematous vesicles when the inflammation is intense. Prolonged inflammation results in scaling and thickening of the skin. Infections in the lesions are common. Eczema has been classified, somewhat artificially, into exogenous and endogenous types, based on whether the disease process is induced by external or internal means. However, in many cases the inducing factors and mechanisms of eczema are unknown (Table E2).

Pathology

Typically, the earliest pathological changes involve spongiosis, i.e. accumulation of oedema fluid between the keratinocytes within the epidermis, and infiltrates of lymphocytes, monocytes, and eosinophils. In chronic cases, thick hard plaques (lichenification) may develop.

Management

Treatment of eczema is symptomatic. Weeping eczematous eruptions should be treated with potassium permanganate and less acute eczema with steroids. Known inducers and aggravating factors should be avoided. Recently, Chinese herbal remedies have been reported to give some benefit.

EFFUSION: An abnormal collection of fluid in a body cavity (pleura, peritoneum, synovial joint). The fluid can be either a transudate or exudate.

Transudates can be caused by: cirrhosis of liver, portal vein obstruction, right heart failure, constrictive pericarditis, Meigs syndrome and malnutrition.

Exudates can be caused by: bacterial peritonitis, tuberculous peritonitis, metastatic neoplasms, mesothelioma and connective tissue disease.

Table E2 Exogenous and endogenous eczema

Type	Inducing factors	Mechanisms
Exogenous		
Irritant contact dermatitis (not all lead to eczematous lesions)	Detergents, mineral oils	Direct skin damage (common in atopic individuals)
Allergic contact dermatitis	Epoxy resins, nickel, chromate, lanolin, perfumes, sticking plasters, topical drugs	Type IV hypersensitivity
Light-induced eczema	Photo-contact allergy, e.g. sunscreen creams; drug eruptions, e.g. chlorpromazine; exacerbation of existing eczema, e.g. atopic dermatitis	Unknown
Endogenous		
Atopic eczema/dermatitis (mainly in children)	Allergic and non-allergic stimuli: dairy products, house dust mite, pollens, danders, wool, etc.	Often high IgE levels but mechanism unknown
Discoid eczema	Unknown	Unknown
Seborrhoeic eczema/dermatitis	*Pityrosporum* yeasts thought to play a role	Unknown (early feature in about 1/3 AIDS patients)
Pompholyx	Onset of warm weather, dermatitis or fungal infections of feet, ingestion of contact allergens, e.g. nickel, and stress	Unknown
Asteatotic eczema (mainly in elderly)	? Reduced epidermal lipids ?, hypothyroidism, uraemia, and dehydration might contribute	

Table E3 Physiochemical properties of transudates and exudates

	Transudate	Exudate
Vascular permeability	Normal	Increased
Protein content	0–1.5 g/dl	1.5–6 g/dl
Protein type	Albumin	All types
Fibrin present	No	Yes
Specific gravity	1.010–1.015	1.015–1.027
Cells	None	Inflammatory cells

The essential differences between the physio-chemical properties of transudates and exudates are shown in Table E3.

EHRLICHIOSIS: An infection with a member of the *Ehrlichia* spp.

Aetiology and risk factors

Ehrlichia is a Gram-negative bacterium closely related to *Rickettsia*. The species most commonly recognized as a human pathogen is *Ehrlichia chaffeensis*, which is transmitted to humans by a tick bite. The animal reservoir is currently unknown. Ehrlichiosis is an apparently rare infection, but it has only recently been recognized as a human pathogen.

Pathology

The bacterium is an obligate intracellular organism parasitizing macrophages, monocytes and neutrophils. It multiplies in the cytoplasm of the target cell and has been found in cells of the reticuloendothelial system (lymph nodes, liver and spleen), in bone marrow and in peripheral blood leucocytes. The effect of the organism on the bone marrow can result in a normocellular picture, myeloid hyperplasia, erythroid hypoplasia, thrombocytopenia, or aplastic anaemia. Focal necrosis of the liver, spleen or lymph nodes may occur and a histiocytic perivascular infiltration is evident in many solid organs. Clinically, infection can range from being asymptomatic to a severe systemic infection. The patient may present with fever, malaise, myalgia, headache and a maculopapular rash. Leucopenia, anaemia, thrombocytopenia and elevated liver transaminases are also present. Complications include pulmonary, central nervous system, renal and disturbed coagulation leading to gastrointestinal haemorrhages. Laboratory diagnosis is by serology or demonstration of the organism by PCR. The organism cannot be grown on artificial media. Treatment is with tetracycline.

ELEPHANTIASIS: see Filariasis.

EMBOLISM: Solid, liquid or gaseous material that is carried within the bloodstream from one area of the circulation to another.

Aetiology and risk factors

Emboli arise from fragments of thrombi, atheromatous plaques, from foreign material introduced through intravenous catheters, from bone marrow elements, fat, air or nitrogen, amniotic fluid or from breakage of tumour within the intravascular spaces.

Pathology

Since the majority of emboli arise from thrombi within the circulating system the word thromboembolism is often used synonymously with embolism. The pathological consequences of emboli depend on which side of the circulation they arise. Emboli arising within the venous system travel though the right side of the heart and end up in the pulmonary circulation as pulmonary emboli. Those that arise in the left side of the circulation block systemic arteries, the clinical effects depending on which organ is involved, e.g. brain, kidney or peripheral vascular system. In addition, the effects of emboli are dependent on their size and origin.

Pulmonary embolism is a recognized complication of deep vein thrombosis. The thrombi are found in the femoral, iliac and popliteal vessels. Depending on the size of the embolus, it may obstruct either the main pulmonary artery, or both pulmonary branches, producing saddle embolisms, or smaller fragments may lodge in the terminal bronchial arteries. The lung has a dual blood supply from the pulmonary artery as well as the bronchial arteries, which arise directly from the aorta. Hence small emboli will only cause infarction if the bronchial supply is also compromised, as happens in cardiac failure. Obstruction to the large pulmonary arteries can have a dramatic effect with cardiac arrest and death (see Fig. T5, p. 247). Once the emboli have lodged in the vascular supply they eventually get organized and the vessel attempts to recanalize. With chronic pulmonary emboli there is a rise in pulmonary artery pressure and hence right ventricular hypertrophy secondary to pulmonary hypertension.

Systemic emboli generally occur because of thrombosis within the heart itself. Patients with atrial fibrillation or following myocardial infarction are at risk of thrombosis within the atrial appendage or within the ventricle. These thrombi break off to produce a shower of emboli that can affect many different organs. Embolization to cerebral circulation may lead to cerebrovascular

E

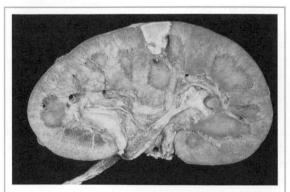

Fig. E1 Kidney showing a wedge shaped cortical infarct as a result of embolism blocking one of the branches of the renal artery. (Reproduced with permission from Lakhani SR, Dilly SA, Finlayson CJ. *Basic Pathology*, 2nd edn. London: Arnold, 1998)

accident (stroke). Embolization also commonly occurs to the kidney where a wedge-shaped renal infarct may appear (Fig. E1). A third common site of embolization is to peripheral arteries of the limbs. Embolization to the mesenteric arteries produces intestinal infarction.

Management
The management consists of rapid diagnosis and anticoagulation. Embolectomy may be necessary in certain situations, especially if there is a large embolus within the pulmonary arteries.

 Cerebrovascular disease; Infarction; Myocardial infarction; Thrombosis

EMPHYSEMA: Permanent enlargement of air spaces distal to the terminal bronchioles. It results from the destruction of the alveolar wall, the most common aetiological factors being smoking and dust inhalation. α1-Antitrypsin deficiency also leads to emphysema.

 Chronic obstructive airways disease (COAD)

EMPYEMA: Pus in the pleural space which can be caused by a variety of different bacteria.

ENCEPHALITIS: Diffuse inflammation of the brain which may often be in association with inflammation of the meninges, when the condition is called meningoencephalitis.

Aetiology and risk factors
Encephalitis is caused principally by viruses. Viruses that cause meningitis (adenoviruses, Coxsackieviruses, enteroviruses) may also cause encephalitis (see Viral meningitis). Encephalitis may

Table E4 Arboviral causes of encephalitis

Aetiology	Vector/Reservoir
Western equine	Mosquito
Eastern equine	Mosquito
Venezuelan equine	Mosquito
Japanese	Mosquito
Murray Valley	Mosquito
St Louis	Mosquito
California	Mosquito
Colorado	Tick
Louping ill	Tick

also be a complication of viruses that cause exanthema (measles, mumps, VZV, rubella; see appropriate entry). Encephalitis is also a principal component of the pathology in some other important viral infections (HIV, rabies, poliomyelitis, progressive multifocal leucoencephalopathy, herpes simplex). Some arboviral (arthropod-borne) viral causes of encephalitis are given in Table E4. Encephalitis may be a complication of *Listeria* meningitis (see Listeriosis) and is the predominant pathology in African trypanosomiasis (sleeping sickness; see Trypanosomiasis).

Pathology
Encephalitis is characterized by an inflammatory cell infiltrate, neuronal degeneration and microglial hyperplasia. The cellular infiltrate is initially with neutrophils followed by monocytes and macrophages, often in a perivascular location (Fig. E2).

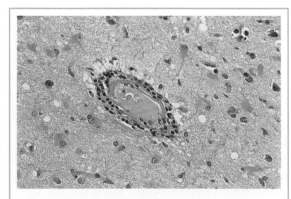

Fig. E2 Histological section of brain showing perivascular inflammatory infiltrate.

Clinically, the patient presents with cerebral dysfunction: focal neurological signs, seizures, disorientation, memory loss, coma with fever, headache, nausea and vomiting. The peripheral white count may be normal, or there may be leucopenia or leucocytosis with a relative lymphocytosis. Lymphocytes are predominant in the cerebrospinal fluid, with a normal glucose and normal or elevated protein concentration.

Laboratory diagnosis is by isolation of the pathogen, serology, or PCR. Treatment is according to the pathogen. Acyclovir is the drug of choice for herpes simplex encephalitis.

ENCEPHALOPATHY: An array of symptoms characterized by drowsiness, confusion, decrease in consciousness, and impairment of higher functions, as a result of cerebral dysfunction.

Encepholopathy can result from infection (meningitis, encephalitis, septicaemia), structural effects (raised intracranial pressure, hydrocephalus), toxins (ammonia, urea), electrolyte imbalances (hyponatraemia, hypernatraemia). If the symptoms are present acutely, an infective or structural cause is the likely suspect. Metabolic causes result in a more chronic form.

Appropriate investigations include CSF examination, serum electrolytes and urea, blood cultures, CT scan, blood pressure measurement and fundoscopy.

ENDOCARDITIS: Infection of the heart valves.

Case

A 65-year-old man complained to his GP of night sweats, malaise and weight loss. The patient had poor dentition and had visited his dentist several times over the past year. He gave a history of rheumatic fever as a child. On examination the doctor noted that the patient had splenomegaly and a heart murmur and was pyrexial (38°C). He also had splinter haemorrhages and proteinuria, with erythrocytes in the urine. The doctor, suspecting bacterial endocarditis, took three sets of blood cultures within the space of an hour and organized an echocardiogram.

> Microbiology: all six blood cultures yielded *Streptococcus sanguis* (Fig. E3). The minimum inhibitory concentration (MIC) of benzylpenicillin was 0.05 mg/ml.
> Echocardiogram: evidence of a valvular vegetation seen (Fig. E4).
> Haematology: Hb 10.1 g/dl; WBC 18 000 × 10^6/l; differential 80% polymorphs; ESR 90 mm/h.

Shortly after starting treatment, the patient developed a right hemiplegia.

Aetiology and risk factors

Bacterial endocarditis can be caused be any bacterium or fungus. The commonest group of

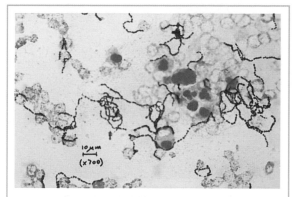

Fig. E3 Gram stain of blood culture showing chains of Gram-positive cocci.

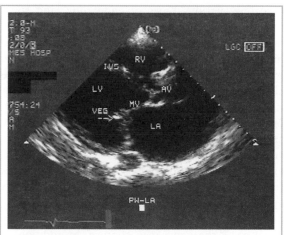

Fig. E4 Evidence of vegetation (veg) attached to mitral valve (MV). (Reproduced with permission from Asmi MH, Walsh MJ. *A Practical Guide to Echocardiography*. London: Chapman & Hall, 1995)

organisms causing the condition are the viridans streptococci of the oral flora. Other important causes of endocarditis are *Staphylococcus aureus* in intravenous drug users and coagulase-negative staphylococci on prosthetic heart valves. The endothelium of the heart can be damaged by turbulent flow, particularly where a high-pressure jet of blood impinges on the endocardium. Such conditions occur in valvular stenosis or regurgitation or some congenital heart defects. One major condition predisposing to valve damage, and thus turbulent flow, is rheumatic fever.

Pathology

Fibrin and platelets aggregate at the damaged endothelium to produce a vegetation (Fig. E5), which may subsequently become colonized by bacteria. Transient bacteraemia occurs frequently, particularly following dental manipulations such as

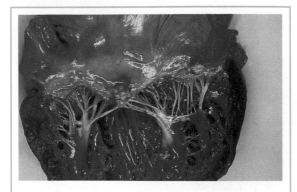

Fig. E5 Section of heart showing vegetations on valve.

Table E5 Diagnosis of endocarditis

Major criteria
- Persistently positive blood culture over a period of 12 hours or three out of four positive blood cultures taken within an hour, all from separate venepunctures at different sites
- Echocardiographic evidence of a vegetation, abscess or dehiscence of prosthetic valve

Minor criteria
- Predisposing factor, e.g. rheumatic fever
- Fever >38°C
- Positive microbiology (but not meeting the above major criterion) or positive serology
- Recognized peripheral phenomena – splinter haemorrhages, Roth spots, Osler nodes, Janeway plaques, glomerulonephritis
- Other echocardiographic evidence consistent with endocarditis but not meeting the major criteria

descaling, various types of endoscopy, and some operations. The organisms may adhere to the fibrinous vegetation on the heart valve and start to multiply in this protected site. Adhesion of the bacteria to the vegetation is mediated by surface characteristics of the organism such as the production of a dextran polymer (by the oral streptococci), or the expression of a fibronectin-binding factor (by *Staph. aureus*). Bacterial metabolism within the vegetation stimulates the valvular endothelium to express tissue thromboplastin, which promotes further fibrin deposition, and the vegetation grows and can lead to further damage to the valve leaflets and thus further haemodynamic disturbance. In some cases the valve may rupture. In addition to these local effects, with the presence of a constant antigenic challenge there is a polyclonal activation of B-cells, leading to the release of pro-inflammatory cytokines (and thus the constitutional symptoms), hypergammaglobulinaemia and immune complex formation. The immune complexes may account for some of the peripheral manifestations of endocarditis, e.g. Osler nodes (painful skin nodules), but may characteristically be deposited in the glomerulus (type III hypersensitivity).

Other complications of endocarditis include myocardial abscess and embolization of the infected vegetation. This may lead to mycotic aneurysms (localized dilation of arteries caused by septic emboli) or to neurological events such as hemiplegia. Endocarditis is diagnosed by a combination of two major criteria, one major and three minor criteria, or five minor criteria, as indicated in Table E5.

Management

Management of endocarditis depends upon the causative organism, as shown briefly in Table E6.

ENDOMETRIAL CARCINOMA: A malignant tumour arising from the endometrial glandular tissue.

Aetiology and risk factors

The tumour is most common after the age of 55 years. It is encountered with increased frequency in women who are obese, have high blood pressure, are infertile and have a history of diabetes.

Table E6 Management of endocarditis

Organism	Antibiotic	Duration
Streptococcus MIC to penicillin <0.1 mg/l	Benzylpenicillin	4 Weeks
	Benzylpenicillin + gentamicin	2 Weeks
Streptococcus or *Enterococcus* MIC to penicillin >0.1 mg/l	Benzylpenicillin (or amoxycillin or vancomycin)	4–6 Weeks
	Benzylpenicillin (or amoxycillin or vancomycin) + gentamicin	2–6 Weeks
Staph. aureus	Flucloxacillin	4–6 Weeks
	Flucloxacillin + gentamicin	1–2 Weeks
MRSA methicillin-resistant *Staph. aureus*.	Vancomycin (or teicoplanin)	4–6 Weeks
	Vancomycin (or teicoplanin) + gentamicin	1–2 Weeks
Coagulase-negative staphylococcus	Vancomycin (or teicoplanin)	4–6 Weeks
	Vancomycin (or teicoplanin) + gentamicin	1–2 Weeks

Pathology

Endometrial carcinoma is an adenocarcinoma since it arises from glandular tissue. There are two broad types:

- those that arise on a background of endometrial hyperplasia as a result of excess oestrogenic stimulation;
- those without associated hyperplasia.

The former are usually well-differentiated carcinomas with a good prognosis. The latter arise in an older age group and tend to be poorly differentiated with a worse prognosis.

Endometrial carcinoma spreads via direct involvement of the myometrium and peritoneal structures, spread to lymph nodes and via the blood occurring later. When it does disseminate, lungs, liver and bone are favoured sites for secondary deposits.

Prognosis depends on stage of disease. Staging is divided into four groups. In stage I, the tumour is confined to the corpus, in stage II, it also involves cervix, stage III means extension outside the uterus but still within true pelvis, and stage IV means distant spread or involvement of bladder or rectum. Most women present with stage I disease and have a 90% 5-year survival.

Management

Surgery with or without radiotherapy is the standard treatment.

 Cervical carcinoma; Diabetes insipidus; Ovarian cancer

ENDOMETRIOSIS: The presence of endometrial glands and stroma outside their normal location within the uterine cavity.

Aetiology and risk factors

It is not clear why endometriosis occurs but three theories have been put forward. In the metaplastic theory it is postulated that endometriosis arises directly from coelomic epithelium. The regurgitation theory suggests that there is retrograde menstruation through the fallopian tubes and hence colonization of the peritoneal surface by endometrial tissues. The vascular dissemination theory suggests that endometriotic tissue disseminates to distant sites such as lung and lymph nodes via the vascular system.

Pathology

Endometriosis occurs in the ovaries, peritoneal surface, laparotomy scars, umbilicus, vagina, vulva and appendix and rarely at distant sites such as lymph nodes. It can result in infertility or dysmenorrhoea, and patients occasionally present with pelvic pain. It is mostly seen in young women in the third and fourth decades.

Morphologically, the endometriosis resembles normal endometrial tissue. When endometriosis occurs in the ovary it results in haemorrhage and in the production of so-called 'chocolate cysts'. Recurrent haemorrhages, particularly when associated with periuterine endometriosis, result in fibrosis and formation of adhesions between the tubes, ovaries and other structures within the peritoneal cavity.

Management

This includes hormonal treatment with oestrogen–progestogen to transform the functioning tissue to decidua and gonadotrophin inhibitory agents. Surgery to remove endometriosis is the mainstay of treatment.

ENDOMYOCARDIAL FIBROSIS: A rare disorder occurring in children and young people, mainly on the African continent. It is characterized by fibrosis of the ventricular endocardium.

ENDOTOXIC SHOCK: Vascular collapse triggered by the lipopolysaccharides (endotoxins) of Gram-negative bacteria. Also known as septic shock*, it is a complication of septicaemia, sometimes secondary to trauma or surgery, and carries a high mortality (up to 50%). It is associated with high levels of inflammatory cytokines, e.g TNF, IL-1.

 Meningococcal meningitis

ENTERIC FEVER: Systemic infection with *Salmonella typhi* or *Salmonella paratyphi*.

 Typhoid fever

EPIDIDYMITIS: An infection of the epididymis which can be caused by a number of bacterial pathogens such as *Chlamydia trachomatis, Neisseria gonorrhoeae, Escherichia coli.*

EPIGLOTTITIS: Acute inflammation of the epiglottis occurring mainly in children and caused by a number of respiratory bacterial pathogens, especially *Haemophilus influenzae*. There is local swelling, which can rapidly lead to respiratory obstruction. The patient shows the typical peripheral neutrophilia of an acute pyogenic infection and the blood culture is nearly always positive. Management is with the appropriate antibiotics but occasionally tracheostomy may be necessary.

ERYSIPELAS: Skin infection caused by *Streptococcus pyogenes*.

 Necrotizing fasciitis

ERYSIPELOID: A pruritic, purplish, usually self-limiting, skin infection caused by *Erysipelothrix rhusiopathiae*. An occupational hazard for gardeners, butchers and fishmongers. Treated with penicillin.

ERYTHEMA CHRONICUM MIGRANS: Spreading erythematous skin lesion following infection with *Borrelia burgdorferi*. Skin manifestation of Lyme disease.

 Lyme disease

ERYTHEMA MULTIFORME: A self-limiting skin condition which appears to be a hypersensitivity reaction to drug or infectious agents.

Aetiology and risk factors
Infections associated with erythema multiforme include histoplasmosis, mycoplasma infections, typhoid and leprosy. Drugs thought to be responsible include sulphonamides, antimalarials, penicillin and salicylates. It is also occasionally seen in malignancies such as lymphomas and collagen-vascular disorders such as systemic lupus erythematosus.

Pathology
The patient presents with skin lesions, which include vesicles and bullae as well as the characteristic target lesions (Fig. E6). These target lesions are composed

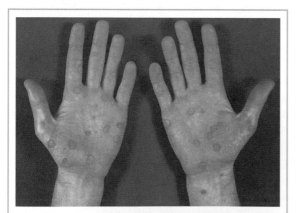

Fig. E6 A patient with multiple lesions of erythema multiforme in the palms. (Reproduced with permission from Toghill, PJ (ed.) *Examining Patients. An Introduction to Clinical Medicine*. London: Edward Arnold, 1995)

of a red macule with a pale centre. The lesions are usually distributed widely throughout the body.

Histologically the target lesion is composed of a central area of necrosis surrounded by a rim of perivascular inflammation. There is also usually an

inflammatory infiltrate at the dermoepidermal junction with degeneration and necrosis of the basal keratinocytes. This necrosis and inflammatory damage is thought to be a result of cytotoxic cell injury. The lymphocytes causing the immune-mediated damage are T-cells of the CD8 type.

A severe form of erythema multiforme with involvement of the eyes is known as the Stevens–Johnson syndrome*.

Management
Management comprises identification of the underlying aetiology and management of that condition.

 Inflammation

ERYTHEMA NODOSUM: An inflammatory reaction of fatty tissue, leading to nodular skin lesions.

Aetiology and risk factors
Erythema nodosum is associated with infections due to β-haemolytic streptococci, tuberculosis,

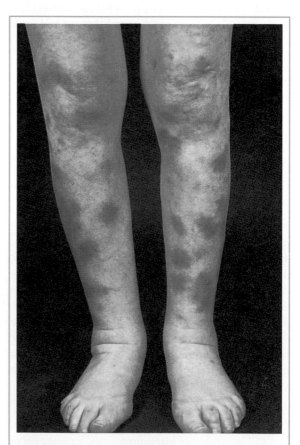

Fig. E7 Patient with erythema nodosum. Note raised, red coloured nodules over the shins. (Reproduced with permission from Toghill, PJ (ed.) *Examining Patients. An Introduction to Clinical Medicine*. London: Edward Arnold, 1995)

leprosy, systemic fungal infections (e.g. histoplasmosis), drug administration with oral contraceptives or sulphonamides, sarcoidosis, malignancies and inflammatory bowel disease.

Pathology

The basic pathology of erythema nodosum is a panniculitis. This usually affects the lower legs and especially the shins (Fig. E7). The disease presents with erythematous nodules, which may be very painful. Histological examination of the lesions shows inflammation involving the subcutaneous fatty tissue. The connective tissue septa, which separate the lobules of fat, are widened due to oedema and fibrin exudation. There is also an acute inflammatory response composed of neutrophils within the septa. The release of lipids from the fat cells attracts a macrophage response. Multinuclear giant cells may also be identified. There is no evidence of vasculitis.

Management

This is symptomatic and treatment is aimed at the underlying condition.

 Inflammation

ERYTHRASMA: A chronic reddish-brown scaling lesion with sharply demarcated edges found in the groin or between the toes that fluoresces red under ultraviolet light and is caused by *Corynebacterium minutissimum*. It is treated with erythromycin.

ESSENTIAL (PRIMARY) THROMBOCYTHAEMIA: A myeloproliferative disorder* characterized by inappropriately high platelet counts.

Patients may present with bleeding or thrombosis*, sometimes both together, due to platelet dysfunction. The high platelet count may also be detected on routine blood count performed for some other reason such as health screening. About a third of patients with ET have an enlarged spleen, but some are hyposplenic due to repeated infarction of the spleen.

It may at first be difficult to distinguish between ET and other 'reactive' causes of thrombocytosis*, particularly after illness or operation, and a period of clinical observation may be required. If reactive, the platelet count will usually reduce with time, but in ET it continues to rise. The disorder may convert to myelofibrosis over a number of years, or more rarely transform to an acute leukaemia.

Reduction of the platelet count to normal levels by cytotoxic agents such as hydroxyurea will usually normalize platelet function. Anticoagulants or aspirin may be required if the presentation has been with thrombosis.

EXANTHEMA: A term generally denoting the transient erythematous skin rashes produced by systemic effects of childhood viral infections.

Aetiology and risk factors

Some viral causes of exanthema are given in Table E7. Several bacterial infections are also associated with skin rashes, such as *Treponema pallidum* (syphilis), *Salmonella typhi* (typhoid fever), *Streptococcus pyogenes* (scarlet fever), *Neisseria meningitidis*, *Rickettsia* (typhus, Rocky Mountain spotted fever), *Borrelia* (erythema chronicium migrans), *Streptobacillus moniliformis* and *Spirillum minus* (rat-bite fever).

Other skin manifestations of infectious disease also occur (see Erythema multiforme, Erythema nodosum).

Table E7 Viral causes of exanthema

Aetiology	Incubation time	Characteristics
Echovirus, e.g. types 1–7, 9, 11, 12, 16 and Coxsackievirus types A5, 6, 9, 16	3–8 Days	Pinkish, evanescent macular rash on body and may occur on palms and soles
Measles	10–12 Days	Reddish macular-papular rash starting on the neck and spreading to the trunk and limbs, coalescing and evolving into a brownish discoloration. Koplik spots present on the oral mucosa adjacent to the molars (enanthema)
Rubella	14–21 Days	Pinkish macular-papular rash beginning on the head and neck and spreading to the trunk over 2–3 days
Chickenpox	14–21 Days	Crops of lesions beginning as macules and evolving to papules, vesicles and pustules appearing on the trunk and spreading to the limbs over a period of about a week
Parvovirus 16	5–10 Days	Bright red cheeks and called 'slapped cheek' disease with lacy pinkish rash on extensor surfaces of limbs
Herpes hominis 6 (exanthema subitum)	5–15 Days	Abrupt appearance of a generalized macular rash lasting 1–2 days

E

Pathology

Rashes caused by viruses are produced either by direct multiplication of the agent in the skin, or by the indirect effects of the inflammatory response on the cells and vasculature of the skin. Keratinocytes and histocytes in the skin are sources of pro-inflammatory cytokines and arachidonic acid metabolites, in response to microbial products. Mast cells found near to skin vessels may also release inflammatory and vasoactive metabolites, all of which contribute to the development of a rash.

Characteristics of various rashes are given in Table E7. The patients often present with a fever and upper respiratory symptoms, which precede the development of the rash. Infections with ECHO or Coxsackie viruses may be part of a picture of aseptic meningitis. Coxsackie A16 and enterovirus 71 are the cause of 'hand-foot-and-mouth' disease* characterized by a vesicular eruption in the mentioned areas. Coxsackieviruses also cause 'herpangina', characterized by vesicular eruptions in the oropharynx that evolve into ulcers. Laboratory diagnosis is by serology. There is no specific treatment.

EXTRINSIC ALLERGIC ALVEOLITIS: An inflammatory granulomatous response in the walls of the alveoli and terminal bronchioles to allergens in inhaled organic dusts (also called hypersensitivity pneumonitis).

Case

A 28-year-old farm worker attended his GP clinic with a headache, non-productive cough and 'flu-like' symptoms. He was given antibiotics. Two weeks later he was admitted as an emergency with fever, dry cough, severe dyspnoea (shortness of breath) and chest pain. On examination, he had mild tachycardia, 'crackling' on auscultation, especially at the lung bases, and some wheezing. A chest radiograph was taken and a blood test carried out. The radiograph showed multiple bilateral small nodules sparing the lung bases. A lung function test showed reduced lung compliance and diffusing capacity. His blood test showed a slightly elevated WBC and his ESR was normal. In view of his occupation, a specialized test was carried out to detect antibodies to fungal and actinomycete antigens; this showed precipitating antibodies to both *Micropolyspora faeni* and *Aspergillus fumigatus*. A diagnosis of farmer's lung was made and he was given a course of steroids and advised to change his job. He returned to his GP, 4 weeks later, reporting an improvement in his health and was found to have normal pulmonary function.

Aetiology and risk factors

Extrinsic allergic alveolitis is caused by hypersensitivity to a variety of different antigens (Table E8).

The pattern of disease in extrinsic allergic alveolitis depends on the intensity of exposure to the

Table E8 Some causes of extrinsic allergic alveolitis

Antigen	Source	Disease
Bacteria		
Micropolyspora faeni, Thermoactinomyces vulgaris	Mouldy hay, straw or grains	Farmer's lung
Thermoactinomyces sacchari	Mouldy bagass (sugar cane)	Bagassosis
Thermophilic actinomycetes	Mushroom compost	Mushroom worker's lung
Streptomyces albus hypersensitivity	Contaminated fertilizer	*Streptomyces* pneumonitis
Fungi		
Aspergillus species	Mouldy barley	Malt worker's lung
	Mouldy tobacco	Tobacco worker's lung
	Compost	Compost lung
Aureobasidium, Graphium species	Redwood bark, sawdust	Sequoiosis
	Contaminated air conditioning	Ventilator pneumonitis
	Contaminated sauna water	Sauna worker's lung
Cryptostroma corticale	Mouldy maple bark	Maple bark stripper's lung
Penicillium casei	Mouldy cheese	Cheese worker's lung
Other		
Serum proteins, usually pigeons and budgerigars	Avian excreta	Bird fancier's lung
Serum proteins, pituitary antigens	Porcine pituitary powder	Pituitary snuff taker's lung
Serum proteins/urine	Rat droppings/urine	Rodent handler's lung
		Laboratory worker's lung
Coffee bean protein	Coffee bean dust	Coffee worker's lung
Isocynates	Chemical industry	Chemical worker's lung

inducing antigen. The case described showed an acute episode but it may occur in a subacute form in which there may be undiagnosed breathlessness, cough, fever and fatigue. Chronic exposure to antigens in susceptible individuals leads to fibrosis (fibrosing alveolitis), which in most cases is irreversible. Interestingly, this is one of the few pulmonary diseases where non-smokers are more susceptible than smokers.

Pathology

In the acute disease there is a type III hypersensitivity reaction in the wall of the alveoli. This 'Arthus' reaction is mediated by circulating IgG antibodies to the inducing antigen. Complement is also deposited at the site of antigen–antibody complex formation.

This patient had high levels of precipitating antibodies, but note that this does not correlate with the presence or severity of the disease, indicating that other factors are important. One of these factors could be the role of T-cells in the pathology (type IV) and increased numbers of T-cells (especially CD8+). The early histological picture of a lesion shows infiltrating mononuclear cells in the alveoli, which often precedes granuloma formation

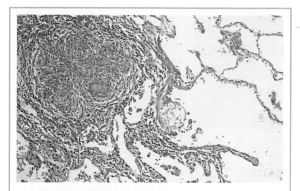

Fig. E8 Lung biopsy showing an intra-alveolar granuloma.

with the presence of macrophages, plasma cells and CD8+ T-cells (Fig. E8). Undoubtedly, T-cells and macrophages play a role in the fibrosis seen after chronic exposure to antigens, probably through the production of cytokines (e.g. IL-1).

Management

Apart from the control of the acute inflammatory response with steroids, the best form of treatment is avoidance.

F

FALLOT TETRALOGY: A form of cyanotic, congenital heart disease in which the children have a combination of ventricular septal defect, over-riding aorta, right ventricular outflow obstruction and right ventricular hypertrophy.

FANCONI ANAEMIA: A congenital form of aplas-tic anaemia*, usually presenting in childhood with progressive pancytopenia. Associated congenital abnormalities are common, particularly skeletal abnormalities of the hands and forearms, micro-cephaly, genital hypoplasia and patchy pigmenta-tion. Failure to thrive and short stature may be presenting complaints.

The underlying genetic defect in this disorder is increased chromosome fragility, with marked sensi-tivity to DNA cross-linking agents. This is the basis of a diagnostic test, in which peripheral blood lymphocytes are exposed to the cytotoxic agent mitomycin C and then assessed for chromosome gaps, breakages and translocations. About one in ten patients go on to develop acute myeloid leukaemia.

Treatment is supportive; bone marrow trans-plantation may be curative.

FARMER'S LUNG A form of extrinsic allergic alveolitis*, triggered by hypersensitivity to the fungus *Micropolyspora faeni* and other actino-mycetes in mouldy hay. Symptoms include fever, cough and dyspnoea, which may lead to interstitial pulmonary fibrosis.

FASCIOLOPSIASIS: Infection with the fluke *Fasciolopsis buski*, one of many intestinal flukes that cause gastrointestinal disease (others are *Metagonimus*, *Gastrodiscoides*). It is endemic in the Far East, Middle East and Africa. Infection is acquired by eating freshwater plants contaminated with the cysts of the organism which excyst in the intestine, mature into adult flukes and attach to the intestinal mucosa. Inflammation occurs at the site of attachment, which may ulcerate, leading to bleeding and iron-deficiency anaemia. The patient may become hypersensitive to adsorption of proteins secreted from the fluke and there may be a peripheral eosinophilia. The patient complains of abdominal pain, diarrhoea, anorexia and vomiting. Symptoms of intestinal obstruction may occur. The laboratory diagnosis is by demonstration of the ova or adult in the faeces or vomit. Treatment is with praziquantel.

FATTY LIVER: Accumulation of lipid within liver parenchymal cells.

Aetiology and risk factors

Fatty change within the liver may be due to excess alcohol ingestion, protein malnutrition, diabetes, pregnancy, congestive cardiac failure, ischaemia, drug treatment with steroids, carbon tetrachloride poisoning, or obesity.

Pathology

Fatty change within the liver is a non-specific reaction to a variety of insults. It may occur adjacent to severely damaged or frankly necrotic tissue. Free fatty acids enter the hepatocytes where they are converted to triglycerides and to choles-terol. Alterations in this normal pathway lead to lipid accumulation within hepatocytes. This process is entirely reversible if the insult causing the fatty change is removed.

There are two forms of fatty infiltration: acute and chronic. The acute form is rare and associated with acute hepatic failure. The microscopic picture is of a microvascular fatty change, the fat accumu-lating in the cytoplasm as small membrane-bound droplets. Chronic fatty change is commoner and associated with chronic alcoholism, malnutrition, and poisoning. The location is macrovascular, since the fat droplets fuse into large aggregates. Liver

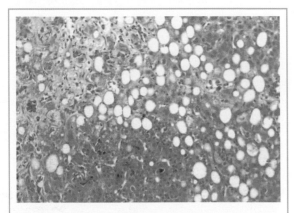

Fig. F1 Histology of liver showing fatty (vacuoles) change. (Reproduced with permission from Lakhani SR, Dilly SA, Finlayson CJ. *Basic Pathology*, 2nd edn. London: Arnold, 1998)

function is usually normal, but gamma glutamyl-transferase (γGT) or alkaline phosphatase may be raised.

Macroscopic examination of the organs affected shows enlargement and yellow discoloration. The organ is usually greasy to the touch. Histologically, the main finding is of vacuoles within the cytoplasm (Fig. F1). These usually begin as small vacuoles but may coalesce to form larger fatty cysts. Liver function is not usually abnormal, but occasionally a raised γGT may be detected.

Management
Treatment is not usually necessary. Removal of the underlying causal agent returns the liver parenchyma to normal.

 Alcoholic liver disease; Cirrhosis

FELTY SYNDROME: An autoimmune condition comprising neutropenia and splenomegaly in patients with rheumatoid arthritis*.

About 1% of patients with rheumatoid arthritis (RA) develop Felty syndrome. There is a strong HLA-DR4 association and often patients have a long history of RA, with high levels of rheumatoid factor and a destructive arthritis with frequent extra-articular manifestations, including vasculitis*. Lymphadenopathy may sometimes be present. The mechanism of neutropenia is through IgG antineu-trophil autoantibodies (type II hypersensitivity), which results in neutropenia through splenic clearance. Splenectomy can be of help in some cases. Bacterial infections are common, especially in those patients with the more severe neutropenia. Nodular regenerative hyperplasia of the liver is sometimes seen.

FIBROCYSTIC CHANGE: A term applied to a spectrum of benign proliferative lesions found within the breast.

Aetiology and risk factors
The most important risk factor is hormonal imbalance. An excess of oestrogens is thought to increase the risk of fibrocystic change. Oral contraceptives, which probably supply a more balanced source of hormones, decrease the risk.

Pathology
Fibrocystic change has in the past been referred to as fibrocystic disease. It comprises a number of different pathologies including cyst formation, increase in fibrous connective tissue, epithelial proliferation that may be atypical or non-atypical, sclerosing adenosis, duct ectasia and apocrine metaplasia within cysts (Fig. F2). Fibrocystic

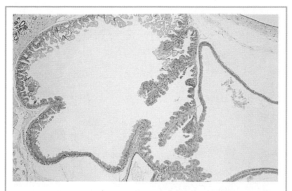

Fig. F2 Histological section of breast showing cyst lined by apocrine epithelium with focal hyperplasia.

change is probably a better term because only some of these lesions are associated with an increased risk of subsequent invasive carcinoma. Cyst, apocrine metaplasia and fibrosis have no sinister implication, but epithelial proliferation, particularly when atypical, carries an increased risk (× 4–5) of subsequent breast carcinoma.

The diagnosis of fibrocystic change is usually made between the ages of 20 and 40 years. It usually presents as a lump. It may also accompany malignant breast disease.

Management
No specific management is required and the diagnosis is usually made on surgical excision of a lump that appears clinically and radiologically benign.

 Breast carcinoma

FIBROIDS: Benign smooth muscle tumours of the uterus. The correct name for the entity is leiomyoma.

Aetiology and risk factors
The tumours are common during reproductive life and tend to regress after the menopause; hence, oestrogen stimulation has been implicated in the aetiology. The cause remains unknown.

Pathology
Leiomyomas are well circumscribed and discrete with a grey-white cut surface (Fig. F3). Tumours may vary in size from very small to extremely large. They tend to occur within the myometrium, just beneath the endometrium (submucosal) or beneath the serosa (subserosal). On microscopic examination, they are composed of bundles of smooth muscle cells arranged in a whorled pattern. Mitotic activity may be seen but is usually sparse. Very rare

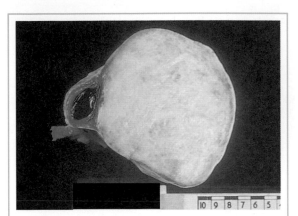

Fig. F3 Macroscopic appearance of a benign leiomyoma with solid white fibrillar cut surface. (Reproduced with permission from Lakhani SR, Dilly SA, Finlayson CJ. *Basic Pathology*, 2nd edn. London: Arnold, 1998)

cases of metastasizing leiomyomas have been described.

Patients usually present with heavy and/or irregular periods, due to enlargement of the area of endometrium. If the tumours are very large, they may produce symptoms related to compression of the bladder. Pregnancy occurring in the presence of uterine leiomyomas may result in spontaneous abortions.

Management
The principal management is surgical excision.

FIBROMA: A benign tumour of fibrous connective tissue.

FIBROMATOSIS: A benign proliferation composed of fibroblasts and myofibroblasts with resultant irregular, poorly defined and nodular proliferation.

Aetiology and risk factors
The aetiology and risk factors are unknown.

Pathology
There are three principal types of fibromatosis: palmar, plantar and penile. The palmar variant is also known as Dupuytren contracture*. There is an irregular and nodular thickening of the palmar fascia which may be either unilateral or bilateral. It produces a flexion contracture usually affecting the fourth and fifth fingers. A similar proliferation occurring on the plantar aspect of the feet is known as plantar fibromatosis. Penile fibromatosis, also known as Peyronie disease, is a nodular proliferation affecting the dorsolateral aspect of the penis. It

may lead to an abnormal curvature of the penile shaft.

Fibromatosis occurs more frequently in males than females.

Management
Fibromatosis may resolve spontaneously; however, surgical excision is sometimes necessary to prevent contractual deformity. It may recur following surgery.

FIBROSARCOMA: A malignant tumour of fibrous connective tissue.

 Sarcoma

FILARIASIS: Infection with one of the filarial tissue nematodes.

Aetiology and risk factors
Filariasis can be caused by *Wuchereria bancrofti*, *Brugia malayi* affecting the lymphatics; *Loa loa* affecting the subcutaneous tissue or *Onchocerca volvulus* affecting the skin and eye. For details see Table F1.

Table F1 Causes of filariasis

Organism	Epidemiology	Disease
Wuchereria bancrofti	Transmitted by the bite of a mosquito and endemic in tropical areas	Elephantiasis
Brugia malayi	Transmitted by the bite of a mosquito and endemic in India and SE Asia	Elephantiasis
Loa loa	Transmitted by the bite of mango fly and endemic in central and west Africa	Calabar swelling
Onchocerca volvulus	Transmitted by the bite of a black fly and endemic in tropical Africa and central America	River blindness

The filarial worms are transmitted by the bite of an arthropod vector and the adult worms mate in the lymphatics (*Wuchereria*, *Brugia*) or subcutaneous tissues (*Loa*, *Onchocerca*).

Pathology
Elephantiasis The adult nematodes live in the lymphatics, periodically releasing microfilariae into the bloodstream and at certain times locating

in the lungs. At the onset of symptoms, the host response against the adult filarial parasite present in the lymphatics leads to lymphangitis and progressively, with further destruction of the lymphatics, to lymphatic obstruction and tissue oedema. Repeated bouts of inflammation lead to granuloma formation, fibrosis and eventual lymphatic obstruction. Clinically, the patient presents with repeated attacks of fever, a marked peripheral eosinophilia and signs of acute inflammation of the lymphatics, particularly in the lower limbs. The lymphatics and spermatic cord are swollen and painful. In chronic disease, lymph leaks into the tissue to give lymphoedema, hydrocele and gross tissue swelling of the lower limbs and scrotum (elephantiasis). Eventually there is fibrosis of subcutaneous tissue with loss of sweat glands.

The presence of microfilaria in the lungs in some individuals leads to the clinical syndrome of tropical pulmonary eosinophilia with wheeze, migrating pulmonary infiltrates and fever. There is a pronounced peripheral eosinophilia. High IgE levels, with specific antifilarial IgG and IgE, are found in the lungs.

Calabar swelling The nematodes are found in the subcutaneous tissue, the female releasing microfilariae into the bloodstream and the life cycle completed in the vector. As with elephantiasis, a host immune and inflammatory response against the filariae in the tissues leads to signs of acute inflammation with erythema and tissue swelling. These swellings appear in various parts of the body as the filariae migrate; this may occur in the eye, giving rise to acute inflammation. Occasionally meningoencephalitis can occur.

Onchocerciasis or river blindness The nematodes are found in nodules in the skin and subcutaneous tissue, the female releasing microfilariae back into the skin, connective tissue or eye. The host immune and inflammatory response to microfilariae of *Onchocerca* are involved in tissue damage to the eye, leading to blindness. The patient complains of firm, non-tender skin and subcutaneous swellings (which contain the nematode) and a pruritic skin rash, which is an allergic response to the filariae. In chronic cases, thickening of the skin occurs with atrophy of the epidermis and separation of the corneum stratum, eventually producing a 'fish-like' skin or hanging folds of lichenified skin. Inflammation in the eye leads to blindness.

Diagnosis is by demonstration of the microfilariae in the blood or tissues and treatment is with ivermectin or diethylcarbamazine.

FISSURE A cleft or groove which may be normal or abnormal. The grooves within the cerebral cortex are normal fissures; however, an ulcer would be an abnormal or pathological fissure.

FISTULA A pathological communication which usually occurs between two internal organs, e.g. a fistula connecting small bowel to large bowel or small bowel to bladder, as may occur in Crohn disease.

FOURNIER GANGRENE: A necrotic lesion of the scrotum and penis caused by bacterial infection.

 Necrotizing fasciitis

FRACTURE: This is defined as a break, generally referring to bone.

Aetiology and risk factors
Bone fractures may arise as a result of trauma, osteoporosis, osteomalacia, or infective or neoplastic diseases of the bone.

Pathology
Fractures can be classified as simple, when they are closed with intact overlying tissues, or compound, when the broken bone penetrates the skin surface. Incomplete fractures are called greenstick. Fractures secondary to metastatic tumour are called pathological fractures (though clearly all fractures are pathological!).

After the fracture, bleeding occurs within the gap, leading to elevation of the periosteum followed by organization with the production of granulation tissue and phagocytosis of dead and dying cells. After a few days, osteoid and cartilage appear at the site. This is referred to as a provisional callus. Over the next week, the amount of fibrous tissue and bony spicules increases and immobilizes the fracture site. The bone content expands to produce a bony callus and remodelling occurs due to the activity of osteoblasts and osteoclasts. Eventually the woven bone is replaced by lamellar bone. If the alignment has been perfect, it may not be possible to see the fracture site.

Factors that affect the healing of a fractured bone include nutritional status, the adequacy of the blood supply, the presence of any foreign material and of any infection, systemic diseases such as diabetes, and the degree of mobility of the fractured ends.

Management
Management includes realignment, if required, together with immobilization using a plaster cast.

 Osteomalacia; Osteoporosis

G

GALLSTONES: Stones which are formed within the gallbladder or, more rarely, within the common bile duct. They are mainly composed of cholesterol, bilirubin and calcium salts. Cholesterol-based stones occur when there is an increase in serum cholesterol and bile salts; these are commonly encountered in obese, multiparous, middle-aged women ('fat, fertile, females in their forties and fifties') (Fig. G1). Oral contraceptives, diabetes

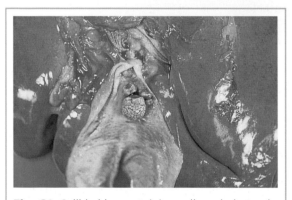

Fig. G1 Gallbladder containing yellow cholesterol stones.

mellitus and terminal ileal disease are other causes of cholesterol stones. Bilirubin stones are uncommon and are associated with chronic haemolytic anaemia such as sickle cell disease, and in some parasitic infestations, most commonly *Clonorchis sinensis*. Gallstones may be silent or cause obstruction in the biliary tract, resulting in cholecystitis, cholangitis, pancreatitis and jaundice, which may be intermittent and associated with fever and upper abdominal pain. The biochemical analysis of these stones is of no clinical value. However, the measurement of serum alkaline phosphatase and γGT are helpful in the management of this condition. Treatment can be either surgical (cholecystectomy; lithotripsy) or medical (chenodeoxycholic acid).

GANGRENE: Black dead tissue, most commonly seen following ischaemia. The tissue may become infected by organisms, in which case it is referred as wet gangrene. In dry gangrene there is no evidence of infection or liquefaction.

GAS GANGRENE: Tissue infection with *Clostridium perfringens* combined with severe systemic toxic manifestations. Typically this follows trauma or even surgery where the organism is inadvertently introduced into tissue having a compromised blood supply and hence poor oxygenation. The organism, which is an anaerobe and is found naturally in the environment and faeces, multiplies in the deoxygenated environment of the compromised tissue, producing many different toxins with proteolytic, haemolytic and cytotoxic action.

Pathology

These and other toxins cause vascular injury and necrosis of muscle and subcutaneous tissue cells. As the organism multiplies in the necrotic tissue, it produces abundant gas as a byproduct of its metabolism. Also the various toxins are absorbed into the circulation where they lead to haemolysis and haemoglobinuria. The patient presents with severe pain at the site of infection, which is blackened and has a thin serosanguinous discharge. Gas in the tissue is revealed on examination by the presence of crepitus. The patient has a high fever and is hypotensive. The urine may have a characteristic 'port-wine' colour due to the haemoglobinuria. Renal failure may ensue. Treatment is by surgical debridement of the necrotic tissue. Hyperbaric oxygen may be useful in management. Penicillin should be given.

GASTRIC CARCINOMA: Gastric carcinoma is a malignant neoplasm arising from the glandular epithelium of the stomach, hence it is an adenocarcinoma.

Case

A 60-year-old man was seen by his GP complaining of tiredness and lethargy. The GP noted that he looked pale and had conjunctival pallor. On questioning, he stated that the symptoms had been gradually getting worse for 9 months. He did not have any abdominal pain and gave no history of haematemesis or melaena. His diet was well balanced although his appetite had deteriorated over the last few months. He knew he had lost weight, as his trousers were now loose on him. He did not have any significant past medical history and was not on any medication.

He was put on iron supplements and was sent for blood tests to the local hospital.

Haematology: Hb 6.5 g/dl with low MCH and MCV; ESR 25.
Blood film: microcytic anaemia.
All other blood tests including the biochemistry were normal.

The patient was referred to a gastroenterologist for further assessment.

Further investigations in hospital were as follows.

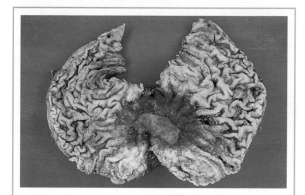

Fig. G2 Gastrectomy specimen showing an ulcer with rolled edges.

Bone marrow aspirate and biopsy: this showed depleted iron stores but no evidence of malignancy.
Chest and abdominal radiographs: normal.
Sigmoidoscopy: normal.
Gastric endoscopy: endoscopy revealed an ulcer measuring 2.0 cm with rolled edges (Fig. G2). A biopsy of the ulcer was taken for histological examination.
Histopathology: moderately differentiated adenocarcinoma.

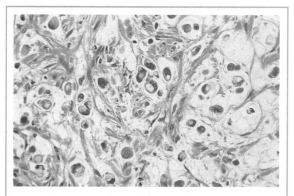

Fig. G3 Histological section showing a classical signet ring carcinoma of the stomach.

The patient underwent full staging with CT scan of the abdomen and bone scan. These investigations were normal. He was referred to the surgeon for further management and subsequently underwent a partial gastrectomy.

Aetiology and risk factors

Risk factors include a positive family history, atrophic gastritis, pernicious anaemia, intestinal type metaplasia and infection with *Helicobacter pylori*.

Pathology

Patients with gastric carcinoma may present in a wide variety of ways ranging from severe and sudden bleed with resultant death to few symptoms apart from general malaise and lethargy. In the first case, erosion of large blood vessels at the base of the ulcer causes massive bleeding. Bleeding may be slow and insidious, in which case patients may present with iron deficiency and symptoms related to the anaemia. Iron deficiency is rare in a man unless he is taking non-steroidal anti-inflammatory drugs that cause gastric erosions or he has an inflammatory or malignant pathology within the gastrointestinal tract. The bowel, from mouth to anus, must be examined. Nutritional deficiency may be responsible but is not a common cause in the Western world.

Classically, the blood picture is of a hypochromic microcytic anaemia with reduced iron stores in the marrow.

Radiological examination is used to rule out other pathology such as disseminated cancer and to exclude cardiac failure, which is a complication of chronic anaemia. Endoscopy and barium examinations are the cornerstone of the investigations. In this case, an ulcer was identified, which on biopsy was malignant.

Gastric carcinomas are, by definition, adenocarcinomas. They may exhibit glandular formation when they are referred to as of 'intestinal type' or they may infiltrate as small groups or single cells when they are designated as of 'diffuse type' (Fig. G3). They first spread locally to involve local lymph nodes but may eventually metastasize to liver, lung and bone.

Management

This is dependent on the size and extent of the tumour. Excision is the primary treatment in localized disease and chemotherapy and radiotherapy may be used to control local and systemic spread.

 Gastritis; Pernicious anaemia

GASTRIC ULCER: Loss of the gastric epithelium with the exposure of the underlying tissue to varying degrees.

 Peptic ulcer

GASTRITIS: Inflammation of the gastric mucosa, which may be acute or chronic.

GASTROENTERITIS: Often used synonymously with the term food-poisoning, denoting an acute infection of the gastrointestinal tract leading to diarrhoea or vomiting.

Aetiology and risk factors

Infection is acquired by ingesting contaminated food or water. However, not all food-borne infections primarily cause gastrointestinal disease, e.g. *Clostridium botulinum* (see Botulism); *Listeria monocytogenes* (see Listeriosis); *Toxoplasma gondii* (see Toxoplasmosis) and *Taenia* spp. (see Tapeworm infection, Cysticercosis). In some food-/water-borne infections, although gastrointestinal symptoms are prominent, they are considered under other entries (see Cholera, Cryptosporidiosis, Giardiasis, Typhoid fever, Yersiniosis). Common causes of gastroenteritis are shown in Table G1.

Table G1 Common causes of gastroenteritis

Viral	Bacterial toxin	Bacterial invasion/ adhesion
Rotavirus	*Staph. aureus*	*Campylobacter*
Adenovirus	*Bacillus cereus*	*Salm. enteritidis*
Calicivirus	*Cl. perfringens*	*E. coli* strains
Small round structured virus		

Pathology

Viral pathogens The viruses are associated with acute onset of watery diarrhoea or vomiting. Infection is spread by the faeco-oral route, from contaminated water or by eating shellfish. With rotavirus there is a villous atrophy of the enterocytes and an associated cell lysis. Both this and the fact that intracellular calcium levels are increased following infection may be related to the development of symptoms.

Toxin-induced disease With *Staphylococcus aureus* and *Bacillus cereus*, preformed toxin contaminating the food (cream, cold meat for *Staph. aureus* and typically rice for *B. cereus*) causes vomiting within 1–5 hours of ingestion. In all cases the individual is usually apyrexial.

Staph. aureus enterotoxins probably act by releasing neuropeptides such as substance P, or by directly stimulating the local vagus nerve ending in the gastrointestinal tract, thereby inducing emesis.

B. cereus produces at least two toxins: one causes emesis and another has haemolytic and dermonecrotic activity, causing diarrhoea.

Cl. perfringens enterotoxin is a pore-forming protein toxin that causes cell lysis and whose main site of action is the ileum.

Enterotoxigenic *E. coli* (ETEC) produce two sorts of toxins: one type of similar structure and action to cholera toxin called heat-labile toxins (LT) and another, which are small peptides and called heat-stable toxins (ST).

Enterohaemorrhagic *E. coli* (EHEC) or verotoxin-producing *E. coli* (*E. coli* O157) is dealt with elsewhere (see Haemolytic uraemic syndrome).

Adhesion-induced disease In enteropathogenic *E. coli* (EPEC), the attachment can lead to actin polymerization at the point of contact and the production by the enterocyte of a 'pedestal' with effacement of the microvilli (attaching and effacing lesion). Adherence may of itself impair brush-border enzymes and lead to diarrhoea, e.g. in *Campylobacter jejuni*.

The mechanism of diarrhoea formation in enteroaggregative *E. coli* (EAggEC) and diffusely adherent *E. coli* (DAEC) is unclear although toxins have been detected in some strains.

Invasive disease Clearly the details will vary according to the specific pathogen, e.g. *Campylobacter*, *Salmonella*, EIEC. Generally, bacteria attach to specific receptors on the surface of the enterocyte by a number of different adhesins, e.g. fimbriae. Adherence of the organism induces proteins in the pathogen, which are necessary for invasion. Similarly the organism may induce the epithelium to release pro-inflammatory mediators, e.g. IL-8 (a powerful chemoattractant for neutrophils) or leukotriene LTB4. The organism may then be taken up into the cell, its attachment subverting the host signal pathway leading to phagocytosis. Alternatively, organisms may be taken up at coated pits by a microtubule-related pathway. Organisms may translocate across the epithelial layer either by direct penetration of the enterocyte or via the gap junction between cells. Once in the lamina propria the organisms can further induce acute inflammation.

Laboratory diagnosis is by electron microscopy (viruses), isolation of the pathogen from the faeces, or serology. Generally, treatment is supportive, although antibiotics may be given for bacterial pathogens if the infection is dysentery-like or there are other medical indications.

GAUCHER DISEASE: An autosomal recessive disorder, caused by the absence or deficiency of the enzyme glucocerebrosidase (cerebroside β-glucosidase), resulting in accumulation of the lipid glucocerebroside in reticuloendothelial cells or neurons in the brain.

There are four forms of the disorder (infantile neuronopathic, juvenile neuronopathic, adult

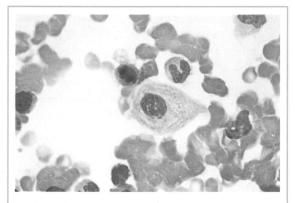

Fig. G4 Gaucher cell in bone marrow aspirate: cytoplasm resembles 'wrinkled tissue paper'.

neuronopathic, and adult non-neuronopathic). As a result of the deficiency of homogentisic acid oxidase, there is an accumulation of glucocerebroside in liver, spleen, bone marrow and brain. The diagnosis is confirmed by demonstration of the deficiency in cultured leucocytes, skin fibroblasts or urine. In addition, glucocerebroside accumulated within reticuloendothelial cells can clearly be seen on bone marrow examination (Fig. G4). Patients with Gaucher disease are prone to bone, joint, and postoperative wound infection. Administration of recombinant glucocerebrosidase corrects at least some features of the disease.

GERM CELL TUMOUR: A tumour derived from the germ cells of the testis or ovary, e.g. seminoma (testis), dysgerminoma (ovary), teratomas.

GESTATIONAL HYPERTENSIVE DISEASE: See Pre-eclampsia.

GIANT CELL ARTERITIS: See Vasculitis.

GIARDIASIS: An intestinal infection with *Giardia lamblia*. The infection is usually acquired by drinking contaminated water or eating raw vegetables irrigated by untreated sewage. The infectious stage is the cyst which, after ingestion, excysts in the duodenum and jejunum, where the trophozoites attach to the mucosa. There is an inflammatory infiltrate in the lamina propria comprising neutrophils and lymphocytes and accompanied by villous atrophy of the mucosa. Functional disturbances occur with disaccharidase deficiency. The clinical presentation can be quite variable in severity. The patient presents with epigastric pain, flatulence, abdominal colic, distension and watery diarrhoea lasting about a week. In chronic infections there are intermittent episodes of diarrhoea with foul-smelling faeces. Severe villous atrophy may occur with consequent malabsorption of fats and vitamins. The patient may have steatorrhoea and weight loss and an abnormal D-xylose absorption test. Laboratory diagnosis is by detection of the characteristic cysts in the faeces or serology. Treatment is with metronidazole.

GINGIVITIS: Inflammation of the gums.

 Periodontitis

GLANDERS: An infection of horses with *Burkholderia mallei*, occasionally occurring in humans after contact with infected horses. The patient may present with septic shock* and widespread abscesses, affecting particularly the skin, subcutaneous tissue and lungs. Laboratory diagnosis is by isolation of the organism and treatment is with an aminoglycoside and co-trimoxazole.

GLANDULAR FEVER: A viral infection with the Epstein–Barr virus (EBV), usually associated with generalized lymph node enlargement which is common in teenagers and young adults. It is also known as infectious mononucleosis, but the increased white cells found in the blood are lymphocytes, not monocytes.

Case

A 19-year-old dental student developed a sore throat and fever, being unable to swallow solid food. She started a course of antibiotics (amoxycillin), but stopped this the following day when she developed an itchy maculopapular rash. The day after that she noted enlargement of cervical lymph nodes and visited the student health clinic. A blood count showed a lymphocytosis with reactive lymphocytes on the blood film (Fig. G5). A Paul Bunnell test was positive and liver function tests showed mildly elevated enzymes. A diagnosis of

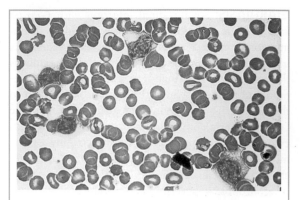

Fig. G5 Blood film in a case of glandular fever showing reactive lymphocytes.

glandular fever was made. Her throat symptoms settled within a week, though she suffered from tiredness for the following month.

Aetiology and risk factors
Infection with EBV is usually acquired by close physical contact ('the kissing disease'). Pharyngitis may be the only presenting symptom, but is usually associated with cervical lymphadenopathy and frequently with a more generalized enlargement of lymph nodes and spleen. Liver function tests are frequently abnormal and some cases may be mistaken for infectious hepatitis.

Pathology
EBV infects epithelial cells lining the respiratory tract and B-lymphocytes through binding to CD21. The reactive lymphocytes found in the blood consist mainly of CD8+ T-lymphocytes reacting against the EBV-infected B-cells. These lymphocytes show morphological changes, indicating that they are in a state of immunological activation (Fig. G5). Sometimes these changes are sufficiently bizarre to raise suspicion of a diagnosis of acute leukaemia, particularly if the platelet count is reduced, as it sometimes is. Similar reactive changes may be found in other viral infections.

One of the serological characteristics of glandular fever is the production of antibodies directed against the cells of other animal species (heterophil antibodies). These may be detected by their reaction with sheep, horse or ox red cells. This reaction forms the basis of a diagnostic test, the Paul Bunnell, or its abbreviated form the Monospot. Non-specific heterophil antibodies, present in normal people, are first absorbed out of the serum with guinea-pig kidney cells. Then the serum is mixed with sheep red blood cells, which agglutinate if the test result is positive. Other viral infections may be associated with heterophil antibodies, but

as these tend to pursue the same clinical course as glandular fever, there is little requirement for the testing of specific antibodies against EBV. A similar clinical picture to glandular fever may be found in toxoplasmosis* and acute HIV* infection.

In patients with the rare X-linked lymphoproliferative (Duncan) syndrome, EBV infection usually leads to either death or the development of lymphoma. Note that EBV is also linked (with malaria) to Burkitt lymphoma*. On the other hand, about 20% of the population acquire EBV without any clinical illness, becoming carriers.

Management
Recovery without specific treatment is the rule, though malaise and easy-tiring may persist for months. Alcohol should be avoided if there is significant derangement of liver function tests. The spleen is softened and enlarged in 50% of cases so contact sport is best avoided during the acute phase because of the risk of rupture.

GLIOMA: A malignant tumour arising from glial cells. Examples are astrocytoma, oligodendroglioma and ependymoma.

Aetiology and risk factors
The aetiology is unknown. There may be a genetic predisposition.

Pathology
The vast majority of primary brain tumours in adults are astrocytomas. The usual presenting signs and symptoms are headaches, seizures and neurological defects.

These tumours are a result of neoplastic transformation of glial cells. The tumours range from low-grade astrocytomas to poorly differentiated and high-grade astrocytomas, which are also known as glioblastoma multiforme (Fig. G6).

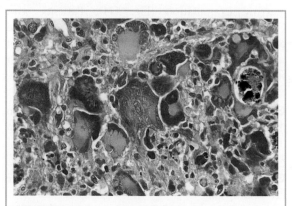

Fig. G6 Numerous bizarre giant cells seen in glioblastoma multiforme.

Oligodendrogliomata constitute about 10–15 % of glial tumours. These tumours are generally seen in the cerebral hemispheres and involve the white matter. They are gelatinous and circumscribed. They may show cystic degeneration and haemorrhage. The tumours contain monomorphic cells in which the nuclei are surrounded by a clear cytoplasm.

Ependymomas are commonest in childhood and can cause hydrocephalus.

Management

Treatment consists of surgical excision although resection of these diffuse infiltrating tumours is extremely difficult. Patients receive radiotherapy and chemotherapy following the resection but prognosis remains poor.

GLOMERULONEPHRITIS: A group of renal diseases in which the lesions are primarily glomerular.

Case

An 11-year-old boy presented at his hospital emergency clinic with periorbital oedema. On examination he was found to have slightly raised blood pressure (160/95 mmHg) and a mild pyrexia. His mother told the GP that he had suffered from a mild sore throat about a week earlier. He was admitted and blood and urine tests were carried out. He was mildly anaemic but his WBC and differential count were normal. Urine analysis revealed proteinuria and haematuria with erythrocyte casts. A throat swab did not show growth other than normal flora. His antistreptolysin O antibody levels were high (1500 IU/ml). Serum C3 was low (0.2 g/l). A creatinine clearance test showed 45 ml/min. He had hypoalbuminaemia (29 g/l) and a proteinuria of 1.8 g/day.

A renal biopsy was not carried out since he had the classical symptoms of post-streptococcal glomerulonephritis (Fig. G7). His blood pressure

gradually dropped and his symptoms diminished. He was discharged after a week.

Aetiology and risk factors

Glomerulonephritis can be classified on either a clinical or pathological basis, the latter being more precise, having better correlation with pathological mechanisms, response to therapy and prognosis (see Table G3 for details of classification, laboratory

Table G2 Sources of antigens responsible for immune-complex-mediated glomerulonephritis (GN)

Antigens	Disease/condition
Exogenous	
1. Infectious agents	
Bacteria	
Nephritogenic streptococci	Poststreptococcal GN, infected surgical equipment, endocarditis, pneumonia, *Yersinia*, syphilis, typhoid, pneumonia
Staphylococcus aureus/albus	
Corynebacterium bovis	
Streptococcus pneumoniae	
Klebsiella pneumoniae	
Yersinia enterocolitica	
Treponema pallidum	
Salmonella typhi	
Mycoplasma pneumoniae	
Viruses	
Cytomegalovirus	CMV infection
Epstein–Barr	Burkitt lymphoma
Hepatitis B	Hepatitis
Measles	Subacute sclerosing panencephalitis
Retrovirus-related antigen	Leukaemia
Fungi	
Candida albicans	Candidiasis
Parasites	
Echinococcus granulosus	Hydatid cysts
Plasmodium malariae	Malaria (quartan)
Plasmodium falciparum	Malaria (malignant tertian)
Schistosoma mansoni	Schistosomiasis
Toxoplasma gondii	Toxoplasmosis
2. Iatrogenic agents	
Toxoids	Serum sickness
Heterologous serum	
Drugs	
Endogenous/Self	
Immunoglobulins	Cryoglobulinaemias
Nuclear antigens	Systemic lupus erythematosus
Tumour antigens	Neoplasia
Thyroglobulin	Thyroiditis
GBM antigen	Goodpasture syndrome

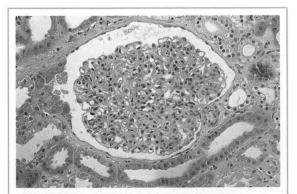

Fig. G7 Post-streptococcal glomerulonephritis. Note the swelling and extreme cellularity of the glomerular tuft.

Table G3 Classification of glomerulonephritis

Type	Laboratory findings	Histological picture
Acute diffuse proliferative GN (post-streptococcal GN; post-infectious GN)	Moderate proteinuria; red blood cells in urine with granular and red cell casts; blood urea and serum creatinine increased and clearance rate of creatinine reduced with post-strep GN; high ASO titre – case described; low serum C3	Diffuse enlargement and increased cellularity of glomeruli; increased number of mesangial and endothelial cells and polymorphs and macrophages present. IF microscopy shows deposition of IgG and C3, giving a granular pattern to the peripheral capillary loops
Crescentic (rapidly progressive) GN	Secondary disease; shows features as above; idiopathic form shows normal or reduced complement levels. Detection of immune complexes/cryoglobulins variable	Diffuse hypercellularity; fibrin associated with crescents
Diffuse membranous GN (idiopathic membranous GN; membranous nephropathy)	Proteinuria and mild microscopic haematuria: serum IC not demonstrable	Diffuse hyaline thickening of capillary walls, no cellular infiltrate. EM shows dense amorphous material in subepithelial region and thickening of BM. IgG and C3 detectable
Mesangiocapillary (membrano-proliferative) GN	Proteinuria (nephrotic syndrome)	Early events – diffuse proliferative change in endothelial and particularly mesangial (types I, II and III) cells, capillary lumen reduced. By EM, irregular deposits (IgG and C3) on subendothelial side of BM (type I), in lamina densa of BM (usually C3: type II) and in both (type III)
Focal GN (primary – IgA nephropathy; secondary – Henoch–Schönlein syndrome, infective endocarditis, poly-arteritis nodosa)	Some patients have nephrotic syndrome	Proliferation, probably of mesangial cells affecting periphery of one or more lobules, variable numbers of glomeruli affected; mesangial deposition of IgA
Lupus nephritis (in SLE)	Serum autoantibodies to dsDNA and nucleoproteins, circulating IC, decreased serum C3, C4 and C1q	Spectrum may be seen; no abnormality to proliferative, diffuse and IC, IgG, IgA, IgM; C3, C4 and C1q deposited in subendothelial location; areas of severe segmental damage with irregular fragments of nuclei is pathognomonic for SLE
Minimal change nephrotic syndrome	Proteinuria, little globulin in urine, hypoalbuminaemia	Normal except for appearance of fixed dilatation of capillaries; EM characteristic fusion of foot processes of epithelial cells; idiopathic, no evidence of IC
Focal glomerulosclerosis (10–30% nephrotic syndrome cases)	Proteinuria, microscopic haematuria common	Most glomeruli look normal but sclerosis in those close to medulla; IgM and C3 deposition in association with sclerotic lesions
Diabetic glomerulosclerosis (in diabetes mellitus)	Proteinuria	Deposition of eosinophilic, hyaline material in mesangium of lobules; may show nodular and diffuse glomerulosclerosis; severe hyalination may occur
Glomerular amyloidosis (in primary and secondary amyloidosis)	Proteinuria, sometimes with nephrotic syndrome	Amyloid deposited around GBM; capillary obliteration may be seen
Chronic glomerulonephritis (cause of renal failure)		Most types of histology; commonest with IgA deposits

findings and histopathology). Most, but not all glomerulitis has an immunological basis and is caused by antigen–antibody complexes deposited on the wall of the glomerular capillaries. Immune complexes may be localized within the glomeruli as the result of

- filtration of circulating immune complexes as they pass through the glomerular capillaries;
- serum antibodies reacting with constituents of the glomerular basement membrane (GBM);
- serum antibodies reacting with non-GBM renal antigens or those absorbed from the serum.

Some of the antigens responsible for the immune complex formation are known (Table G2).

Pathology

In the case described above, the acute nephritic episode was caused by an unidentified 'nephritic' strain of *Streptococcus*. Culture of the organism from throat swabs is only positive in about one-third of cases. Infections of the skin can also lead to this condition, which occurs most frequently in children of school age and usually resolves in time. It is more serious in adults, and more often progresses to chronic renal failure. It is thought that anti-streptolysin O antibodies form complexes that are deposited in a granular distribution in the glomeruli (see Table G3). These result in a type III hypersensitivity reaction, which results in acute damage to the glomeruli leading to hypertension and its consequences (see Fig. G7). In Goodpasture syndrome the antigen comes from the glomerulus itself, and the hypersensitivity reaction is of type II.

Antibody–antigen interactions in the kidney show a number of major histological features:

- increased cellularity due to proliferation of mesangial cells and polymorph infiltration;
- thickening of the GBM due to either deposition of large immune complexes in the subepithelial area, with swelling of endothelial and epithelial cells, or prolongation of mesangial cells between the endothelial and basement membrane;
- crescent formation due to fibrin stimulating the endothelial cells lining Bowman's space. This, together with infiltrating polymorphs, compresses the glomerular tuft, giving rise to a crescentic appearance.

More often than not most of the glomeruli are affected but there may be only some and this is described as focal or segmental. In some cases the glomerulonephritis is idiopathic, with no detectable antibodies or complement.

The mechanisms by which antibody–antigen complexes cause glomerular injury and the consequences of the induced nephritis are shown in Fig G7. Damage occurs through:

- complement activation
- attraction of macrophages which produce a variety of mediators and neutrophils which degranulate on ingestion of complexes or on attachment to antigen bound to the basement membrane
- activation of the clotting and kinin systems.

Management

There is little that can be done for the acute form of glomerulonephritis described in this case and it usually resolves. Up to 30% of cases can develop progressive renal disease up to 10 or more years later. The majority of the non-acute post-infectious cases are treated with steroids. Chronic glomerulonephritis is a common cause of renal failure requiring renal transplantation*.

 Amyloidosis; Goodpasture syndrome; Hypersensitivity; IgA nephropathy; Renal failure

GLUCOSE-6-PHOSPHATE DEHYDROGENASE (G6PD) DEFICIENCY:

Sex-linked inherited deficiency of G6PD, an essential enzyme in the production of reducing power via NADPH. Reducing power is required for protection of the red cell from oxidant damage. Abnormally functioning variants of the enzyme are found in the Mediterranean, West Africa and SE Asia. Oxidant stress may be provided by drugs such as antimalarials, sulphonamides and salicylates. Some foods, particularly fava beans, may also precipitate haemolysis, as may infections. The clinical manifestations depend on the type of abnormal enzyme. They include chronic haemolytic anaemia, acute intravascular haemolysis after oxidant stress, and neonatal haemolytic jaundice. The oxidized haemoglobin precipitates in the red cells where it may be seen as Heinz bodies in reticulocyte preparations. Blister cells may be seen on the blood film.

The diagnosis may be confirmed by assay of the enzyme in red cells, but young red cells have increased enzyme activity, so the assay may not be reliable during a haemolytic crisis when the reticulocyte count is increased. Treatment is to avoid factors that precipitate haemolysis. During acute haemolysis, blood transfusion may be required, and increased fluids to maintain a good output of urine to prevent renal tubular damage.

Heterozygotes for G6PD deficiency show a degree of protection against severe malaria.

GLUTEN-SENSITIVE ENTEROPATHY:

Damage to intestinal mucosa with resultant malabsorption due to an allergic reaction to gliadin protein.

 Coeliac disease

GLYCOGEN STORAGE DISEASES: A group of autosomal recessive disorders characterized by hypoglycaemia due to the deficiency of a specific enzyme involved in the metabolism of glycogen. At least 12 enzyme defects have been described.

Table G4 shows the major glycogen storage diseases.

Table G4 The major glycogen storage diseases

Type	Enzyme defect
I – von Gierke disease	Glucose 6-phosphate
II – Pompe disease	α1,4-Glucosidase
III – Cori disease	Amylo-1,6-glucosidase
IV – Anderson disease	Amylo-1,4→1,6-transglucosidase
V – McArdle disease	Muscle phosphorylase
VI – Hers disease	Liver phosphorylase
VII – XII	

Pathology

Two major effects are seen as a result of the deficiency of specific enzymes:
- the intracellular deposition of glycogen which, when it involves the hepatic cells, causes hepatomegaly, fibrotic changes and subsequently liver failure, and when the myocardial cells are involved, causes cardiac failure;
- hypoglycaemia as a result of failure to break down liver glycogen and depletion of glucose stores.

The liver, kidney and gut are involved in type I, the heart is the most commonly affected in type II. Severity varies, types III, V and VI being mild, type I severe and types II and IV lethal.

Liver function tests are abnormal in most cases of glycogen storage disease. Type IV is associated with cirrhosis. Hyperuricaemia is prominent in types I, III and IX. The diagnosis is made by the demonstration of the enzyme deficiency in leucocytes in types II, III and IV, whilst in the other types this is demonstrated in the liver.

Management

The mainstay is maintenance of blood glucose concentrations. In cases with significant hepatic involvement that might progress to hepatic tumours, a liver transplantation may be the only treatment available.

GOITRE: A swelling of the thyroid gland which may be unilateral or bilateral and smooth or knobbly (Fig. G8). It may occur in euthyroid, hypothyroid or hyperthyroid states. A full thyroid profile (FT4, FT3, TSH) should be carried to help

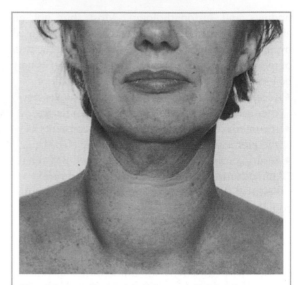

Fig. G8 A patient with a large colloid goitre. (Reproduced from Browse NL. *An Introduction to the Symptoms and Signs of Surgical Disease*, 3rd edn. London: Arnold, 1997)

ascertain the cause of this swelling. If a thyroid carcinoma is suspected, a serum thyroglobulin measurement is also necessary.

 Thyrotoxicosis

GONORRHOEA: An infection with *Neisseria gonorrhoeae*. A sexually transmitted disease.

Case

A 35-year-old heterosexual male attended his GP complaining of pain on micturition and a discharge from his penis. Suspecting the patient may have gonorrhoea, the GP referred the patient to the Sexually Transmitted Diseases clinic. The patient admitted having unprotected sex within the past few days. A list of the patient's contacts was obtained and a swab was taken for microscopy and culture.

Microbiology: a Gram stain showed numerous pus cells with intracellular Gram-negative diplococci (Fig. G9). *Neisseria gonorrhoeae* was cultured from the pus.

Aetiology and risk factors

Neisseria gonorrhoeae is a Gram-negative diplococcus and an obligate human pathogen. The organism is very susceptible to desiccation and is only transmitted by sexual contact. Asymptomatic carriage can occur and this more frequently occurs in females. These asymptomatic carriers are impor-

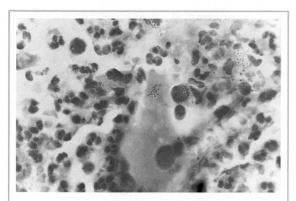

Fig. G9 A Gram stain showed numerous pus cells with intracellular Gram-negative diplococci.

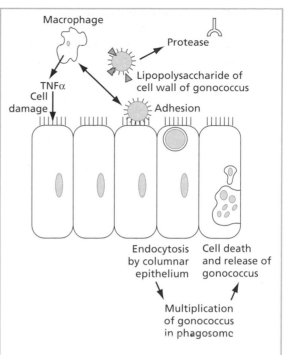

Fig. G10 Diagram showing pathogenesis of gonorrhoea.

tant in the spread of disease and infected patients should have all their contacts traced and screened. After transmission of the organism during sexual contact, it adheres to columnar epithelium of the urethra, cervix, oropharynx or rectum by means of pili. Pili are short hair-like projections on the surface of the bacillus, composed of proteins, which may vary in composition (antigenic variation) or expression (phase variation). Such mechanisms are important in avoidance of the immune system by the infecting organism. The genetic mechanisms underlying antigenic variation are similar to those generating antibody diversity in humans. Homologous recombination occurs between duplicated segments of the pilin gene to produce a chimeric molecule, which is then expressed. The potential variety is so large that during an infection protective immunity does not develop. Additionally pilin expression can be turned on or off depending upon the local circumstances. Other surface components such as lipopolysaccharide or outer-membrane proteins (OMP), e.g. porin, opacity proteins, can similarly be variably expressed and may, like the pili, determine whether the gonococcus is phagocytosed or not. Variations in the porin are also related to serum resistance of the gonococcus and it is a major target of vaccine production. Gonococci also produce an IgA protease that may help it to avoid the host's immune defences. Also, the organism may be taken up by the columnar epithelium by endocytosis and thus avoid the host defence mechanisms (Fig. G10).

Pathology

The organism multiplies locally on the mucosal surface and is shed in oral or genital secretions. The organism may spread to the fallopian tubes and cause pelvic inflammatory disease (PID)*, or spread via the bloodstream to set up distant infected foci,

e.g. arthritis. Factors determining the outcome of disease include expression of specific OMP, e.g. sialylation of the carbohydrate of the LPS, and host factors, e.g. hypocomplementaemia. Damage to cells is caused by stimulation of the production of pro-inflammatory cytokines by the LPS. Diagnosis is by isolation of the organism from specimens.

Management

Management is with β-lactams, e.g. ampicillin. It is important that contacts are traced and offered treatment.

GOODPASTURE SYNDROME: An autoimmune disorder affecting the lungs and kidneys.

Aetiology and risk factors

This is a rare disorder found in about 1 per 100 000 of the population and most often in young or middle-aged men. The cause is unknown, but smoking increases the risk of development of the disease and there is some evidence that it may develop following a recent viral infection.

Pathology

Patients usually present either with breathlessness and cough with bloody sputum (haemoptysis), or with blood in their urine (haematuria). They may also complain of non-specific chest pain, fatigue and foamy urine. A chest radiograph reveals extensive alveolar shadowing due to pulmonary haemorrhage.

Pulmonary haemorrhage causes an increase in gas transfer and particularly KCO. The haemorrhage is the result of autoantibodies to alveolar basement membrane, which results in local bleeding in the lung. Autoantibodies to kidney basement membrane result in crescentic glomerular nephritis leading to proteinuria (hence the foamy urine) and to haematuria. The autoantibody-mediated damage is classified as a type II hypersensitivity and is mainly caused by complement activation by the basement membrane-bound autoantibodies and release of proteolytic enzymes, etc., by polymorphs. Pulmonary bleeding is the most common cause of death.

Management

Since this is an acute disease, treatment should be prompt:
● plasma exchange
● treatment with immunosuppressive drugs.
Both treatments have greatly improved prognosis.

Hypersensitivity

GOUT: An arthritic condition occurring as a result of deposition of sodium urate crystals in joints, as a result of elevated blood uric acid.

Case

A 45-year-old company director presented in the early hours of the morning to the casualty department with a painful left big toe. He had been out the night before at a dinner gala. The pain had occurred suddenly and the toe was red, swollen and exquisitely tender. Routine biochemical tests including serum uric acid and liver function were requested. His results returned with normal serum electrolytes, urea and creatinine concentrations. He had an elevated serum uric acid of 0.68 mmol/l and γGT of 80 IU/l.

Aetiology and risk factors

Primary gout is predominantly a disease of men. It is common in the middle-aged, high social class, overweight individual who indulges plentifully in alcohol. In addition, there is usually a strong family history of gout. Secondary gout occurs in diseases where there is excessive breakdown of purines (increased nucleic acid turnover), e.g. leukaemia, myeloproliferative disease, psoriasis, carcinomatosis, cytotoxic drug use. The biochemical abnormality in primary and secondary gout is hyperuricaemia, resulting from overproduction (high dietary intake, increased purine synthesis, increased nucleic acid turnover) or decreased renal clearance of uric acid (chronic renal disease, drugs, poisons and hyperparathyroidism).

Pathology

The case described here is the typical presentation of primary gout; the attack usually occurs early in the morning, precipitated by either a surgical operation, starvation, thiazide diuretic use, or excessive alcohol. In this case it was alcohol, which explains why in addition to an elevated serum uric acid he had an elevated γGT. The big toe is the commonest site of attack. Other joints can be involved but the joints of the lower limb are the most commonly affected. In the majority of attacks only one joint is affected. The joint is usually red, warm and swollen and very tender (Fig. G11). There are a number of associated features seen in patients with gout; there may be gouty tophi in the ear lobes or around joints. However, these occur much later in the disease process. There is a high incidence of vascular disease, hypertension and renal disease in these patients.

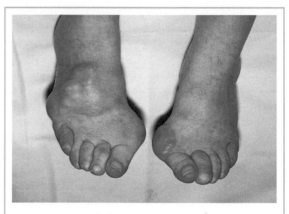

Fig. G11 Chronic gouty swellings of the feet. (Reproduced with permission from Toghill, PJ (ed.) *Examining Patients. An Introduction to Clinical Medicine.* London: Edward Arnold, 1995)

The diagnostic test is aspiration of the joint and examination of the synovial fluid using polarized light microscopy to identify negatively birefringent urate crystals. An elevated level of serum uric acid confirms the diagnosis.

Management

In acute attacks, treatment is with an NSAID or, if contraindicated, colchicine. To prevent attacks, purine-rich food should be avoided, and weight and alcohol intake reduced. Aspirin, which increases uric acid, should be avoided. Allopurinol can be used prophylactically to reduce uric acid.

GRAFT-VERSUS-HOST DISEASE (GVHD): An immunological attack against the recipient's tissues mediated by immunocompetent donor lymphocytes. This is most commonly seen following stem cell transplantation*. The disorder is usually classified as acute or chronic, depending on whether it occurs more than 3 months after the transplant, though there is a large overlap.

Pathology

Clinical manifestations of GVHD Tissues that express large amounts of HLA antigens are those that are most commonly affected, though no organ system is immune. These organs are skin, liver and intestine. In the skin a maculopapular erythematous rash, or diffuse erythema is most commonly seen. In severe cases this may progress to blistering and peeling. Skin rashes are common in the post-transplant period, particularly as allergic manifestations of drugs, but unlike these fixed drug eruptions, GVHD commonly affects the skin of the soles and palms. Acute GVHD usually appears about 2 weeks after bone marrow transplantation, coinciding with myeloid engraftment. GVHD of liver and intestine are usually seen after the skin effects. In the intestine diarrhoea is the usual symptom. This is characteristically green in colour, and can be severe enough to result in dehydration and intestinal bleeding. Painless jaundice is the usual first manifestation of liver GVHD. A fall in blood counts is also commonly seen in the presence of GVHD.

In cases of diagnostic difficulty, it is possible to biopsy affected tissues such as skin (Fig. G12) or rectal mucosa to confirm GVHD. However, the histological appearances are rarely typical.

In chronic GVHD, a scleroderma-like picture may develop, with pigmentation. Diverted by the immunological battle against the recipient's tissues, the transplanted immune system fails to mount an effective defence against micro-organisms, so that there is an increased incidence of difficult infections such as cytomegalovirus pneumonitis.

Relationship between GVHD, graft failure and graft-versus-leukaemia effect Removing the T-cells from a bone marrow graft lessens the chances of GVHD developing, as these are the main immunological mediators of the attack against the recipient's tissues. The T-cell removal may be done *in vitro* or *in vivo* using monoclonal antibodies against T-cell or other lymphoid antigens. The disadvantage of T-cell depletion is that graft failure (rejection) is more likely, though the chances of this happening can be decreased by an effective conditioning regimen to suppress the recipient's immunity completely.

The effectiveness of bone marrow transplantation in curing malignant haematological diseases such as leukaemia is not only due to the powerful conditioning regimen killing residual leukaemic cells in the recipients marrow. There is also an ongoing immunological action by the transplanted immunological cells against malignant cells in the recipient. Thus T-cell depletion of donor marrow reduces the incidence of GVHD, but also increases the likelihood of leukaemia relapse. In addition, patients who have evidence of GVHD are less likely to suffer a relapse of their leukaemia. This immunological action is termed graft-versus-leukaemia (GVL) effect and is the subject of intensive investigation to determine whether it might be possible to remove particular subpopulations of T-lymphocytes from the graft in order to get GVL without GVHD.

Third-party GVHD Immunocompetent lymphocytes from cellular blood product transfusion may settle in an immunodepressed recipient's tissues, proliferate, and cause inadvertent GVHD. Fortunately, this is a rare occurrence, but when seen it is usually fatal. Prevention is by irradiating cellular blood products that are being transfused to immunocompromised recipients.

Management of GVHD

Obtaining a good HLA match between the donor and recipient guards against the development of GVHD, and GVHD is almost never seen in syngeneic or autologous transplants. Where there is a risk of GVHD, T-depletion of the donor marrow decreases the incidence of GVHD (see above).

Most allograft recipients are treated with the immunosuppressive drug cyclosporin for several months after their transplant in order to prevent

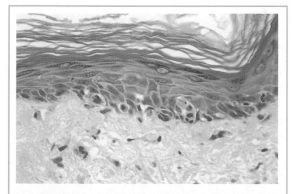

Fig. G12 Apoptotic basal cells (colloid bodies) in the basal layer of epidermis characteristic of GVHD.

GVHD. The majority of such patients develop some manifestation of GVHD, though this is often mild skin GVHD not requiring treatment. When significant GVHD develops, immunosuppression with steroids such as prednisolone forms the mainstay of treatment.

GRANULOMA: A collection of macrophages sometimes surrounded by a rim of lymphocytes.

 Tuberculosis

GRAVES DISEASE: An autoimmune disease characterized by the presence of thyroid stimulating antibodies in the blood, causing hyperthyroidism.

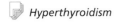 *Hyperthyroidism*

GUILLAIN–BARRE SYNDROME: A post-infectious peripheral neuropathy.

Aetiology and risk factors
The principal recognized cause is a gastrointestinal infection with the Gram-negative enteric pathogen *Campylobacter jejuni*, although it can follow infections with *Mycoplasma pneumoniae*, some viral infections such as VZV, CMV, EBV, or vaccination (e.g. rabies). In 50–75% of cases, the illness presents 1–3 weeks after a gastrointestinal or respiratory illness.

Pathology
In the case of *Campylobacter jejuni*-associated disease, the core structure of the lipopolysaccharide of the micro-organism has an identical sugar component to that of gangliosides found in neurons. Antibodies produced by the host against the lipopolysaccharide and cell wall proteins cross-react with these gangliosides and myelin proteins (Fig. G13).

Initially there is oedema of the neuron with infiltration by lymphocytes, followed by macrophages and subsequent segmental demyelination. *Campylobacter* is mainly associated with axonal degeneration and minimal inflammation presenting as primarily a motor neuropathy, although it is also found in association with the more usual sensori-

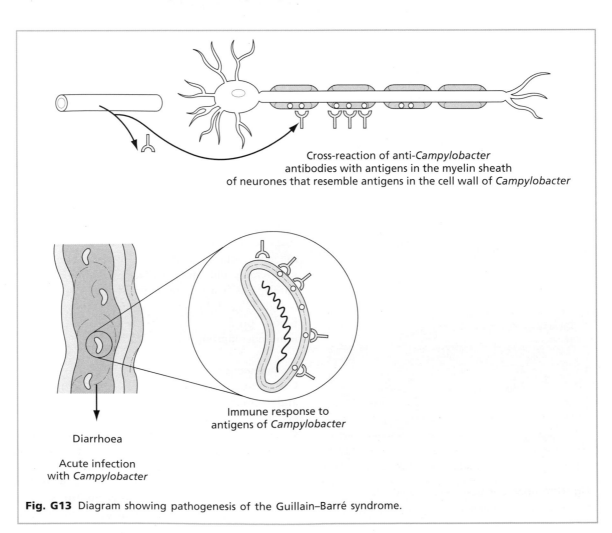

Fig. G13 Diagram showing pathogenesis of the Guillain–Barré syndrome.

motor picture of demyelination presenting with symmetrical numbness, paraesthesia and ascending paralysis. The nerve conduction velocity may be considerably reduced. The paralysis starts in the limbs and spreads to the trunk and even muscles of respiration. In Miller–Fisher syndrome, there is paralysis of the III, IV and VI cranial nerves presenting as ophthalmoplegia, areflexia and ataxia. There is eventual clinical recovery in most patients, although up to 20% may have residual damage and there is a 5% mortality rate. The diagnosis is clinical but may be supported by nerve conduction studies. The cerebrospinal fluid protein content is frequently elevated. Treatment is supportive.

GUMMA: A granulomatous chronic inflammatory destructive lesion of tertiary syphilis which can occur in any organ.

 Syphilis

GYNAECOMASTIA: An enlargement of the male breast which may be unilateral or bilateral, a benign condition accounting for 70% of male breast disorders.

Aetiology and risk factors
Gynaecomastia occurs physiologically in the neonatal period and puberty; other causes regarded as pathological include: drugs (spironolactone, oestrogens, cimetidine, digoxin), liver cirrhosis, malnutrition, testicular, lung, liver, kidney and feminizing adrenal tumours, testicular tumours (oestrogensecreting), choriocarcinoma, primary and secondary hypogonadism, hyperthyroidism, hyperparathyroidism, chronic renal failure, haemochromatosis, cirrhosis and Klinefelter syndrome.

Pathology
Several mechanisms can cause this condition: atrophy or destruction of the testis, increased oestrogen, prolactin and gonadotrophin levels. In each case there is an imbalance in the oestrogen and androgen concentrations in the male. In neonates, gynaecomastia results as a result of exposure to maternal hormones, whilst in puberty it is as a result of an imbalance in oestrogen and androgen levels. In both these instances, the condition resolves itself. Histologically, it is characterized by proliferation of the ducts of the breast and the surrounding stroma. A moderate degree of epithelial hyperplasia is also present. If a pathological cause is suspected, in addition to a history and clinical examination, estimations of serum testosterone, oestrogen, LH, FSH, SHBG (sex-hormone-binding globulin), prolactin, TSH, urea, creatinine, calcium and liver function tests will be helpful. Other investigations that may aid in making a diagnosis include a skull and chest radiograph, pituitary and adrenal function tests and karyotyping.

Management
Usually no treatment is required. Surgical excision is carried out for cosmetic reasons or to rule out malignancy.

G

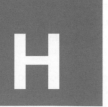

HAEMANGIOMA: A benign tumour of blood vessels, also known as an angioma.

HAEMOCHROMATOSIS: A condition resulting from an excess of iron in the body.

Case
A 45-year-old man presented at the general medical outpatient clinic with a chronic history of weight loss, lethargy and non-specific symptoms. He also provided some history of polyuria despite not drinking a lot of fluid. On clinical examination the only significant finding was the fact that he appeared tanned despite no history of recent travel. A panel of blood investigations were requested which included full blood count, serum electrolytes and urea, blood glucose and liver function tests. All these tests were within normal limits. His urine dipstick test was positive for glucose and a fasting blood glucose was requested: the result was 10 mmol/l. After further consultation with other physicians, it was suggested that his iron status should be assessed. The results revealed an elevated serum iron and ferritin, with decreased serum transferrin. The total iron-binding capacity was decreased.

A diagnosis was made of haemochromatosis and a liver biopsy was scheduled. In the meantime he was treated with venesection.

Aetiology
Haemochromatosis can be either primary or secondary. **Primary** haemochromatosis is a familial disease with an autosomal recessive dominance. It results from an abnormal gene located on chromosome 6 and is closely linked with the HLA system and occurs clinically in homozygotes. **Secondary** haemochromatosis occurs from iron overload due to either:
- increased dietary intake of iron
- increased iron infusions from repeated transfusions
- liver disease or
- chronic haemolytic anaemias.

Pathology
When excessive amounts of iron accumulate in the body, it is deposited in various tissues such as the pancreas, myocardium, skin and endocrine glands. Deposition in the pancreas results in pancreatic islet cell destruction and diabetes. The above patient had glycosuria and a high blood glucose. His unexpected tan was a result of the deposition of melanin in the skin, giving it a slate-grey appearance ('bronze diabetes'). Iron deposition may also affect the pituitary (hypopituitarism), heart (cardiomyopathy, heart failure), spleen (splenomegaly), adrenal (Addison disease), testes (atrophy), and joints (arthritis). In the liver, excess iron deposition results in cirrhosis and failure, portal hypertension and, in severe cases, hepatoma. The liver disease is usually exacerbated by excessive alcohol ingestion.

The diagnosis of haemochromatosis is suggested by increased serum iron and ferritin, and saturation of iron-binding protein. It is confirmed by demonstration of excess iron in the liver from a percutaneous biopsy (Fig. H1) and by PCR for the abnormal gene.

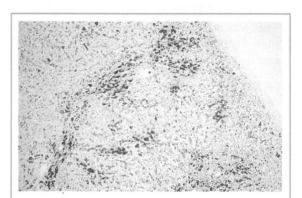

Fig. H1 Section of liver showing iron accumulation stained in blue.

Management
Management is mainly by repeated venesection, diabetes and heart failure being treated by conventional methods. Desferrioxamine is also used prophylactically in patients at risk of developing heamochromatosis.

HAEMOLYTIC ANAEMIA: Anaemia* due to a reduced red cell life span.

Destruction of red cells may occur within the circulation (intravascular) or within the reticuloendothelial system (extravascular). In severe cases of haemolysis both mechanisms may operate.

Aetiology and risk factors
Intravascular haemolysis Some causes of intravascular haemolysis are:
- acute haemolytic blood transfusion reaction
- microangiopathic haemolytic anaemia*

- paroxysmal cold haemoglobinuria
- acute haemolysis associated with G6PD deficiency.

Extravascular haemolysis Some causes of extravascular haemolysis are:

- warm autoimmune haemolytic anaemia*
- cold agglutinins*
- sickle cell disease*
- delayed haemolytic blood transfusion reaction
- hypersplenism*
- hereditary spherocytosis*.

Congenital causes of haemolysis These may be divided into membrane defects, defective red cell metabolism and abnormalities of haemoglobin.

Membrane defects include hereditary spherocytosis*, elliptocytosis and abetalipoproteinaemia.

Defective red cell metabolism may involve impaired reducing power or impaired energy production. Reducing power is needed to maintain haemoglobin in the reduced state, since oxidation of haemoglobin results in its precipitation within the red cell and removal of the red cells by the spleen. Glucose-6-phosphate deficiency* impairs reducing power and makes the red cell more susceptible to oxidant damage. Energy is required to maintain the normal shape and flexibility of the red cell membrane and to power the ion pump responsible for transferring sodium into and potassium out of the cell. In pyruvate kinase deficiency, defective energy production from the glycolytic pathway results in haemolysis.

Haemoglobin defects resulting in haemolysis include the thalassaemias* and haemoglobinopathies such as sickle cell disease*.

Pathology

General features of haemolytic anaemias The anaemia is normocytic or macrocytic in type. If a reticulocyte stain is performed, an increased number of reticulocytes may be found in the blood, reflecting increased marrow activity with erythroid hyperplasia in an effort to compensate for the red cell destruction. On the conventionally stained blood film, polychromasia ('many colours') may be noted – in fact just a grey tinge to the normal staining of red cells, reflecting their youth. Spherocytes may be present in any cause of haemolysis but are particularly common in warm autoimmune haemolytic anaemia* and hereditary spherocytosis*. Other clues to the cause of the haemolysis, such as fragmented cells in microangiopathic haemolytic anaemia* and sickled cells in sickle cell disease*, may be seen on the blood film.

The body has several means of conserving haemoglobin released in the circulation and preventing its loss through the glomerulus into the urine. Initially, free haemoglobin will bind to haptoglobin. This is carried to the liver to be unloaded, so no haptoglobins are left in the circulation; thus low haptoglobin levels are a sensitive marker of intravascular haemolysis. Free haemoglobin may then bind to albumin, forming methaemalbumin, which may be detected by the Schumm test. When available albumin is saturated, free haemoglobin will pass through the glomerulus. The renal tubular cells may ingest some of this haemoglobin. They are then shed at a later date into the urine, when they may be detected by staining a urinary deposit for iron. Such positive urinary haemosiderin may be a useful indicator of previous intravascular haemolysis. Appearance of haemoglobin in the urine (haemoglobinuria) must be distinguished from bleeding into the urinary tract (haematuria). This may be most conveniently done by microscopic examination of a urine specimen for intact red cells.

Removal of red cells from the circulation by the reticuloendothelial system and its associated phagocytes allows the haemoglobin to be reprocessed. Increased production of bilirubin results in jaundice. The bilirubin is prehepatic, unconjugated, water insoluble, so does not appear in the urine. Hence haemolytic jaundice is sometimes called acholuric jaundice, in contrast to post-hepatic jaundice due to biliary obstruction when the bilirubin has been conjugated and will appear in the urine. Increased porphyrins from the breakdown of haem are excreted into the bile. In cases of chronic haemolysis pigment, gallstones* may be formed. In the bowel porphyrin breakdown products undergo a number of chemical changes, and are reabsorbed into the bloodstream to appear in the urine as urobilinogen. This may be detected by a sensitive dipstick test.

HAEMOLYTIC DISEASE OF THE NEWBORN: A

neonatal condition in which antibody directed against red cell antigens, usually anti-D, crosses the placenta and destroys fetal red cells. This may result in intrauterine death from high output cardiac failure associated with severe anaemia, pleural effusions and ascites – hydrops foetalis. Milder cases are associated with neonatal haemolytic anaemia. The high levels of unconjugated bilirubin found in the serum may stain the basal ganglia of the brain, resulting in long-term neurological dysfunction. This is termed kernicterus.

The mother's immune system will usually have been sensitized to make anti-D by previous red cell transfusions or small transplacental haemorrhages during previous pregnancies. This is an important reason why Rhesus D-negative women in the reproductive age group should not be transfused with Rhesus D-positive red cells. In recent years a programme of anti-D prophylaxis has been successful in reducing the incidence of haemolytic disease of the newborn. Rhesus D-negative mothers receive intramuscular injections of anti-D during pregnancy and immediately after delivery of a Rhesus D-positive baby. This destroys any fetal Rhesus-positive red cells that have passed across the placenta before they can sensitize the maternal immune system. A Kleihauer fetal cell test is performed on the maternal blood after birth to estimate the amount of fetal red cells that have entered the maternal circulation, in case more than the standard amount of anti-D (500 units) should be needed (Fig. H2). Approximately 4 ml of packed fetal red cells will be removed by 500 units of anti-D.

With the reduction in the incidence of haemolytic disease of the newborn due to anti-D, other antibodies are becoming more important, such as anti-c and anti-Jk[a] (Kidd blood group system). Although anti-A and anti-B are usually IgM antibodies that do not cross the placenta, some mothers may develop 'immune' IgG antibodies that may cause ABO haemolytic disease of the newborn. Although common, this is usually mild.

It is difficult to assess the severity of haemolytic disease *in utero*. The level of maternal antibodies provides some guidance. When high levels are present, amniocentesis may be performed to measure bilirubin level in the amniotic fluid. If high for the stage of pregnancy, then intrauterine transfusion may be performed using an amnioscope and ultrasound guidance. After delivery, mild cases may be treated by phototherapy and more severe ones by exchange transfusion via the umbilical vein.

HAEMOLYTIC URAEMIC SYNDROME: Usually a post-infectious complication leading to a microangiopathic haemolytic anaemia*, thrombocytopenia* and renal failure. It may also occur in association with non-infectious causes.

Aetiology and risk factors

The best recognized infective cause of HUS is a gastrointestinal infection with *E. coli* O157 although it may follow other infections, e.g. *Shigella*, HIV. Infection with *E. coli* is often acquired by consuming undercooked hamburgers but may be associated with other foods. Typically it occurs in children less than 3 years and patients over 60 years of age.

Pathology

There is widespread endothelial injury in the renal microvasculature and in some cases this may extend to many organs of the body, in which case the condition is known as thrombotic thrombocytopenic purpura*. Both conditions may occur in the absence of infection in relation to, for example, drugs, neoplasia, pregnancy, or be idiopathic, and both illnesses may represent a spectrum of severity or pathogenesis.

In relation to *E. coli* there is frequently an episode of diarrhoea, often bloody, followed by the renal and haematological abnormalities about a week later. *E. coli* O157 produces one of a family of closely related verotoxins inhibiting protein synthesis in affected cells. Pathologically the main damage occurs in the glomerular or preglomerular microvasculature where there is a thrombotic microangiopathy or intimal proliferation and consequent stenosis. The endothelial damage may be due directly to the verotoxin or may be the result of the release of free radicals and cationic proteins from activated neutrophils and the production of pro-inflammatory cytokines. The patients present with diarrhoea, often bloody, followed by anaemia and renal failure. There is microscopic haematuria and proteinuria. Occasionally the protein loss may be severe enough to cause a nephrotic syndrome*. There may be cerebral signs, e.g. fits, coma. There is peripheral neutrophilia, thrombocytopenia and evidence of fragmented cells. The Coombs test is negative. Serum albumin may be decreased and urate increased due to haemolysis. Haptoglobin levels are reduced. The treatment is supportive and the patient may require dialysis.

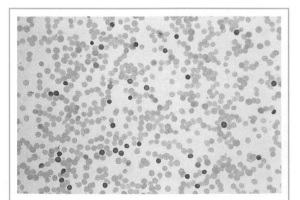

Fig. H2 A strongly positive Kleihauer fetal cell test. The maternal cells are pale ghosts due to haemoglobin A having been washed out by an acid buffer. The fetal cells stain more deeply as their content of haemoglobin F is resistant to acid elution.

HAEMOPHILIA: Inherited deficiency of coagulation factors VIII (haemophilia A) or IX (haemophilia B or Christmas disease).

Aetiology and risk factors

The inheritance of haemophilia A and B is sex linked, males being affected, females asymptomatic carriers. However, only about two-thirds of patients with haemophilia exhibit the classic inheritance pattern, either because they have a new mutation or there is no family to express the inheritance pattern.

Pathology

Clinical manifestations of haemophilia frequently present when the child starts to try to walk and is subject to minor falls. However, bleeding from the umbilical stump at delivery may occur and minor surgery such as circumcision may result in prolonged bleeding. Recurrent haemarthrosis may lead to fibrosis and stiffness of the joint (ankylosis) and to secondary bony arthritic changes.

A coagulation screen will show a prolonged activated partial thromboplastin time (APTT) in keeping with a defect in the intrinsic coagulation system, a normal prothrombin time and normal thrombin time. APTT on mixtures of patients' and normal plasma shows no prolongation unless an inhibitor of factor VIII or XI has developed, which is unusual before treatment. To confirm the diagnosis, measurement of factor VIII and IX levels should be performed. Nature overprovides us with coagulation factors and severe haemophiliacs have less than 1% of normal levels (less than 1 unit/dl.)

Female carriers of haemophilia or Christmas disease have modestly low but asymptomatic levels of coagulation factors. If the factors are measured by an immunological rather than a functional method, then levels will be found to be higher, reflecting the fact that in many cases of haemophilia a defective coagulation factor is produced which is measured in an immunological assay but not a functional (clotting) assay. To detect carriers the appropriate Y chromosome may be traced through families by restriction fragment length polymorphism.

Management

The mainstay of treatment is early intravenous administration of appropriate coagulation factor concentrates for the treatment of bleeding episodes. In haemophilia A, factor VIII concentrate is appropriate, in Christmas disease factor IX. With experience haemophiliacs may recognize the early symptoms of a bleed before clinical signs become evident. Severe haemophiliacs may be trained to self-administer coagulation factor concentrate at the earliest sign of a bleed or even prophylactically several times a week. Supportive treatment with concentrate is also required to cover dental treatment and orthopaedic operations. Physiotherapy, particularly hydrotherapy, helps to maintain mobility.

Complications of treatment include viral transmission from blood products, notably HIV infection. Donors of coagulation factor concentrates are screened for hepatitis B, hepatitis C and HIV carriage but every few years new pathogens are discovered, contaminating blood products. Most coagulation factor concentrates are treated by heat and detergent to inactivate viruses. Recombinant coagulation proteins, made by inserting the appropriate gene into bacterial or animal cells, are now becoming available and should be free of infective risk. Haemophiliacs, and all regular recipients of blood products, should have subcutaneous immunization against hepatitis B but should not receive intramuscular injections because of the risk of haematoma formation.

Bleeding that is external may be treated by fibrinolytic inhibitors such as tranexamic acid, but internal bleeding such as haemarthrosis should not be treated in this manner as this will result in resolution by fibrosis. In mild haemophiliacs, administration of the ADH analogue DDAVP (desmopressin) causes release of stored factor VIII from stores in endothelial cells. DDAVP is of no use in Christmas disease and is less effective with each dose in haemophilia as the factor VIII stores become exhausted. Regular opiate administration for control of pain may result in addiction.

HAEMORRHAGIC ANAEMIA: Anaemia* induced by bleeding. The haemoglobin level is initially normal after acute haemorrhage, but drops over the succeeding hours and days as fluid passes into the circulation from the tissues. An increased reticulocyte count may then be found as the bone marrow attempts to compensate for the red cell loss. Chronic loss of red cells may lead to iron-deficiency anaemia*.

HAEMORRHAGIC DISEASE OF THE NEWBORN: Bleeding in the neonatal period associated with deficiency of the vitamin K-dependent coagulation factors II, VII, IX and X. These factors are manufactured in the liver and the disorder is commoner in premature babies with immature livers. Commercial infant milk formulae contain added vitamin K, so haemorrhagic disease is commoner in breast-fed babies. Presentation may

H

be with bleeding from the umbilical cord stump, generalized bruising or intracerebral bleeds, which may be fatal or cause long-term disability. The prothrombin time and APTT are both significantly prolonged in affected cases.

Management

A single injection of vitamin K shortly after delivery or repeated oral doses of vitamin K are protective and should be routinely administered. There has been some suggestion that babies who have had intramuscular vitamin K may be at increased risk of childhood malignancy, though this has now largely been discounted and there is no excuse not to give oral vitamin K to babies at risk.

HAEMOSIDEROSIS: A condition of iron overload usually applied to iatrogenic iron overload secondary to repeated red cell transfusions. There is increased haemosiderin in the bone marrow and a high ferritin level in the serum. Other causes of iron overload are haemochromatosis*, sideroblastic anaemia* and chronic congenital haemolytic anaemia.

HAIRY CELL LEUKAEMIA: A rare chronic B-cell lymphoproliferative disease most often seen in elderly males, involving a type of lymphocyte found in small numbers in normal blood. As the name suggests, this is characterized by numerous surface cytoplasmic projections resembling hairs (Fig. H3). The cytoplasm is relatively voluminous and the nucleus may contain nucleoli; sometimes these cells are termed 'fried egg cells'.

Clinically, the disorder is characterized by significant splenomegaly without marked lymphadenopathy. The blood shows cytopenias, including a macrocytic anaemia in many cases and a monocytopenia. Bone marrow aspirate frequently shows a dry tap and trephine biopsy is often necessary for diagnosis.

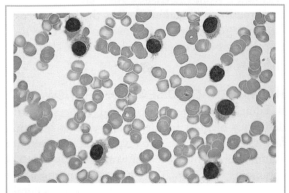

Fig. H3 Abnormal lymphocytes in hairy cell leukaemia.

The disorder is important to recognize because it is easily confused with chronic lymphocytic leukaemia* or splenic lymphoma with villous lymphocytes but differs from these disorders in treatment and prognosis. HCL responds well to the cytotoxic agent 2-CDA and to interferon and splenectomy, but does not respond well to the alkylating agents.

HAMARTOMA: A malformation in which there is an abnormal mixture of otherwise normal tissue elements.

HAND-FOOT-AND-MOUTH DISEASE: An infection mainly of children caused by Coxsackievirus A (types 5, 10 and 16), B (types 2 and 5) and enterovirus type 71 which presents as a sore throat and fever. Ulcers appear in the mouth and vesicles develop on the palms of the hands and soles of the feet.

 Exanthema

HAND–SCHÜLLER–CHRISTIAN DISEASE: A malignant neoplasm arising from Langerhans cells (histiocytes) derived from bone marrow.

 Histiocytosis X

HASHIMOTO THYROIDITIS: An chronic inflammatory condition of the thyroid, usually with an enlarged gland (goitre).

Aetiology and risk factors

This is an autoimmune disease with a probable genetic susceptibility. It is weakly associated with HLA-DR4 and DR5 and is considerably commoner in women. Autoantibodies to thyroid peroxidase and to thyroglobulin are present, as well as antibodies that stimulate thyroid growth.

Pathology

There are two main variants, an atrophic variant and one in which patients present with goitre. In the latter type, there is diffuse enlargement of the thyroid (Fig. H4). The thyroid parenchyma is diffusely involved by chronic inflammatory cells including lymphocytes, plasma cells and macrophages, with the formation of germinal follicles. The thyroid follicles undergo oncocytic change (Hurtle cells). In the atrophic variant, there is more fibrosis and less lymphoid infiltrate.

About 50% of the patients develop hypothyroidism, although occasionally hyperthyroidism may occur ('hashitoxicosis'). Patients with Hashimoto thyroiditis are at an increased risk of lymphoma.

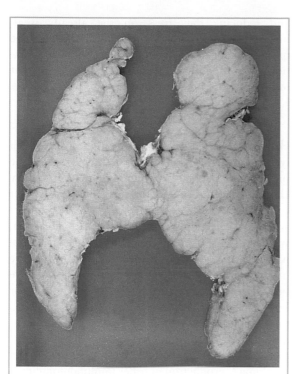

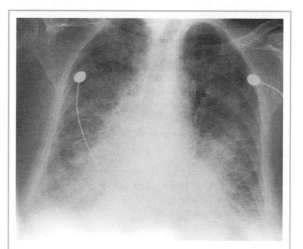

Fig. H5 Chest radiograph showing interstitial and alveolar pulmonary oedema and cardiomegaly. (Reproduced with permission from Curtis J, Whitehouse G. *Radiology for the MRCP*. London: Arnold, 1998)

Fig. H4 Macroscopic appearance of Hashimotos thyroiditis with diffuse enlargement of the gland.

Management

Hypothyroidism is treated by hormone replacement therapy. A large or painful goitre may require surgical removal.

 Goitre; Hypothyroidism; Non-Hodgkin lymphoma

HAY FEVER: The commonest form of allergy, a type I (IgE-mediated) hypersensitivity to environmental antigens, usually of plant or animal origin.

 Allergy

HEART FAILURE: Inability of the heart to maintain an adequate cardiac output due to 'pump failure'. It may be *congestive* (right-sided), resulting in venous congestion, or *biventricular*, resulting in both pulmonary and peripheral oedema.

Case

A 63-year-old man presented to the cardiology clinic complaining of increasing shortness of breath (SOB), tiredness and exhaustion over the past 3 months, his exercise tolerance having dropped to just 100 metres. He also experienced SOB at night and was unable to lie flat, needing three or four pillows to be comfortable. He had woken up on a number of occasions gasping for breath.

His past medical history included a myocardial infarction 3 years previously and a 'mild stroke' 6 months later. His current medication included aspirin 100 mg/day and a thiazide diuretic.

On examination, he was found to be mildly SOB at rest. His pulse was 110/min and his blood pressure 100/80 mmHg. His peripheries were cold and he had pitting peripheral oedema. The jugular venous pressure was raised to 7 cm above the sternal notch. Auscultation of his chest revealed widespread inspiratory crackles.

A chest radiograph confirmed pulmonary oedema and cardiac failure (Fig. H5).

Blood tests showed a Hb of 11g/l and urea of 26 mmol/l, creatinine of 50 mmol/l and abnormal liver function tests with a raised AST and alkaline phosphatase.

The cardiologist made a diagnosis of worsening cardiac failure due to ischaemic heart disease. He advised a low salt diet and changed his medication to include an ACE inhibitor (calcium antagonist).

Aetiology and risk factors

Cardiac failure results from 'pump failure' and hence anything that damages the myocardial tissue may be implicated. The causes include hypertension, myocardial ischaemia and infarction, myocarditis, pericardial effusion and tamponade.

Pathology

Table H1 shows the common causes of cardiac failure.

The symptoms and signs relate to accumulation of fluid within the lung and serous cavities due to venous congestion (Fig. H5). Inability of the heart

Table H1 Common causes of cardiac failure

Right-sided	Left-sided
Left-sided failure	Ischaemic heart disease
Chronic pulmonary disease	Hypertensive heart disease
Tricuspid valve disease	Aortic valve disease
Congenital heart disease	Mitral valve disease
Pulmonary hypertension	Myocarditis
Pulmonary embolism	Cardiomyopathy
	Amyloidosis
	High-output conditions

Low-output	High-output
Myocardial disease from ischaemic heart disease, myocarditis, cardiomyopathy, amyloidosis and arrhythmias	Anaemia
Increased pressure load from systemic hypertension and valve stenosis	Valve incompetence
Cor pulmonale	Thyrotoxicosis
	Fever
	Arteriovenous malformation
	Paget disease of bone
	Beri beri

to pump blood efficiently and to maintain a cardiac output sufficient for the needs of the body leads to back pressure and pulmonary venous congestion. Fluid transudate leaks out into the pleural cavity and into alveolar spaces, leading to increasing shortness of breath. This also accounts for orthopnoea (SOB on lying flat) and the need for many pillows at night. Although the failure usually starts with the left ventricle, the right ventricular function will also deteriorate with time due the high pulmonary venous pressure so that eventually there will be biventricular failure. The right-sided cardiac failure results in congestion of the liver, ascites and peripheral oedema.

The decreased cardiac output also has an effect on the systemic circulation and hence organs such as the brain, kidneys and the heart itself. With decreasing output, in a man who is already an arteriopath (previous myocardial infarct and cerebrovascular accident, CVA), there is a risk of a further CVA. The kidneys are also very likely to show ischaemic changes and this is reflected in the raised urea and creatinine. The combination of acidosis that results from renal impairment, the coronary atheroma, and the decreased output also puts an extra strain on the myocardium and the patient is at risk of a further myocardial infarction or fatal arrhythmia.

Management

The important management issue relates to controlling his cardiac failure by improving renal function and reducing the stress on the already weak myocardium. The vicious cycle that is set up can be quite resistant to treatment. Sometimes a combination of a myocardial stimulant and a drug that improves renal function may be required.

 Atheroma; Hypertension; Myocardial infarction

HEAVY CHAIN DISEASES: A group of rare B-cell lymphoproliferative disorders characterized by the production of defective immunoglobulin heavy chains, not attached to their corresponding light chains. Heavy chain diseases may be best understood as a related process to Bence Jones myeloma, where only light chains are produced by the malignant plasma cells. In heavy chain disease, the immunoglobulin component produced may have been destined for incorporation in an IgG, IgA or IgM molecule. The corresponding heavy chains may therefore be γ, α, or μ. They will be detected as a monoclonal protein in serum, urine, or sometimes as a component of amyloid deposits. As in myeloma*, production of other immunoglobulins is depressed, with resulting hypogammaglobulinaemia.

α-Chain disease is the commonest, being found mainly in children and young adults. The major sites of IgA production are the intestine and lungs, so not surprisingly α-chain disease is most commonly found at these sites. Just as *Helicobacter* infection may predispose to lymphoma of the stomach, so other enteric infections may predispose to α-chain disease. Thus the disorder is commonest in areas of the world where chronic enteric infections are endemic, such as the Mediterranean and Middle East. Severe malabsorption due to mucosal infiltration may be found in early stages of the disease, and tumours of malignant B-cells in the intestine in later stages. Like *Helicobacter*-induced lymphoma, early stages of the disease may respond to antibiotic therapy.

ε-Chain disease resembles a rapidly progressive form of myeloma, except that lymph nodes, spleen and liver are often involved and the malignant plasma cells often spill into the blood. Many patients have a history of chronic autoimmune disorders such as rheumatoid arthritis* or system lupus erythematosus*.

HENOCH–SCHÖNLEIN PURPURA: Also known as anaphylactoid purpura; a relatively common form of vasculitis* involving small blood vessels in a number of organs and characterized by non-thrombocytic purpura of the skin (especially around joints) (Fig. H6), arthralgia, gastrointestinal

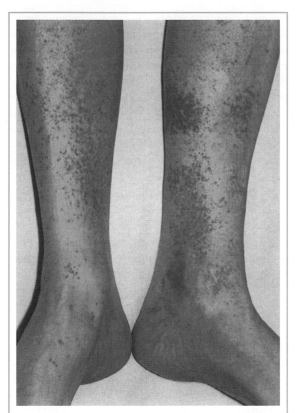

Fig. H6 Purpura in patient with Henoch–Schönlein disease. (Reproduced with permission from Toghill, PJ (ed.) *Examining Patients. An Introduction to Clinical Medicine*. London: Edward Arnold, 1995)

pain and glomerulonephritis. Platelets and the coagulation system are normal.

Children between 4 and 10 years old are commonly affected, often with a history of upper respiratory tract infection or of hypersensitivity to certain foods. The most important manifestation of this disease is nephritis, renal failure being the main cause of death. However, in most cases the renal failure is mild and transient, usually with complete recovery. Histologically, the glomerulonephritis* is focal with irregular, granular deposits of IgA, C3 and fibrin in the glomeruli. Deposits of IgA and C3 (often outside the purpuric areas) are also found in the skin and are diagnostic for this condition. Joints and the gastrointestinal tract are also commonly involved. The seasonal nature of the condition is consistent with a role for specific antigen(s). The immunological and clinical similarities between this condition and IgA nephropathy suggest that they are two forms of the same disease, IgA nephropathy lacking the multisystem involvement. The available data are consistent with an immune-complex and complement-mediated pathogenesis for this disease.

Steroid treatment is only partially effective but does seem to control the skin and gastrointestinal pain.

HEPATIC (LIVER) FAILURE: Hepatic failure is a clinical syndrome that results when there is extensive liver disease involving over 80% of the organ. This can be either acute or chronic. The clinical features of hepatic failure are foetor hepaticus, jaundice, portal hypertension, spider erythema, hypogonadism, flapping tremor, spider naevi and ascites.

Aetiology and pathology
Acute liver failure can result from liver cell necrosis as a result of viral hepatitis, toxic drugs (paracetamol, halothane, isoniazid, methyldopa) and chemicals. The condition is characterized by jaundice (because hepatocytes are unable to metabolize the bilirubin produced), hypoglycaemia (failure of glucogenesis), coagulation defects (failure of synthesis of clotting factors, electrolyte abnormalities (hyponatraemia, hypokalaemia), hepatic encephalopathy and hepatorenal syndrome (failure of detoxification) and elevation of liver enzymes (AST, ALT, LDH) in serum. Although there is a high mortality, some patients recover completely.

Chronic liver failure results from cirrhosis*, which is characterized by fibrosis and nodular regeneration. The effects are the same as those seen in acute liver failure, including endocrine changes caused by abnormal catabolism of hormones: gynaecomastia, testicular atrophy, telangiectasia (increased oestrogen), salt and water retention (aldosterone) and foetor hepaticus.

Other causes of hepatic failure include: Budd–Chiari syndrome, acute fatty liver of pregnancy, carbon tetrachloride, Weil and Wilson* diseases.

Management
Management involves correction of bleeding disorders with transfusion with blood products, treatment of infection with antibiotics, and control of hypoglycaemia. In patients with a poor prognosis, liver transplantation should be considered.

HEPATITIS B INFECTION: Infection with hepatitis B virus.

Case
A 36-year-old intravenous drug user presented at the clinic complaining of generalized malaise and joint pains, nausea and pain over the right side of his abdomen. He had noticed that he was passing dark urine. On examination the patient was tender over the liver and was mildly jaundiced. A full

blood count, liver function tests and serology for hepatitis viruses were requested.

> Chemistry: ALT 600 U/l; AST 800 U/l; Alk P 300 U/l; BR 68 mmol/l
> Haematology: Hb 13 g/dl; WBC 8000 × 10⁶/l; differential, 50% lymphocytes; INR normal
> Microbiology: HBsAg positive; anti-HBsAg negative; IgM anti-HBc positive; IgG anti-HBc negative; HBeAg positive; anti-HBeAg negative

The patient made an uneventful recovery and 6 months following the acute infection, repeat serology showed persistence of HBsAg, HBeAg and lack of anti-HBeAg, indicating that he had become a high-risk carrier:

> Microbiology: HBsAg positive; anti-HBsAg negative; IgM anti-HBc negative;
> IgG anti-HBc positive; HBeAg positive; anti-HBeAg negative

Aetiology and risk factors

Hepatitis B is a double-stranded DNA virus consisting of a nucleocapsid core surrounded by an outer envelope of the surface antigens (HBsAg) comprising surface proteins (e.g. p39) on which resides the domain which binds to the HBV receptor found on liver cells. The nucleocapsid comprises the DNA associated with a DNA polymerase and the core antigen (HBcAg). HBeAg is similar (in primary sequence) to the HBcAg but is transcribed from a different location on the HBV genome and has a different secondary structure to the HBcAg and is therefore antigenically distinct.

Pathology

After attachment to the hepatocyte, the virus is taken up into the cell and the uncoated DNA transported to the cell nucleus where it is converted to a fully double-stranded DNA template, which is used for transcription of viral RNAs, using the host cell RNA polymerase. The viral RNAs are then used as templates for producing further HBV DNA, and as mRNA for producing the surface and core antigens and viral polymerase. Mature HBV is then released from the hepatocytes. Hepatitis B is not a cytopathic virus and the damage to hepatocytes is thought to be mainly by virus-specific CD8+ T-cells. Hepatitis B is transmitted by blood products or infected excreta and typically infects IVDUs, homosexuals and sex workers. It is an occupational hazard for health care workers, particularly in tropical countries where the virus is hyperendemic and where transmission frequently occurs to the neonate during birth. Transmission may also occur in association with blood transfusion in countries that do not screen donors. Histopathologically, the findings are identical to those found with other viral hepatitides (see Viral hepatitis). Complications of acute infection include fulminant hepatic failure and the development of a chronic carrier state. Complications of the latter are cirrhosis and hepatocellular carcinoma.

Management of disease may include treatment with interferon-α, which is thought to reduce the risk of viral persistence. Prevention is by vaccination, using yeast-derived recombinant HBsAg. Other preventive measures include screening all donor blood and the avoidance of multiple needle use.

HEPATOCELLULAR CARCINOMA: A malignant tumour arising from liver cells.

Aetiology and risk factors

Hepatocellular carcinoma is strongly associated with hepatitis B virus infection (HBV). Other risk factors include cirrhosis* (and hence all causes of cirrhosis, e.g. alcohol abuse, α1-antitrypsin deficiency, etc.) and exposure to aflatoxin, a product of *Aspergillus flavus* which can contaminate stored grain.

Pathology

Hepatocellular carcinomas arise from liver cells and may be unifocal, multifocal or diffuse. Males are affected more often than females. They range from well-differentiated tumours to anaplastic carcinomas, which may be difficult to identify as liver cells. The well-differentiated tumours grow in trabeculae or cords and may form glandular structures. The fibrolamellar variant occurs in a younger age group (20–40 years), is not associated with HBV or cirrhosis, and has a better prognosis than conventional hepatocellular carcinoma.

The tumour is particularly common in South East Asia and Africa and it is believed that a combination of HBV infection, exposure to aflatoxin, and genetic predisposition combine to produce the high incidence. The HBV infection is often due to vertical transmission, resulting in a very high risk of carcinoma by adulthood.

Patients either present with symptoms and signs related to cirrhosis or due to non-specific symptoms such as abdominal pain, weight loss and general malaise. Occasionally, gastrointestinal bleeding due to varices is the presenting symptom.

Although raised levels of AFP are detected in two-thirds of the patients, this is by no means specific for the disease, being also encountered in germ cell tumours, cirrhosis, liver cell necrosis and neural tube defects. However, it is a sensitive indicator of recurrence in treated patients. Serological markers of HBV infection are often present. Rarely, the tumour cells may secrete ectopic erythropoietin, causing polycythaemia*.

Management

Surgical resection of unifocal tumours may be possible. Infarction of tumour may also be attempted by cannulation of the supplying vessels and introducing beads to block the blood flow. The prognosis of hepatocellular carcinoma is poor. Immunization against HBV may be the best way to prevent the disease in areas with a high incidence of HBV infection.

 Cholangiocarcinoma; Cirrhosis

HEREDITARY ANGIOEDEMA: The commonest deficiency affecting the complement system, an autosomal dominant defect leading to absence of an inhibitor of the complement component C1s, which normally regulates inflammatory responses. Typically there are also low levels of C2 and C4, due to overactivation of the 'classical' pathway. There are recurrent attacks of swelling of subcutaneous and mucosal tissue, lasting a few days, which may lead to laryngeal or intestinal obstruction. Treatment includes various drugs that stimulate C1 inhibitor synthesis (e.g. danazol) or inactivate plasminogen (e.g. tranexamic acid).

HEREDITARY HAEMORRHAGIC TELANGIEC-TASIA: Also known as Osler–Weber–Rendu disease, this is an autosomal dominant inherited condition of small blood vessels characterized by multiple fragile superficial knots of capillaries, particularly on the mucous membranes of the mouth, nose, oropharynx and surrounding skin. These cause local bleeding problems, which may result in iron deficiency. Management is by local cauterization, a useful application of laser therapy.

HEREDITARY SPHEROCYTOSIS: An autosomal dominantly inherited deficiency of red cell membrane proteins spectrin or protein 4.1. Portions of red cell membrane are removed by the macrophages of the reticuloendothelial system, resulting in the formation of spherocytes (Fig. H7). The general features of haemolytic anaemia* will be present and the blood film shows similar appearances to warm autoimmune haemolytic anaemia*; however, the direct antiglobulin test is negative. Where there is doubt about the presence of sphero-

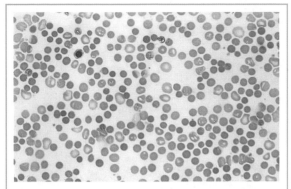

Fig. H7 Blood film in hereditary spherocytosis showing the majority of red cells are spherocytes.

cytes on the blood film, the osmotic fragility test can provide confirmation. In this test the red cells under investigation are suspended in different concentrations of hypotonic saline solution. Water will cross the semipermeable red cell membrane to dilute the contents of the red cell to the same osmotic pressure as the surrounding saline. Normal red cells can expand to accommodate the extra fluid but spherocytes will burst.

In vivo the spherocytes are destroyed in the spleen and splenectomy will usually correct the anaemia, though the blood film abnormalities persist.

HERPANGINA: Infection with Coxsackievirus A (types 1–10), B (types 2–5) and Echovirus 6, 9, 16, 17, which presents as a sore throat, fever and faucial ulcers.

HERPES SIMPLEX ENCEPHALITIS: Encephalitis caused by herpes simplex virus.

Case

A 50-year-old female complained of feeling generally unwell with a high temperature and a headache. On the following day her friend noticed a change in her behaviour and she had an epileptic seizure. On admission to hospital the patient was comatose. A CT scan and lumbar puncture were performed.

Microbiology: CSF clear with 300 WBC, predominantly lymphocytes; 100 erythrocytes; protein 0.6 g/l; glucose 4.1 mmol/l ; blood glucose 5.6 mmol/l
PCR: herpes simplex virus detected
Radiology: MRI scan showed features consistent with herpes simplex encephalitis (Fig. H8)

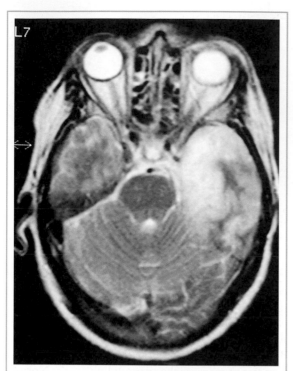

Fig. H8 CT scan shows evidence of a lesion in the left temporal lobe, which is consistent with herpes encephalitis. (Reproduced with permission from Curtis J, Whitehouse G. *Radiology for the MRCP*. London: Arnold, 1998)

The patient was started empirically on acyclovir pending the results of the lumbar puncture.

Aetiology and risk factors

Herpes simplex virus is a double-stranded DNA virus that comprises two strains, HSV-1 and HSV-2. The genome of herpesviruses in general consists of long and short unique sequences which have palindromes at each end. These unique sequences may be present in either orientation to yield four separate genomic arrangements. Genotypically, HSV-1 and HSV-2 have about 50% homology but are antigenically different. The viruses are transmitted by direct contact with oral secretions (HSV-1) or genital secretions (HSV-2). Transmission can be from an infected lesion or from an asymptomatic excretor. Binding and penetration of the herpesvirus is mediated by viral envelope glycoproteins (gp C, D and B) which attach to a cell surface receptor such as heparan sulphate.

Pathology

Viral replication occurs at mucocutaneous surfaces prior to entry of the virus into nerve axons and replication in sensory ganglia. The virus undergoes a lytic cycle, replicating within the cell nucleus and inducing the formation of characteristic intranuclear inclusions. Multinucleate giant cells may be

seen, caused by cell fusion induced by the virus as it buds from cell to cell. Local replication induces the formation of a vesicle containing oedema fluid, degenerate cells and free virus; accumulation of inflammatory cells to the area changes the vesicle to a pustule. Virally infected cells are killed by cytotoxic T-cells, via either necrosis or apoptosis. Primary infection is accompanied by a fever, sore throat, vaginal or urethral discharge, regional lymphadenopathy and painful vesicles at the site of inoculation. Subsequently, the virus enters the sensory nerves and remains latent in the sensory ganglia. Here the virus does not replicate but is maintained in a latent phase by viral mRNA, which inhibits viral replication. Reactivation of HSV may occur in response to a variety of stressful stimuli.

Herpes encephalitis, which characteristically affects the temporal lobes, may be a primary infection or may follow reactivation. Virus probably enters the CNS from the sensory trigeminal ganglia. Expression of intracellular adhesion molecules (e.g. ICAM-1) is increased in brain microvasculature by HSV and is responsible for the infiltration of the lesion by lymphocytes.

The symptoms of encephalitis are the result of necrosis of the nerve cells. Laboratory diagnosis may include:

- electron microscopy (although the herpes viruses look identical and thus VZV cannot be distinguished from HSV);
- histology, to demonstrate multinucleate giant cells with eosinophilic intranuclear inclusions;
- immunofluorescent stain of vesicle scrapings;
- culture;
- PCR.

Management

Treatment is with acyclovir or famciclovir.

HIDRADENITIS: Anaerobic or staphylococcal infection of the sweat glands, often with multiple draining sinuses.

HIRSCHSPRUNG DISEASE: Congenital megacolon arising as a result of the absence of ganglion cells within the muscle wall and submucosa of the bowel.

Aetiology and risk factors

The aetiology is unclear but the disease is associated with Down syndrome and with neurological abnormalities, suggesting a generalized defect of neural crest development.

Pathology

Hirschsprung disease is more common in males than females. The rectum is the main segment of the bowel affected by the disorder, but the proximal bowel may be affected to a variable extent. Absence of myenteric plexuses and hence ganglion cells leads to proximal dilatation and hypertrophy of the bowel. The colon may be massively dilated (megacolon). If the bowel wall becomes thin, there is a risk of bowel perforation.

The disease usually presents during the neonatal period because of a failure to pass meconium. Diagnosis is made on colonic biopsy using immunocytochemistry to demonstrate the lack of ganglion cells.

Management
Treatment is surgical, with removal of the aganglionic segment.

 Down syndrome

HISTIOCYTOSIS X:
An old term for Langerhans cell histiocytosis, which describes a group of proliferative disorders of histiocytic cells.

Aetiology and risk factors
The aetiology is unknown, although it is thought to represent a reactive proliferation due to defects in T-cell immunoregulation.

Pathology
Histiocytosis X has been subdivided into three categories, Letterer–Siwe syndrome, Hand–Schüller–Christian disease and eosinophilic granuloma, representing different expressions of the same disorder.

Letterer–Siwe syndrome occurs before the age of 2 years and the principal clinical feature is of cutaneous lesions affecting the trunk and scalp. Patients may also have enlargement of liver, spleen and lymph nodes. Destructive bone lesions may also be present. Involvement of the bone marrow leads to anaemia and thrombocytopenia with recurrent infections. Without treatment it is usually rapidly fatal.

Eosinophilic granuloma principally involves the medullary cavities of bones. A combination of histiocytes and eosinophils, together with other inflammatory cells, are present. Common sites of involvement include the ribs and femur. This variant of histiocytosis usually follows an indolent course and may resolve spontaneously. The Hand–Schüller–Christian variant of histiocytosis describes a combination of bone involvement, diabetes insipidus and exophthalmos due to a proliferation involving these sites. It may undergo spontaneous regression.

Management
Some forms of histiocytosis undergo spontaneous regression but chemotherapy and radiotherapy may also be useful in treating these disorders.

HISTOPLASMOSIS:
A systemic infection with the fungus *Histoplasma capsulatum* or *Histoplasma duboisii*.

Aetiology and risk factors
Histoplasmosis is endemic in the central–southern half of North America and Africa, respectively. The fungus is inhaled as spores from the environment, typically bird or bat infected areas, where it is found in the soil.

Pathology
In the alveoli the spores replicate in the macrophages (Fig. H9).

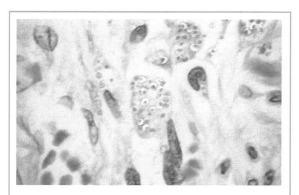

Fig. H9 Histoplasma in macrophages.

The yeast spreads from the lungs to the reticuloendothelium system and other areas of the body. Granulomata are formed at sites of localization and eventually become calcified. In a host who has contained the infection, waning CD4 T-cell levels can allow reactivation of disease. The disease may follow one of the following courses:
- remain asymptomatic
- an acute pulmonary infection resembling influenza
- a chronic pulmonary infection with cough, fever, weight loss and pulmonary cavitation resembling tuberculosis
- disseminated disease affecting the bone marrow, liver and spleen.

Disseminated disease presents with non-specific symptoms similar to chronic pulmonary disease although there may be focal signs and symptoms referable to local granuloma formation and tissue destruction, e.g. oropharyngeal ulceration, Addison disease*, or meningitis. Hepatosplenomegaly is common and the patient may be anaemic and pancytopenic. Alternatively, if the host response is ineffective, disseminated disease can present as an acute condition similar to endotoxic shock* with anaemia, pancytopenia and hepatosplenomegaly. Complications include pericarditis, erythema nodosum, choroiditis, mediastinal fibrosis and a histoplasmoma. Fibrosis of the mediastinum can lead to superior caval compression and the 'single coin' lesion of a histoplasmoma in the lungs has to be differentiated from a neoplasm.

In the African variety the most frequent presentation is skin and bone lesions, often with sinus formation. The cellular reaction is a combination of acute inflammation and granuloma leading to tissue destruction. The patients present with chronic ulceration of the skin and chronic discharging sinuses. Diagnosis is by histology, serology, (both antibody and antigen detection) and isolation of the fungus. Epidemiologically the skin test may be used. The treatment is usually amphotericin or itraconazole.

HIV: Human immunodeficiency virus(es), responsible for the acquired immunodeficiency syndrome (AIDS). Because of their tropism for T-lymphocytes, macrophages and other immunological cells, their main effects are on resistance to infection.

 Acquired immunodeficiency syndrome (AIDS)

HODGKIN DISEASE: A malignant proliferation of lymphoid tissue with characteristic histological and clinical features distinguishing it from other (non-Hodgkin*) lymphomas.

Case

A 17-year-old youth was referred to the surgical department after he noticed a swelling in the left side of his neck. On examination he had multiple enlarged rubbery nodes in the left anterior and posterior triangles and in the left supraclavicular fossa. On specific enquiry he admitted to a month's

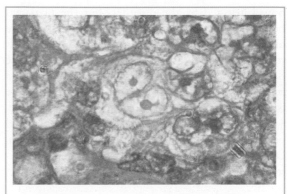

Fig. H10 The Reed–Sternberg cell is a giant cell, commonly binucleate, with prominent 'owl's eye' nucleoli.

history of drenching night sweats and his mother stated that he had lost weight over the last few months.

A cervical lymph node was biopsied under general anaesthetic. Histology demonstrated classical features of nodular sclerosing Hodgkin disease, including numerous Reed–Sternberg cells (Fig. H10).

Staging investigations were undertaken, including a CT scan of chest and abdomen, which demonstrated enlarged mediastinal and hilar lymph nodes (Fig. H11).

Blood count showed a mild normocytic anaemia (Hb 11 g/dl) and an increase in neutrophils, eosinophils and platelets. The ESR was considerably elevated (100 mm/h).

Aetiology and risk factors

The Reed–Sternberg and Hodgkin cells are the malignant cells of the disease though they are often

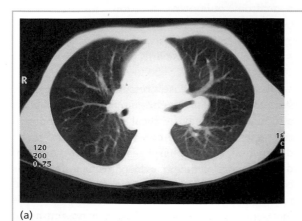

(a)

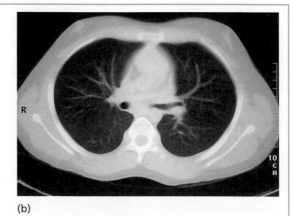

(b)

Fig. H11 CT scan of chest showing enlarged mediastinal and hilar lymph nodes at diagnosis (a) and after three cycles of treatment (b).

outnumbered by other cell types, particularly lymphocytes, macrophages, plasma cells and fibrous tissue. In most cases the Hodgkin cells can be shown to have Epstein–Barr virus incorporated in their genome. It is likely that the transforming effects of EBV, incompetently handled by a primitive lymphoid cell, are responsible for many cases of Hodgkin disease.

Pathology

Four basic histological types of Hodgkin disease are recognized, based on the type of cellular reaction to the Hodgkin cells. Most frequently there is a fibrous reaction to the presence of the Hodgkin disease tissue, resulting in broad bands of interlocking fibrous tissue dividing up the more cellular areas of the lymph node This is termed nodular sclerosing (NS) Hodgkin disease (Fig. H12).

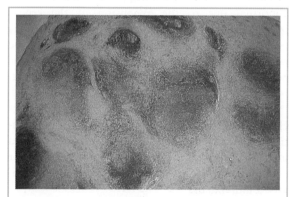

Fig. H12 Lymph node involved with Hodgkin disease. Nodular sclerosis subtype showing extensive fibrosis (pink material).

Sometimes this subdivision is further subdivided into type I and type II, depending on the morphology of the Hodgkin disease cells.

An alternative, but much rarer cellular reaction is the infiltration with large numbers of reactive lymphocytes found in lymphocyte-predominant (LP) Hodgkin disease.

Sometimes the degree of lymphoid infiltration may raise suspicion of a non-Hodgkin lymphoma*. Some lymphoid infiltration is usually present. When it is absent, the disease is classified as lymphocyte-depleted (LD) Hodgkin disease. As with most histological classifications of disease, intermediate forms exist, particularly mixed cellularity Hodgkin disease.

In general those subtypes associated with a cellular reaction around the Hodgkin disease cells – lymphocyte-predominant and nodular sclerosing variants – are associated with a better prognosis.

Table H2 Clinical staging of Hodgkin disease

Clinical stage	Involvement of
I	One anatomical lymph node group
II	Two or more lymph node groups on one side of the diaphragm
III	On both sides of the diaphragm
IV	Spread to non-lymphoid tissues such as liver or bone marrow

Clinical staging of Hodgkin disease

Hodgkin disease starts in a lymph node and spreads to other nodes in the anatomical group and then to surrounding groups. The clinical staging of Hodgkin disease includes clinical examination and CT scans of chest and abdomen. The clinical staging of Hodgkin disease into four groups is shown in Table H2. The spleen is classed as an honorary lymph node for the purposes of this classification.

Cytokines produced by the Hodgkin tissue result in a number of systemic symptoms, particularly fever, night sweats and weight loss. If these symptoms are present, the clinical staging number has the suffix B added, if they are absent then suffix A. Thus the patient described above is clinical stage IIB. Sometimes Hodgkin disease may spread from an involved lymph node directly into contiguous tissues such as lung. This situation is not considered as prognostically poor as spread to anatomically distant non-nodal tissue so is given the suffix E.

Management

Localized disease is treated by radiotherapy. More generalized disease is treated by combination chemotherapy. Which stages receive which modality of treatment varies between countries and institutions. The majority of cases are cured with modern management. Relapsed or refractory disease usually responds to high-dose chemotherapy with autologous stem cell rescue.

HOOKWORM INFECTION: Infection by one of the intestinal nematodes, e.g. *Ancylostoma duodenale*. They have a similar life cycle to *Strongyloides* spp. (see Strongyloidiasis). The worms attach to the intestinal mucosa by their mouthparts, causing local trauma, and feed on the blood from the host, leading to a microcytic hypochromic picture of iron-deficiency anaemia and hypoproteinaemia. There is a peripheral eosinophilia with low serum iron and elevated serum transferrin. The worms move to different locations in the intestine, the severity of symptoms depending on the worm burden. The patient presents with colicky abdominal pain, anaemia and oedema. A pulmonary eosinophilia syndrome is also produced as the larvae migrate through the lungs. Some species of nematode cannot complete the life cycle in the human host, e.g. the dog hookworm *Ancylostoma braziliensis*, and these give rise to a pruritic, erythematous serpiginous, migrating lesion as the larvae move through the skin (cutaneous larva migrans*). Laboratory diagnosis is by demonstration of the ova in the faeces and management is with oral iron or blood transfusion and albendazole or mebendazole.

HORMONE-SECRETING TUMOURS: See Ectopic hormone production.

HOSPITAL-ACQUIRED INFECTION: Also called nosocomial infection, an infection acquired by a patient whilst in hospital. There are several different definitions, mainly clinically based, but differing with respect to timing and the system under investigation.

Aetiology and risk factors
Overall, the hospital-acquired infection rate is about 10% in the UK. Organisms commonly associated with nosocomial infection are *Staphylococcus aureus*, *Staphylococcus epidermidis*, *Enterococcus faecalis*, *Acinetobacter calcoaceticus*, *Pseudomonas aeruginosa*, *Stenotrophomonas maltophilia*, *Klebsiella pneumoniae* and other members of the *Enterobacteriaceae*. Increasingly, these organisms are multi-antibiotic resistant. Predisposing factors are the abrogation of the normal defence mechanisms of the body by virtue of age, disease, or treatment such as chemotherapy, antibiotics, surgery or the use of endotracheal tubes, venous and arterial lines and urinary catheters. Patients in particular areas of the hospital such as the ITU, are commonly susceptible to nosocomial infection, and the commonest organ systems involved are the urinary tract, skin and respiratory tract. Infection may be with the patient's normal flora (endogenous infection) or by an organism acquired from the hospital environment (exogenous infection), the principal sources being another infected patient or a member of staff. Infection can be acquired directly by contact, via the air or food, or indirectly from some piece of contaminated equipment. Perhaps the most important vehicle of transmission is the hands of staff members. The elementary principles of prevention of hospital-acquired infection were laid down by Florence Nightingale and Ignatz Semmelweis, i.e. source isolation, an adequate distance between beds, and hand-washing. Because of medical advances since that era, an additional factor in the control of infection would be adequate disinfection or sterilization of medical equipment.

HUMAN PAPILLOMA VIRUS: See Cervical carcinoma.

HUNTINGDON DISEASE: A progressive neurodegenerative disease affecting patients between the ages of 20 and 50 years. The main pathological finding is loss of GABAergic neurons of the caudate nucleus of the basal ganglia. It is transmitted in an autosomal dominant fashion. Patients present with uncontrolled, jerky hyperkinetic movements and dementia. The CSF is normal.

The molecular basis of the disease is expansion of the trinucleotide CAG in exon 1 of a gene which has been localized to chromosome 4. The gene produces a protein, huntingtin, which becomes abnormal due to the expansion of the repeat sequences. The normal function of huntingtin has not been fully characterized, but it appears to be associated with the cytoskeleton and is required for neurogenesis. Accumulation of the abnormal protein leads to cell death.

HYALOHYPHOMYCOSIS: A term denoting infections with non-pigmented moulds commonly found in soil and causing skin, eye, sinus, subcutaneous or disseminated disease, usually in immunocompromised individuals.

HYDATID DISEASE: Disease caused by the tapeworms *Echinococcus granulosus* or *Echinococcus multilocularis*.

Aetiology and risk factors
These pathogens have a worldwide distribution with endemic foci in the UK. The normal transmission cycle is between sheep and carnivores, e.g. dogs, which harbour the adult worm in their intestine, shedding ova into the environment, where they are eaten by herbivores. Humans acquire the disease by direct transmission from infected dog faeces or by eating contaminated vegetables.

Pathology
In the intermediate host (sheep, human) the ova hatch into an oncosphere which penetrates the intestinal wall, entering the portal circulation and being carried to the liver or lungs. Occasionally they pass through the lungs to be disseminated to any organ in the body, e.g. brain, bone. The oncosphere, if not phagocytosed and destroyed by the host, develops into a cyst containing scolices from which adult tapeworms can develop if ingested by

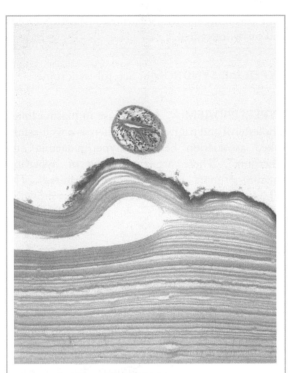

Fig. H13 Scolex of hydatid in cyst.

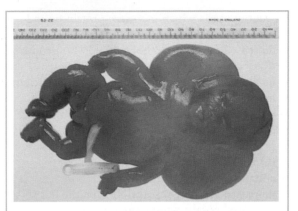

Fig. H14 Eighteen weeks old hydropic fetus with Turners syndrome. (Courtesy of R. Scott, UCLMS; reproduced with permission from Lakhani SR, Dilly SA, Finlayson CJ. *Basic Pathology*, 2nd edn. London: Arnold, 1998)

a carnivore (Fig. H13). The cyst slowly enlarges and may remain asymptomatic or present with signs of a space-occupying lesion, depending on the site of localization (e.g. a palpable abdominal mass, jaundice due to obstruction of the biliary system, epilepsy if localized in the brain, or cough and chest pain if in the lungs). Complications include erosion by the cyst into the gallbladder or bronchus, secondary infection with bacteria, or rupture into a viscus. If the cyst ruptures, an acute anaphylactic reaction can occur, due to sensitization to the cyst antigens. There is usually a peripheral eosinophilia and the cyst can be localized radiologically (plain radiograph, ultrasound or CT scan). Laboratory diagnosis is by serology and treatment is a combination of albendazole and surgery.

 Cysticercosis; Tapeworm infection

HYDATIDIFORM MOLE: A disorder characterized by cystic dilatation of the chorionic villi and with trophoblastic proliferation, following fetal death *in utero*. Its importance lies in the fact that is it a precursor of choriocarcinoma*.

HYDROPS FETALIS: A fetus with generalized oedema and ascites as a result of circulatory failure. There are numerous causes including cardiac malformations, chromosomal abnormalities (e.g. Down syndrome*), thoracic malformation (e.g.

diaphragmatic hernia), α-thalassaemia, fetal infections (e.g. toxoplasmosis and cytomegalovirus infection), and twin–twin transfusions (Fig. H14).

HYPERCALCAEMIA: Hypercalcaemia is used to describe the biochemical state of a patient's serum or plasma when the 'corrected' total calcium is > 2.62 mmol.

Aetiology and risk factors
There are a number of conditions that can raise the total serum calcium concentration:
- artefactual: hyperproteinaemia, dehydration, prolonged tourniquet application, hyponatraemia (< 120 mmol/l);
- endocrine: hyperparathyroidism, Addison disease, thyrotoxicosis, hypothyroidism, acromegaly, Cushing syndrome, phaeochromocytoma, VIP, MEN;
- malignant disease: breast carcinoma, lung carcinoma, renal carcinoma, Hodgkin lymphoma, non-Hodgkin lymphoma, multiple myeloma, adult T-cell lymphoma, Burkitt lymphoma;
- granulomatous disease: sarcoidosis, tuberculosis, mycoses, berylliosis;
- drugs: lithium, oestrogens, vitamin A toxicity, thiazide diuretics, milk-alkali (Burnett) syndrome;
- others: acute renal failure (polyuric phase), porphyria, hypophosphatasia, familial hypocalciuric hypercalcaemia, idiopathic hypercalcaemia of infancy and immobilization.

Pathology
The following mechanisms have been identified to help raise serum calcium in the body and are employed by the various conditions suggested:

H

- venous stasis which increases protein bound fraction of calcium;
- increased parathyroid hormone (PTH) production;
- increased renal tubular reabsorption of calcium;
- increased bone resorption;
- lytic bone disease;
- ectopic production of 1,25(OH)$_2$D;
- production of osteoclast-activating factors (OAFs), cytokines, PTHrP;
- enhanced sensitivity to PTH;
- increased calcium absorption from the gut;
- increased renal calcium absorption.

The resultant clinical effect of hypercalcaemia in the body is that of weakness, lassitude, weight loss, mental changes, nausea, vomiting, constipation, abdominal pain, polyuria, dehydration, renal calculi, renal failure, corneal calcification and short QT interval on ECG.

Management

Blood
Bone profile (calcium, albumin, phosphate, alkaline phosphatase)
Electrolytes and urea
Parathyroid hormone (PTH)
Thyroid hormones (T4, T3 and TSH)
Angiotensin-converting enzyme (ACE)
Protein electrophoresis
Vitamin D metabolites [1,25(OH)$_2$D, 25(OH)$_2$D]
Parathyroid hormone-related protein (PTHrP)
Bone marrow examination
Urine: calcium (24 hour)
Radiological: bone scan, chest radiograph

In patients with mild symptoms, improve oral rehydration (2–3 l/24 h). In patients with severe symptoms, give i.v. saline 3–4 litres over 24 hours. Calcitonin 100–200 units, 12-hourly s.c. and prednisolone 10–20 mg, 8-hourly p.o. are useful in the short term. Diphosphonates, mithramycin and phosphates can also be given but only by experienced medical staff.

HYPEREOSINOPHILIC SYNDROME: Increased numbers of eosinophils in the blood and bone marrow and their infiltration into tissues without evidence of preceding inflammation or allergy.

It affects mainly men between 20 and 50 years of age. Eosinophil infiltration is typically into the lungs (Loeffler syndrome), liver, spleen, central nervous system and the heart where it is associated with cardiomyopathy. Treatment is with steroids and/or hydroxyurea.

HYPER-IgE SYNDROME: See Job syndrome.

HYPERLIPIDAEMIA: An increase in plasma lipids (cholesterol and triglycerides). There is a well-established association between hyperlipidaemia and atheroma*. There are two types of hyperlipidaemia, primary and secondary (acquired). The WHO classification of hyperlipidaemia is shown in Table H3.

Table H3 WHO classification of hyperlipidaemia

Type	Lipoprotein abnormality	Major lipid abnormality
I	Chylomicrons	↑ Triglycerides
IIa	LDL	↑ Cholesterol
IIb	LDL, VLDL	↑ Triglycerides, cholesterol
III	IDL	↑ Triglycerides, cholesterol
IV	VLDL	↑ Triglycerides

Table H4 Causes of primary and secondary hyperlipidaemia

Primary hyperlipidaemia	Secondary hyperlipidaemia
Lipoprotein lipase deficiency (AR)	Hypothyroidism
Familial hypercholesterol-aemia (AD)	Nephrotic syndrome
Familial mixed lipo-proteinaemia (AD)	Diabetes mellitus
Familial type III hyper-lipidaemia (AR)	Systemic lupus erythematosus
Familial triglyceridaemia	Alcoholism
Familial combined hyperlipidaemia	Increased dietary fat Cholestasis Drugs: thiazides, oestrogens, β-blockers Obesity

AD, autosomal dominant; AR, autosomal recessive.

Table H4 shows the causes of primary and secondary hyperlipdaemia.

The clinical features of hyperlipidaemia are xanthelasmas (cholesterol deposits on the eyelid), premature arcus in the eye, xanthomas (cholesterol deposits in the skin and tendons). In some rare instances, pallor of small retinal vessels due to lipaemia retinalis is present.

Management

Management is usually with the use of lipid-lowering medication such as bile acid sequestrants, fibrates and HMG-CoA reductase inhibitors. In those patients with secondary hyperlipidaemia, treatment of the cause is the first line of action.

HYPERPARATHYROIDISM (PRIMARY): A condition caused by single or multiple parathyroid adenomas or by parathyroid hyperplasia.

Case

A 45-year-old woman complained of severe abdominal pain. Her past medical history showed that she had been treated for 'depression' and had suffered from bouts of abdominal discomfort, vomiting and constipation for the last 2 years. On examination, there were no abnormal findings. The following investigations were requested: a full blood count, electrolytes, urea, bone profile, liver profile, amylase and an abdominal radiograph. She returned the next day to the clinic. The significant findings were elevated serum calcium (corrected) of 2.85 mmol/l and a low serum phosphate of 0.65 mmol/l. A further group of investigations were requested which revealed a normal serum angiotensin-converting enzyme, normal thyroid function and a normal plasma parathyroid hormone (PTH).

An abdominal radiograph revealed that she had a renal calculus in her left kidney.

Aetiology and risk factors

This condition occurs in about one case per thousand persons. It occurs at any age, affecting both genders, but more commonly in women. It is usually caused by one of the following: adenoma, carcinoma or diffuse hyperplasia. The majority result from an adenoma, usually affecting one gland and often an incidental finding during laboratory screening.

Pathology

The excessive production of parathyroid hormone from the adenoma leads to an increase in serum calcium and a decrease in serum phosphate. Therefore patients may present with symptoms of hypercalcaemia*, although a large proportion present without symptoms.

The striking biochemical abnormalities in this patient are the elevated serum calcium, expected in patients with hyperparathyroidism, and the low phosphate level, a result of the phosphaturic action of PTH (not always seen). The normal serum PTH in this patient confirmed the diagnosis of hyperparathyroidism, since a normal individual with high serum calcium would have a suppressed PTH level. The serum alkaline phosphatase was increased in this patient, a finding seen in about a third of the patients with the condition.

The clinical symptoms are a reflection of the accumulation of calcium in the body. The neuropsychiatric symptom displayed in this patient was depression; gastrointestinal symptoms were vomiting and constipation. In this patient the abdominal pain was a result of renal colic from renal stones, which was identified on the plain abdominal radiograph. These stones usually contain calcium phosphate or calcium oxalate. Some patients experience severe bone pain, due to increased bone turnover and progressive loss of bone mineral. Patients with hyperparathyoidism are often wrongly diagnosed as having a malignancy or psychiatric condition.

Management

If treatment is required, surgical removal of the abnormal parathyroid gland is indicated.

HYPERSENSITIVITY: A general term for reactions or diseases due to undesired immune responses. The widely used Gell and Coombs classification subdivides it into five categories (see Table H5).

HYPERSPLENISM: Enlargement of the spleen, resulting in increased sequestration of white cells,

Table H5 Categories of hypersensitivity

Type	Principal mechanism(s)	Examples
I: Immediate	IgE; mast cell degranulation	Hay fever, penicillin allergy
II: Antibody-mediated; cytotoxic	IgG; complement, phagocytes	Rhesus incompatibility, transfusion reactions
III: Immune complex- mediated	Antigen–antibody complexes; neutrophils; macrophages	Post-streptococcal nephritis, systemic lupus erythematosus
IV: Delayed; cell-mediated	T-cells; cytokines	TB granuloma, transplant rejection
V: Stimulatory	Antibody to hormone receptors	Thyrotoxicosis

red cells and platelets. The spleen is normally responsible for the removal of blood cells at the end of their life span and this function is exaggerated as a result of hypertrophy of that organ. Any cause of splenomegaly may result in hypersplenism but significant sequestration of blood cells is only found when the spleen is palpably enlarged.

Causes of splenomegaly include cirrhosis* with portal hypertension, myelofibrosis, chronic congenital haemolytic anaemias*, chronic lymphoproliferative disorders, storage diseases such as Gaucher, and tropical splenomegaly.

HYPERTENSION: A persistently raised blood pressure in excess of 140/95 mmHg.

Case

A 45-year-old man was referred to a cardiologist for investigation of hypertension following a routine medical examination for life insurance.

He had no symptoms related to his hypertension, and no family history of heart disease. He smoked 20 cigarettes per day but did not consume alcohol. He was a director of an advertising agency and described his job as 'very stressful'.

On examination, he was overweight, weighing 102 kg. His blood pressure, using a large sphygmomanometer cuff, was 170/110, with a pulse rate of 100 beats/min. There were no other physical findings of note and in particular, there was no femoral delay in his pulse, there were no carotid or abdominal bruits, and his retina did not show evidence of papilloedema or haemorrhage.

He was sent for blood tests, ECG, chest radiograph and abdominal ultrasound. Routine haematological and biochemical investigations and 24-hour urinary vanillylmandelic acid (VMA) levels were all normal.

Abdominal ultrasound: normal kidneys and renal vessels. Adrenals normal.
ECG: sinus rhythm, 95 beats/min. Left ventricular hypertrophy. No evidence of left ventricular strain.

The cardiologist treated the man with an antihypertensive calcium antagonist. His follow-up was satisfactory initially and he was discharged to the care of his general practitioner. He subsequently defaulted and was lost to follow-up.

Four years later while sitting in a business meeting, he developed severe headache and collapsed. He was rushed to hospital but was dead on arrival. Resuscitation was unsuccessful. A postmortem examination was carried out.

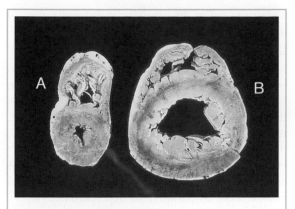

Fig. H15 Macroscopic appearance of the heart following severe hypertension. The section in (b) shows massive left ventricular hypertrophy compared to the section in (a).

Postmortem report: The body was that of a middle-aged man. No external findings of note. Internal examination showed an enlarged heart weighing 650 g. There was marked left ventricular hypertrophy (Fig. H15). The aorta and major vessels showed evidence of moderate atheroma. The lungs were heavy and oedematous and weighed 720 g and 750 g. Examination of the brain showed evidence of intracerebral bleed in the region of the middle cerebral artery due to rupture of a microaneurysm. The kidneys were slightly small and weighed 80 g and 90 g and showed evidence of ischaemic scarring.
Cause of death:
- 1a: intracerebral haemorrhage due to
- 1b: rupture of microaneurysm due to
- 1c: hypertension.
Associated with:
- 2: heart failure.

Aetiology and risk factors

A large proportion of hypertension is due to unknown causes, i.e. it is idiopathic. This is also sometimes called primary hypertension. Secondary hypertension may be a result of coarctation of the aorta, renal disease, endocrine abnormalities and in particular adrenal tumour (phaeochromocytoma*), or steroid therapy.

Pathology

The blood pressure normally varies as a physiological response to demands on the cardiovascular system. Hypertension refers to a persistent rise in blood pressure which remains high even at rest. It may cause no symptoms or may present with headaches and symptoms related to complications

H

including heart failure, cerebrovascular disease and renal ischaemia. It is not unusual for hypertension to be discovered incidentally during medical examinations for insurance purposes. It is a treatable disease either in primary and secondary form and an effort should be made to discover secondary causes. Idiopathic hypertension is unusual in young people, so it is important to rule out potentially treatable causes such as renal artery stenosis and phaeochromocytoma. If all potentially secondary causes have been ruled out, it is referred to as primary or idiopathic.

There are a number of treatment options and although some antihypertensive drugs have serious side-effects such as mood changes and impotence, it is possible to find suitable drugs for most patients. Failure of treatment compliance and uncontrolled hypertension can have serious long-term complications on the vascular, renal and cerebrovascular systems. Complications include left ventricular hypertrophy, atheroma and aneurysm formation, cardiac failure, myocardial infarction, retinal disease with papilloedema and haemorrhage, cerebrovascular haemorrhage and infarction, renal ischaemia and infarction. In this particular case, death was sudden and catastrophic due to rupture of microaneurysms in the brain. These occur in patients with hypertension and are called Charcot–Bouchard aneurysms.

With proper control of the blood pressure, many of these complications can be avoided or delayed for long periods.

Management
This is with antihypertensive medication. Additional and alternative approaches include weight reduction, reducing salt intake and relaxation techniques to reduce stress, including yoga. Whether these 'stress-relieving' methods are really useful is still debatable.

 Cerebrovascular disease; Myocardial infarction; Renal failure

HYPERTHYROIDISM: Overactivity of the thyroid, generally due to Graves disease (diffuse thyroid hyperplasia) but occasionally to toxic adenomata or nodules, or to anti-TSH antibody transferred from mother to neonate.

 Thyrotoxicosis

HYPERVISCOSITY: Abnormally viscous plasma or blood. Plasma hyperviscosity is a clinical syndrome of platelet-type bleeding, oedema, confusion and cardiac failure in association with a high plasma

viscosity. This is usually due to a high concentration of paraprotein in the blood, and is found in Waldenström disease and myeloma*. Both the concentration and type of immunoglobulin molecule are important, plasma viscosity being seen more frequently with IgM and IgA (large) molecules than with IgG (small) molecules.

Plasma viscosity may be simply measured by forcing a known volume of plasma through a narrow capillary tube under constant pressure and comparing the time for its passage with that of water. Normal plasma viscosity is approximately 1–2 mPa. In inflammatory conditions associated with increased levels of acute phase proteins such as fibrinogen in the blood, the plasma viscosity may be raised, but in plasma hyperviscosity syndrome results over 4 mPa are usually found.

Elevated blood viscosity may be due to an increased red cell count (polycythaemia*) or a grossly elevated white cell count, particularly found in chronic myeloid leukaemia*. However, the term hyperviscosity syndrome is usually reserved for plasma hyperviscosity. Blood transfusion should be avoided, if possible, in patients with plasma hyperviscosity, as increasing the red cell count and haematocrit may elevate whole blood viscosity and precipitate circulatory failure.

Plasma exchange is an effective treatment for plasma hyperviscosity. Often the removal of as little as a litre of plasma can make a significant difference to viscosity as the graphical relationship between plasma viscosity and paraprotein concentration is not linear.

HYPOGAMMAGLOBULINAEMIA: Decreased serum antibody levels leading to increased susceptibility to infection; patients with hypogammaglobulinaemia usually suffer from pyogenic infection. The cause is usually a genetic defect of B-cells which fail to develop into plasma cells, but it can also be acquired, particularly in low-grade B-cell lymphoproliferative disorders. It is treated with human gammaglobulin injection.

 Antibody deficiency; Immunodeficiency

HYPOPARATHYROIDISM: The result of low or absent secretion of parathyroid hormone from the parathyroid glands.

Aetiology and risk factors
Hypoparathroidism may be congenital or acquired. Acquired causes include: accidental removal of the parathyroid glands during neck surgery, autoimmune disease (a rare disorder with slight female predominance, associated with other autoimmune

diseases), infiltrative conditions and hypomagnesaemia (severe decrease in magnesium blocks parathyroid hormone release from the parathyroid glands). The congenital causes include congenital absence, which occurs when there is failure of the third and fourth branchial arches in development, and is associated with thymic agenesis and deficiency of cellular immunity in Di George syndrome*. There is also a rare inherited disorder (pseudohypoparathyroidism) characterized by a lack of end-organ response to parathyroid hormone. There are normal serum parathyroid hormone levels but no response, as a result of abnormal binding of parathyroid hormone to its target receptors.

Pathology
Hypoparathyroidism is characterized by low serum calcium (ionized) giving rise to paraesthesia, tetany, convulsions (in children) and laryngeal spasm. Muscular contractions such as Trousseau's sign and Chvostek's sign are seen. Ocular changes include cataract and papilloedema. Calcification in the basal ganglia and other soft tissues also occur. The lack of renal excretion of phosphate due to deficient parathyroid hormone results in increased levels of serum phosphate. Alkaline phosphatase levels are normal.

Management
Treatment consists of correction of the abnormality where possible, with the administration of vitamin D analogues and adequate calcium intake and, if necessary, magnesium replacement.

HYPOTHYROIDISM: A condition occurring as a result of underactivity of the thyroid gland itself (primary hypothyroidism) or from hypothalamic–pituitary disease (secondary hypothyroidism).

Case
A 55-year-old woman presented in the outpatient clinic with a history of increasing tiredness. She reported that she had been active until about 5 years ago when she realized she just wanted to 'sit down and do nothing'. She had also noticed that she felt the cold more than others around her and some of her friends said she seemed to have aged quickly. Examination of her notes revealed that she had been diagnosed as depressed 4 years ago and placed on antidepressants. On clinical examination her hair was coarse and her eyebrows were thinning (Fig. H16). Clinical examination revealed a full abdomen, a pulse rate of 50 beats/min (bradycardia) and slowing of the ankle tendon reflexes.

A thyroid screen was requested in addition to routine biochemistry and haematological tests.

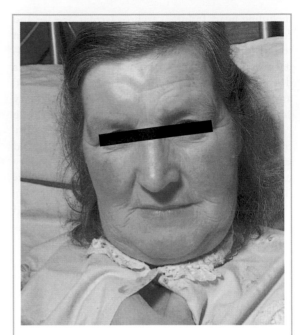

Fig. H16 A patient with hypothyroidism. Note thinning of the hair, loss of outer third of eyebrows, 'peaches and cream' complexion, thickening and heaviness of the eyelids. (Reproduced from Browse NL. *An Introduction to the Symptoms and Signs of Surgical Disease*, 3rd edn. London: Arnold, 1997)

The biochemistry test results revealed normal electrolytes, urea and creatinine concentrations. Her thyroxine (TT4) was 48 nmol/l (low) and TSH was 50 mU/l. Haematology test results revealed a normocytic anaemia.

Aetiology and risk factors
Primary hypothyroidism is the commoner form, and may be congenital, due to defects of hormone synthesis (iodine deficiency, dysmorphogenesis, antithyroid drugs), or to autoimmunity, infection, or a tumour, or may result from surgery or irradiation. In practice, about 95% of cases are autoimmune. Secondary hypothyroidism is rare and may be due to hypopituitarism or isolated TSH deficiency.

Pathology
As in the case described, the lack of adequate circulating thyroid hormones results in a reduction of physiological mechanisms (cellular metabolism, protein synthesis, potentiation of β-adrenergic effects and insulin antagonism) producing a reduction in metabolic rate and activity, slow reflexes, constipation, bradycardia, coarse brittle hair, and cold intolerance. In addition, patients with hypothyroidism may have myxoedema (accumulation of

mucopolysaccharides in face and extremities – Fig. H16). In some patients, psychotic manifestations are evident and they have psychomotor retardation; this patient had a history of depression. Anaemia (normochromic, normocytic) is sometimes a feature, due to decreased erythropoiesis. Hypothyroid patients may also have pleural or pericardial effusions and increased cholesterol levels.

The diagnosis of hypothyroidism is based on a reduced serum level of the thyroid hormones T3 and T4. However, these may fall only in extreme hypothyroidism; therefore, the most sensitive test in primary hypothyroidism is an elevated TSH concentration. In secondary hypothyroidism, the TSH is low. It is also important to test for thyroid autoantibodies; however, they are probably not responsible for the pathology, with the exception of the thyroid-stimulating antibodies.

Management
This is based on replacing thyroid hormones, using thyroxine, measuring the TSH to monitor treatment. Care should be taken with patients with heart failure. T3 replacement is used in some patients.

IDIOPATHIC THROMBOCYTOPENIC PURPURA (ITP): A low platelet count due to autoimmune peripheral platelet destruction.

Case

A 44-year-old housewife and cleaner was referred from the gynaecology department with a 3-month history of menorrhagia, nosebleeds and bruising. There was no significant previous medical history but she took an average of four Anadin tablets a week for migrainous headaches. On examination she was noted to be pale, with bruising of both thighs and venepuncture sites. The gynaecologist had found the following blood count:

WBC 4.6 × 10⁹/l
RBC 3.58 × 10¹²/l; Hb 9.4 g/dl; Hct (ratio) 0.294
MCV 82 fl; MCH 26.3 pg
MCHC 32.0 g/dl; RDW 12.9 %

The blood film confirmed the thrombocytopenia and the minor red cell changes of polychromasia and hypochromia considered to be compatible with a haemorrhagic anaemia. Bone marrow aspirate was performed which showed megakaryocytes to be increased in number, with normal morphology. There was modest increase in erythroid cells and absent iron stores in keeping with chronic haemorrhage. A diagnosis of idiopathic thrombocytopenic purpura was made.

Aetiology

Although most cases of idiopathic thrombocytopenia are autoimmune, they are usually described as 'idiopathic' as it is difficult to perform the necessary immunological tests to prove an immune basis for the disorder. The patient's platelets can be labelled with a fluorescent antiglobulin reagent and analysed by flow cytometry to demonstrate that they are coated with autoantibody, but if the patient is severely thrombocytopenic then impractically large amounts of blood may be required for the test. The patient's plasma can be allowed to react with test platelets from normal individuals, but these test platelets may lack the antigens present on the patient's own platelets and in any case free antiplatelet antibody may not be present in the patient's plasma. For these reasons ITP is usually a diagnosis of exclusion in cases of peripheral platelet consumption, although it is the commonest cause of thrombocytopenia*.

Immune destruction of platelets may be associated with other disease processes. Particularly in children, it may follow viral infections, including glandular fever*. There is an association with chronic HIV infection and acquired immunodeficiency syndrome (AIDS)* and this should be considered when taking the history as the immunosuppressive management of the ITP may require modification in the context of HIV.

Like most autoimmune processes, ITP is commoner in women, and is associated with systemic lupus erythematosus*. The presence of antinuclear factor antibodies should be sought in every case, as SLE is a multisystem immune disease requiring treatment of more than the platelet count. A drug history is important, as some drugs are associated with immune platelet destruction, particularly quinine (often prescribed for night cramps in the elderly) and its relative, quinidine, used in the treatment of cardiac arrhythmias.

Although the spleen may be slightly enlarged in some cases of ITP, if this organ is clinically palpable then the thrombocytopenia is likely to be due to a disease other than ITP.

Pathology

The symptoms are those of platelet-type bleeding into skin (purpura*), and mucous membranes, as described in the case above. Because the circulating platelets in ITP are mostly young and have a good haemostatic ability, bleeding manifestations may be surprisingly few until the platelet count drops below 20 × 10⁹/l (normal 140–500 × 10⁹/l). Trauma and operation will be associated with increased risk of haemorrhage. Aspirin and the non-steroidal anti-inflammatory drugs may severely impair platelet function, worsening bleeding in ITP. Anadin, in the case history given above, is a proprietary compound preparation containing aspirin.

Cytology

The blood count will usually be normal in ITP except for the thrombocytopenia. Sometimes, if significant haemorrhage has occurred, there may be a haemorrhagic anaemia*, as in the case described above. Chronic haemorrhage may lead to the microcytic, hypochromic anaemia of iron deficiency. The red cell morphology should be carefully examined for the presence of helmet cells and red cell fragments seen in thrombotic thrombocytopenic purpura*, haemolytic uraemic syndrome* and disseminated intravascular coagulation*. Blood film examination allows artefactual thrombocytopenia due to EDTA-induced platelet clumping to be excluded. The platelets found in the circulation in ITP are relatively young and therefore large. Staining for RNA and analysis by flow cytometry will show an increase in reticulated platelets.

Bone marrow aspirate will show normal or increased numbers of megakaryocytes, but this investigation gives only a rough indication of megakaryocyte numbers. A bone marrow trephine biopsy improves the quantification of megakaryocytes but is associated with an increased risk of bleeding from the biopsy site and results are not available for a few days. There may be increased numbers of young, immature, small, megakaryocytes. Most importantly, bone marrow biopsy will fail to reveal any significant marrow disease which may be a cause of the thrombocytopenia, such as leukaemia*, myelodysplasia or bone marrow infiltration.

Management

Many cases of ITP are discovered accidentally as a result of blood counts done for health screening or other purposes. If the platelet count is over 100×10^9/l, no treatment is indicated. At levels below 50, particularly if bleeding symptoms are present, immunosuppression is appropriate. The initial treatment is with steroids. If these fail, splenectomy improves the condition in about two-thirds of patients, but places the patient at slightly increased risk of septicaemia with capsulated organisms such as *Pneumococcus* and *Haemophilus influenzae* unless prophylactic long-term penicillin and appropriate immunizations against these organisms are given. Alternative immunosuppressants such as azathioprine may help in some cases.

High doses of intravenous immunoglobulin will produce a temporary improvement in the platelet count in the majority of patients. This will allow recovery from a haemorrhagic emergency or cover a surgical procedure such as splenectomy.

It is best to avoid transfusion of platelet concentrates except in haemorrhagic emergency, as they will be destroyed in a similar fashion to the patient's own platelets and may also sensitize the patient against donor HLA antigens, making them refractory to future random platelet transfusions. Treatment with aspirin and NSAIDs should be avoided in view of their antiplatelet action.

IgA NEPHROPATHY: Also called Berger disease, this is a form of focal glomerulonephritis presenting as haematuria linked to infections and strenuous exercise.

It usually presents as recurrent episodes of macroscopic haematuria following upper respiratory tract infections or strenuous exercise, mainly affecting older children and young adults. Unlike post-streptococcal glomerulonephritis, there is usually a shorter time period between infection and haematuria. Acute nephritis, hypertension and nephrotic syndrome are infrequent forms of presentation. Renal biopsies show focal glomerulonephritis* with focal and mesangial proliferation and prominent deposits of IgA and complement (Fig. I1). There is a strong association between IgA nephropathy and HLA-DR4. The source of IgA is thought to be an abnormal immune response to invading microbes at mucosal surfaces.

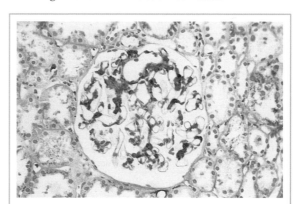

Fig. I1 Glomerulus showing granular deposition of IgA in the capillary loops. This is detected using enzyme-labelled anti-IgA and standard immunohistochemical methodology.

IMMUNE COMPLEX DISEASE: A general term for type III hypersensitivity* diseases, usually associated with antibody responses to persistent antigenic stimulation, which may be exogenous (e.g. serum sickness; post-streptococcal nephritis) or endogenous (such as DNA). For reasons that are not fully understood, antigen–antibody complexes in these conditions become trapped in small blood vessels, particularly of the kidney and skin, instead of being phagocytosed as usual.

IMMUNIZATION: The induction of protective immunity against a particular ('specific') infection. Immunization may be active, using an antigen or antigens from the infecting organism to induce specific T- and/or B-cell memory, or passive, using preformed antibody to transfer immunity.

Table I1 Current immunization practice

Disease	Type of vaccine	Normal administration
Tetanus	Toxoid	3 doses, 2–6 months
Diphtheria	Toxoid	3 doses, 2–6 months (with tetanus)
Pertussis	Killed bacteria	3 doses, 2–6 months (with tetanus)
Polio	Killed or attenuated virus	3 doses, 2–6 months
Measles	Attenuated virus	2 doses, 12–18 months
Mumps	Attenuated virus	2 doses, 12–18 months
Rubella	Attenuated virus	2 doses, 12–18 months
Tuberculosis	Attenuated bacteria (BCG)	10–14 years (at birth in tropics)
Hepatitis B	Recombinant HBV antigen	3 doses
Hepatitis A	Killed virus	Travellers to endemic areas
Yellow fever	Attenuated virus	Travellers to endemic areas
Typhoid	Killed bacteria	Travellers to endemic areas
Cholera	Killed bacteria	Travellers to endemic areas
Rabies	Killed virus	Post-exposure; high risk
Meningitis	Polysaccharide	Travellers; epidemics
Pneumococcal pneumonia	Polysaccharide	High risk; elderly
Haemophilus	Polysaccharide	1 year
Influenza	Killed virus	High risk; elderly
Varicella	Attenuated virus	High risk; immunocompromised

Table I2 Some examples of passive immunization

Disease	Source of antiserum	Normal administration
Tetanus	Immune human; horse	Post-exposure
Diphtheria	Immune human; horse	Post-exposure
Rabies	Immune human	Post-exposure + vaccine
Varicella	Immune human	Immuno-compromised
Snakebite		Post-exposure
Hypogamma-globulinaemia	Pooled human	Monthly

Immunodeficiency diseases are classified into two major groups. **Primary** immunodeficiency diseases result from a disorder intrinsic to the immune system, usually manifest themselves in early childhood, are of genetic origin (i.e. congenital) and are rare. **Secondary** immunodeficiency diseases arise due to influences external to the immune system, e.g. infections themselves, immunosuppressive drugs or ongoing disease processes, and are relatively common. These are often called acquired immunodeficiency diseases.

Primary defects can occur in both the natural (phagocytes and complement) and adaptive immune systems (B- and T-cells) (see Table I3).

Table I3 Primary immunodeficiencies

Stem cell deficiencies
  Reticular dysgenesis

Phagocytic deficiencies
  Chronic granulomatous disease (CGD)
  Leucocyte adhesion deficiency (LAD)
  Chediak–Higashi syndrome

Complement deficiencies
  Deficiencies of most complement components and C1 inhibitor deficiencies

T-cell deficiencies
  Severe combined immunodeficiency (SCID)
  Di George syndrome
  Nezelof syndrome
  Ataxia telangiectasia
  Wiskott–Aldrich syndrome
  'Bare' lymphocyte syndrome

B-cell deficiencies
  X-linked agammaglobulinaemia
  Common variable immunodeficiency
  IgA deficiency
  IgG subclass deficiency
  Immunodeficiency with increased IgM
  Transient hypogammaglobulinaemia of infancy

Active immunization, sometimes called vaccination, is given routinely for some infections, and in special circumstances for others, as shown in Table I1. Several others, not listed, are still on trial (e.g. HIV, *E. coli*, leprosy, malaria). Note that, whilst living attenuated vaccines are usually more potent, they cannot be given to immunocompromised individuals.

Passive immunization is used mainly post-exposure, when there is no time for active immunity to develop (Table I2).

IMMUNODEFICIENCY: The failure or absence of effective immune system components or responses, leading to an increased susceptibility to infection.

In general, the type of infection in an immuno-deficient patient reflects the particular cell type(s) or molecule(s) which are defective. Thus defects in B-cells (i.e. antibody), complement or phagocytes would be more likely to result in infection with encapsulated (pyogenic, pus-forming) bacteria. On the other hand, defects in T-cell immunity lead to infections which are ubiquitous and to which we normally develop good immunity. These 'opportunistic infections'* include a variety of fungi, viruses and intracellular bacteria. The cellular and molecular bases of the primary deficiencies are described under the separate disease entries. The causes of acquired immunodeficiency diseases are listed in Table I4.

Table I4 Major causes of secondary immunodeficiencies

Malnutrition
  Protein, calorie, elements such as zinc and iron

Loss of components of the immune system
  Antibodies – burns, nephrotic syndrome
  Lymphoid cells – intestinal telangiectasia

Immunosuppression caused by:
  Drugs: cytotoxic drugs used to treat tumours, to prepare for transplants, and treat patients with chronic inflammation, e.g. corticosteroids, cyclophosphamide, azathioprine, cyclosporin, methotrexate
  Infections: malaria, measles, HIV
  Tumours: many tumours produce immunosuppressive substances, e.g. cytokines
  Stress: there is good evidence for a role of stress hormones in immunity

Management
Apart from antibiotics where appropriate, the most effective form of treatment is pooled gammaglobulin for antibody deficiencies*. Bone marrow transplantation has been successful for many of the primary immunodeficiencies. A few cases of T-cell deficiency have been treated with thymus grafting. Vaccination with live vaccine preparations is highly dangerous in T-cell deficiency. In secondary immunodeficiency, treatment is directed at the underlying cause.

INFARCTION: Death of tissues by necrosis as a result of vascular insufficiency, resulting from e.g. atheroma, thrombosis or embolism.

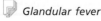 *Myocardial infarction*

INFECTIOUS MONONUCLEOSIS: Caused by Epstein–Barr virus, also called glandular fever.

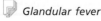 *Glandular fever*

INFLAMMATION: The mechanism by which the body deals with an injury or insult.

Aetiology and risk factors
Causes of inflammation include mechanical injuries, ischaemic damage, infection with bacteria, viruses, fungi and parasites, injuries due to exposure to chemicals, extremes of temperature, radiation injury and injury sustained secondary to immunological mechanisms.

Pathology
Inflammation is divided into acute and chronic types. The cardinal features of inflammation include redness (rubor), heat (calor), swelling (tumor), pain (dolor) and usually some loss of function. The pathology underlying these features is based on vasodilatation, which causes the redness and heat. The swelling is caused by increased permeability of the vessels leading to formation of an inflammatory exudate. Pain noted during inflammation is possibly a result of tissue distension and production of chemical mediators.

Acute inflammation The principal mediators of acute inflammation are the arachidonic acid-derived prostaglandins and leukotrienes, mast-cell derived products such as histamine, and the complement and kinin systems. The principal cells of acute inflammation are the polymorph leucocytes. There are also systemic effects, for example the increase in acute phase proteins and fever. Acute inflammation may resolve, or it may become chronic. Examples of acute inflammation include acute appendicitis and lobar pneumonia.

Chronic inflammation Chronic inflammation differs from acute inflammation in that it is more prolonged and the chief cells involved are the lymphocytes, macrophages and plasma cells. There is also formation of granulation tissue with development of new blood vessels and fibroblasts with resultant fibrous scarring. Granulomatous inflammation is a specific type of chronic inflammation in which granuloma formation occurs. A granuloma is a collection of macrophages, sometimes with a rim of lymphocytes around them. Examples of chronic inflammation include chronic peptic ulceration and tuberculosis.

Management
Management is of the underlying condition and of the symptoms and signs of inflammation.

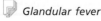 *Appendicitis; Bronchopneumonia; Pneumococcal pneumonia; Rheumatoid arthritis; Sarcoidosis; Syphilis; Tuberculosis*

INFLAMMATORY BOWEL DISEASE: Chronic inflammatory damage of unknown aetiology. The term is principally used in relation to Crohn disease* and ulcerative colitis*.

INFLUENZA: A respiratory illness caused by the influenza or parainfluenza virus. The term is also commonly used to indicate an infection with one of the other respiratory viruses (rhinovirus, coronavirus, adenovirus) causing a common cold, with coryza, nasal congestion, and sore throat. There is little viraemia with these viruses and the local symptoms are caused by the release of local inflammatory mediators such as bradykinin.

Aetiology and risk factors

The influenza virus is represented diagrammatically in Fig. I2.

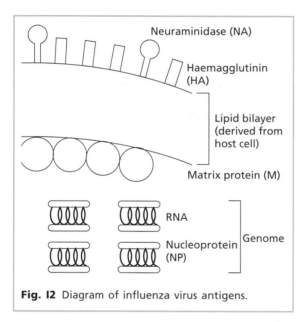

Fig. I2 Diagram of influenza virus antigens.

Influenza characteristically occurs in epidemics or pandemics. There are three main types of influenza virus, A, B and C, based upon the nucleoprotein (NP). The other principal antigens of the virus are the haemagglutinin (H1, H2, H3...) and neuraminadase (N1, N2...). The former is important for adhesion of the virus to the host cell receptor whereas the latter aids the adhesion process by removing sialic acid from respiratory mucus, preventing viral aggregation; it may also be involved in release of the virion from the host cell. Important antigenic variation occurs in both these molecules, particularly in influenza A, but also to some extent in B. Influenza viruses are designated by the type, the origin of isolation, the strain, the year of isolation, and the haemagglutinin (H) and neuraminidase (N) types, e.g. H5N1. Antigenic shift refers to major changes in H or N due to

hybridization of the human with animal viruses, usually in the Far East. This produces new combinations of antigens, and its appearance correlates with pandemics as the global population have no immunity. Antigenic drift refers to minor changes in H or N that occur more frequently, with some reduction in effective immunity.

Pathology

Infection with the influenza virus causes a viraemia and release of interferons, giving rise to the systemic symptoms of malaise, fever, headache and myalgia. The influenza virus also replicates locally in the respiratory epithelium, causing necrosis of ciliated cells and disrupting mucus clearance, resulting in pharyngitis, coryza and nasal congestion similar to the other respiratory viruses. In children influenza virus can also cause croup (laryngotracheitis, principally caused by parainfluenza virus) and in immunocompromised patients, particularly, influenza virus can cause pneumonia. Complications of influenza include secondary bacterial pneumonia, myocarditis, Reye syndrome and the Guillain–Barré syndrome*. Laboratory diagnosis is by serology or viral isolation and management is symptomatic or with amantadine. Prevention is by a killed vaccine, but its effectiveness is limited by the antigenic variation mentioned above, and it is currently only used in high-risk patients.

INHERITED METABOLIC DISEASE (IMD): An inherited condition due to absence or modification of a specific protein as a result of an enzyme defect in a metabolic pathway. Most such conditions have an autosomal mode of inheritance.

Some inherited metabolic disorders are:
- amino acid disorders: maple syrup urine disease, tyrosinaemia type I, homocystinuria, phenylketonuria;
- urea cycle disorders: carbomoyl phosphate synthetase deficiency, ornithine carbomoyl transferase deficiency, citrullinaemia, arginosuccinic acidaemia;
- organic acid disorders: methylmalonic acidaemia, propionic acidaemia, isovaleric acidaemia, glutaric aciduria type II, fatty acid oxidation defects;
- carbohydrate disorders: galactosaemia, glycogen storage disease type I, fructose-1,6-diphosphate deficiency, hereditary fructose intolerance;
- congenital lactic acidosis: phosphoenolpyruvate carboxykinase deficiency, pyruvate carboxylase deficiency, electron transport chain defects;
- peroxisomal disorders: Zellweger and pseudo-Zellweger syndromes, neonatal adrenal leucodystrophy;

- purine and pyrimidine disorders: sulphite oxidase and xanthine oxidase deficiency, adenosine deaminase deficiency;
- lysosomal storage disorders: GM1 gangliosides, Niemann–Pick disease type C, Krabbe leucodystrophy, Wolman disease, Pompe disease;
- others: Menkes syndrome, congenital adrenal hyperplasia.

Pathology

Symptoms usually develop within the first week of life after milk feeding is initiated. The biochemical basis of these disorders is wide-ranging, most of the clinical symptoms and signs occurring as a result of a lack of an enzyme involved in the synthesis of a product. This produces a decreased formation of the product, an accumulation of the substrate and increased formation of other metabolites.

The diagnosis of some of these disorders may be suggested by certain features from the clinical examination, e.g.

- smell: sweet and sickly smell (amino acid and organic acid disorders);
- cataract: galactosaemia;
- hyperventilation: as a result of metabolic acidosis (organic acid disorders);
- hyponatraemia: congenital adrenal hyperplasia;
- neurological deficits: urea cycle disoders;
- unexplained hypoglycaemia, hypocalcaemia, metabolic acidosis, and abnormal liver function tests are important pointers to the suggestion of IMD.

When IMD is suspected the initial important laboratory tests that need to be performed include:

- plasma ammonia
- plasma lactate
- urine and plasma amino acids
- urine organic acids

More recently, antenatal diagnosis of IMD can be done in high-risk families using fetal tissue obtained by chorionic villus biopsy. Specific enzyme measurements are made in cultured amniocytes and metabolites are measured in the supernatant. More specific tests are used for individual IMDs.

INTRACRANIAL HAEMORRHAGE: Bleeding within the intracranial cavity, usually within the brain substance itself and often due to vascular disease. Bleeding may also take place between the layers covering the brain, e.g. subarachnoid, subdural.

IRON-DEFICIENCY ANAEMIA: A microcytic hypochromic anaemia* due to iron deficiency.

Aetiology

Iron deficiency is the commonest cause of anaemia world wide. Most iron in the body is in red cells as haemoglobin, so blood loss has a frequent association with iron deficiency. In Western countries, bleeding associated with menorrhagia is the commonest cause; in developing countries, a combination of nutritional deficiency and blood loss associated with hookworm infection is frequent.

Increased requirements for iron such as in the growth spurt of childhood or repeated shortly spaced pregnancies may precipitate iron-deficiency anaemia in a person with borderline iron status. Because iron-deficiency anaemia may be a presenting feature of gastric or colonic carcinoma, which are associated with chronic blood loss, the cause of the iron deficiency should be carefully sought. Resection of the carcinoma before spread has occurred to other organs may be curative. Investigations such as faecal occult blood testing, gastroscopy and colonoscopy may be appropriate.

The most bioavailable form of iron is in red meat, so vegetarians and the poor who cannot afford meat are at increased risk of iron deficiency.

Pathology

The clinical features are mainly those of anaemia*. In addition, changes in nails and hair may be found, brittle, spoon-shaped nails (koilonychia) being characteristic but rare. As in megaloblastic anaemia patients may complain of sore mouths, painful splitting at the corners of the mouth (angular stomatitis) being most characteristic. Very rarely these mucosal changes may affect the oesophagus, with the formation of an oesophageal web (Plummer–Vinson syndrome).

Iron is required mainly for the manufacture of haem. In addition, iron acts as a coenzyme for several enzymes in the respiratory chain. This may explain the tiredness felt by patients with iron deficiency, which may be out of proportion to the degree of anaemia, particularly in polycythaemic patients who are treated by venesection and become iron deficient but with a normal haemoglobin level.

The blood count shows microcytic hypochromic anaemia with low MCV and MCH. Blood film confirms the count with pale staining red cells and some red cells having a cigar or pencil shape (Fig. I3) being characteristic. Sometimes target cells may be seen. The platelet count may be increased, even if the anaemia is due to nutritional anaemia rather than bleeding. The white cell count is usually normal.

The assessment of iron status

The differential diagnosis of a patient with iron deficiency includes thalassaemia* trait, sideroblastic

Fig. I3 Blood film in iron-deficiency anaemia showing hypochromic red cells and occasional pencil cells.

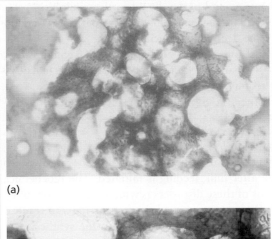

(a)

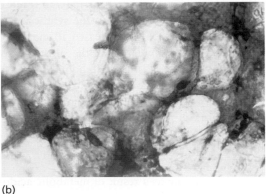

(b)

Fig. I4 (a) Bone marrow particles stained for iron. In iron deficiency no blue staining iron is found, contrasting to normal iron stores (b).

anaemia and the anaemia of chronic disease. Various measurements to confirm iron deficiency are available, all of which have their drawbacks:

- serum iron. This measurement will be low in iron deficiency and high in iron overload. False elevation of serum iron may be found if iron tablets are consumed on the day of the test. Low serum iron may be found in anaemia of chronic disease.
- total iron-binding capacity (TIBC). This serum measurement reflects transferrin levels in the blood, which are elevated in iron deficiency. May be falsely increased in pregnancy and oestrogen administration.
- transferrin saturation. This is calculated by dividing serum iron by TIBC. It provides a more informative measurement than either test done singly. The serum transferrin saturation is decreased in iron deficiency and increased in iron overload.
- serum ferritin. A major transport and storage form of iron this is reduced in iron deficiency and increased in iron overload. False elevations may be found in inflammatory illness, when ferritin acts as an acute phase reactant, and in hepatitis when ferritin is released from damaged liver cells.
- bone marrow aspirate with staining for iron using Perls stain (Fig. I4). This is probably the gold standard for assessing body iron stores, but too invasive for application in every case! It is possible to have absent iron stores but no anaemia if the iron from broken-down red cells is efficiently reused, but patients with iron deficiency will not have stainable iron in their bone marrow.
- transferrin receptor. Cells that require iron express increased amounts of transferrin recep-

tors. These may be detected in the plasma and are increased in iron deficiency. This is a relatively new test for the investigation of iron deficiency, but it shows promise.

There will be some patients in whom the diagnosis of iron deficiency remains in doubt despite the above investigations. In such cases it is justifiable to give a trial of oral iron for a few weeks to see if an improvement in haemoglobin level or MCV occurs. If no improvement occurs, iron should not be continued long term because of the risk of iron overload.

Management

Oral iron treatment will restore the haemoglobin levels to normal in the majority of cases. In the event of gastric intolerance or constipation/diarrhoea with oral iron, it is still usually possible to continue treatment with a lower dose. A good response to oral iron treatment is represented by an increment in haemoglobin level of 1 g/dl per week.

Parenteral iron is usually given by intramuscular injection and is painful. It may also stain the skin, so should be injected into the gluteal region rather than the arm. Treatment of the cause of the iron deficiency may also be required, for example hormonal regulation of menorrhagia.

ISCHAEMIA: Decrease in oxygen supplied to tissues due to vascular insufficiency.

ISOSPORIASIS: A gastrointestinal infection with *Isospora belli*, which appears to be principally a human pathogen. Development of the coccidian parasite occurs in the enterocytes following penetration by sporozoites, which undergo schizogony (asexual reproduction), becoming merozoites. Sexual reproduction produces oocysts, which are the infective form passed with the faeces. The organism principally affects the immunocompromised, e.g. AIDS patients, causing persistent diarrhoea. Laboratory diagnosis is by demonstration of the protozoa in the faeces and management is with co-trimoxazole, pyrimethamine or furazolidone.

J

JAUNDICE: a yellowish discoloration of the skin and sclera, which occurs as a result of deposition of excessive bilirubin (serum bilirubin >50 µmol/l).

Aetiology and risk factors

Jaundice can be classified into three types according to cause – haemolytic, hepatocellular or obstructive – or to the type of bilirubin that is present, i.e. conjugated or unconjugated.

The main causes of jaundice are:
- haemolytic: congenital spherocytosis, haemolysis, ineffective erythropoiesis;
- hepatocellular: Gilbert syndrome, prematurity, Crigler–Najjar syndrome, drugs, viral hepatitis, cirrhosis*;
- obstructive: Dubin–Johnson syndrome, Rotor syndrome, viral hepatitis, alcoholic liver disease, drugs, pregnancy, primary biliary cirrhosis*, gallstones*, bile duct stricture, carcinoma of the head of the pancreas, biliary atresia and sclerosing cholangitis.

Pathology

In haemolytic jaundice, increased bilirubin is delivered to the liver as a result of red cell breakdown, giving rise to an unconjugated hyperbilirubinaemia; as this is not water soluble it does not appear in urine. Laboratory tests' findings reveal a low haemoglobin, decreased haptoglobins, and increases in serum unconjugated bilirubin and urinary urobilinogen. Other liver function tests are usually normal.

In hepatocellular jaundice, the liver is the main cause (defective hepatic uptake of bilirubin and abnormal conjugation) and the excess bilirubin present is mainly conjugated. In the pre-icteric phase, the laboratory tests show an increase in serum AST, ALT, urinary bilirubin and urobilinogen. In the icteric phase that follows, the laboratory tests show an increase in bilirubin, AST and ALT. In addition, there is a moderate increase in the serum alkaline phosphatase and no urinary urobilinogen.

In obstructive jaundice, there is obstruction or impaired excretion of bilirubin (cholestasis*); the laboratory tests' findings are similar to those seen in the icteric phase of hepatocellular jaundice.

Management

Treatment is of the underlying condition.

JOB SYNDROME: A condition displaying repeated cutaneous infections similar to those of chronic granulomatous disease* but with normal neutrophil function, eosinophilia and raised IgE levels. It is probably identical to hyper-IgE syndrome.

JUVENILE CHRONIC ARTHRITIS: A spectrum of arthritic conditions with an onset before 16 years of age and with a duration of greater than 3 months; sometimes used to define a group of seronegative arthritides in children.

There are three subgroups of juvenile chronic arthritis (JCA):

Table J1 Subgroups of juvenile chronic arthritis

Subgroup	Systemic	Pauciarticular		Polyarticular
		Boys	Girls	
Age of onset	<5 years	Usually older	Young	Any age
Gender	M=F	–	–	F>>M
Clinical features	Systemic	Lower limbs esp. hips	Often large joints affected; chronic uveitis (50%) associated with ANA	Symmetrical arthritis of small joints
% Cases[†]	15		50	10
Other information	Protracted course	Family history; ANA negative, HLA-B27 positive in some with overlap with JAS	Occasionally severe	Severe in 15% of cases

ANA, antinuclear antibodies.
†Percentage of cases of all childhood arthritides.

- juvenile rheumatoid arthritis (JRA): a similar disease to that seen in adults and occurring in older children (mainly girls). It has the same HLA-DR4 associations as adult RA and can progress to extra-articular disease, including nodule formation and vasculitis. Patients are mostly positive for rheumatoid factor. This represents about 10% of JCA cases.
- juvenile ankylosing spondylitis (JAS): similar to adult AS with HLA-B27 associations; occurs in older boys; seronegative. The lower limb joints can be affected. JAS represents about 15% of JCA cases.
- juvenile chronic arthritis: the majority of the cases of childhood arthritis (75%) which are seronegative and are further divided into three subgroups according to their symptoms on presentation (Table J1).

The systemic form of the disease is closest to that originally described by Still and diagnosis is made clinically since there are no known HLA or serological associations.

Treatment of aggressive disease is with a combination of steroids and cytotoxic drugs such as chlorambucil. Overall treatment of chronic juvenile arthritis is symptomatic to relieve pain, prevent contractures and deformities, and encourage normal physical and emotional development. To this end, treatment includes physical therapy, drug treatments (NSAIDs) and corticosteroids for more aggressive treatment. Surgery may also be required to improve joint function.

 Juvenile rheumatoid arthritis; Rheumatoid arthritis; Seronegative arthritides; Still disease

JUVENILE RHEUMATOID ARTHRITIS: A similar disease to adult rheumatoid arthritis* with an onset prior to 16 years of age, representing about 10% of the cases of chronic arthritis in children. Girls are mainly affected, and patients are commonly seropositive for rheumatoid factor. The pathology is similar to that seen in the adult form of the disease.

K

KALA AZAR: Systemic infection with *Leishmania donovani*.

 Leishmaniasis

KAPOSI SARCOMA: A malignant neoplasm of blood vessels. It is associated with immunosuppression and in particular AIDS. It is believed to be due to the newly described herpes virus, HHV8.

KAWASAKI SYNDROME: A self-limiting disease of unknown aetiology characterized by an arteritis involving small and medium-sized arteries. It is associated with mucocutaneous lymph node syndrome. Children under 4 years of age are characteristically affected. It manifests with fever, oedema of hands and feet, skin rash, and enlargement of cervical lymph nodes. Patients may develop cardiac complications including coronary artery aneurysms and myocardial infarction.

 Arteritis; Myocardial infarction

KELOID: A raised scar in which there is excessive deposition of collagen.

Aetiology and risk factors
The aetiology remains unknown. Keloids are more common in black people than Caucasians. There appears to be a genetic susceptibility.

Pathology
The morphology of keloids is that of excess collagen deposition within the dermis during the healing process. Between the thick bands of collagen, there are fibroblasts and myofibroblasts running parallel to the collagen bundles. Scattered mast cells may also be present.

One of the commonest locations is the ear lobe (Fig. K1), although keloid may also occur at any site.

Management
Since the cause remains unknown, keloid is very difficult to treat. Surgical excision is sometimes carried out but may result in reformation of the keloid.

 Inflammation

KLINEFELTER SYNDROME: The commonest sex chromosome abnormality (47,XXY), occurring in 1 in 500–600 live male births.

It is caused by non-disjunction of the X chromosome in the mother of an affected child, producing a male child with an extra chromosome (47,XXY). There are a number of patients with this syndrome with more than two X chromosomes (48,XXXY or

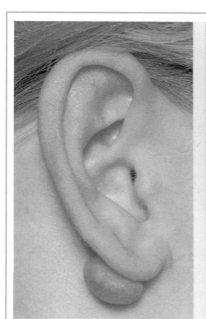
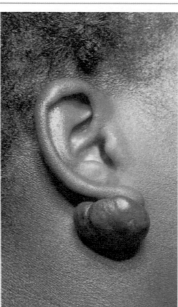

Fig. K1 Patients with keloid scars at the site of ear piercing. (Reproduced from Browse NL. *An Introduction to the Symptoms and Signs of Surgical Disease*, 3rd edn. London: Arnold, 1997)

49,XXXXY). The additional X chromosome disrupts the normal testicular development and the testes remain small and unable to produce spermatozoa. The patient is phenotypically male with tall stature, gynaecomastia, hypogonadism, and a low testosterone level (see Fig. C12, p. 58). Diagnosis is based on finding Barr bodies in buccal scrapings and karyotyping analysis.

KRUKENBERG TUMOUR: Bilateral metastasis to the ovary from a primary mucin-secreting gastric adenocarcinoma.

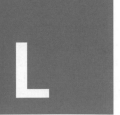

LAMBERT–EATON SYNDROME: A type of paraneoplastic syndrome* that arises in association with small cell carcinoma of the lung. Patients have proximal muscle weakness and autonomic dysfunction, producing a myasthenia-like syndrome.

LANGERHANS CELL HISTIOCYTOSIS: See Histiocytosis X.

LARYNGEAL CARCINOMA: A malignant neoplasm arising from the squamous epithelium of the larynx.

Aetiology and risk factors
These include smoking, alcohol, exposure to asbestos, infection with human papilloma virus (HPV), particularly type 16, and irradiation.

Pathology
Patients usually present with hoarseness of the voice. Approximately two-thirds of the tumours are confined to the larynx at the time of presentation. The tumours are squamous cell carcinomas and those arising from the vocal cords are generally well differentiated and have a slow rate of growth. They rarely metastasize. By contrast, those tumours arising above or below the vocal cords tend to be less well differentiated and behave more aggressively. Rarely, tumours arise from the mucus glands in the larynx and are therefore adenocarcinomas.

Management
Surgery is used to excise the tumour and radiotherapy is used to prevent recurrence. The patients are prone to infection and ulceration of the larynx and this may precipitate pneumonia.

 Lung carcinoma

LEGIONNAIRES DISEASE: A systemic disease caused by *Legionella* species, usually *Legionella pneumophila*, in which pneumonia is a major feature.

Case
A previously healthy 45-year-old man who smoked heavily was admitted to hospital with a diagnosis of pneumonia shortly after returning from a holiday abroad. The patient had received a 5-day course of amoxycillin from his GP with no effect on the clinical condition. The patient was pyrexial and complained of headache, dyspnoea and cough. Although he was producing some sputum, it did not appear purulent. Examination of the chest revealed crepitations and basal consolidation. A blood and sputum culture was taken, together with blood for serology, urine for *Legionella* antigens and routine urea and electrolytes, and a chest radiograph performed. The patient was started empirically on cefuroxime and erythromycin.

Microbiology:
- sputum culture – upper respiratory tract flora only;
- blood culture – no growth after 48 hours
- *Legionella* RMAT (rapid microagglutination test) positive.

Haematology: Hb 13 g/dl; RBC 4.2×10^{12}/l; WBC $14\,000 \times 10^6$/dl; polymorphs 80%; Plt 200×10^9/l.

Radiology: chest radiograph showed consolidation of both lower lobes.

Chemistry: Na 120 mmol/l; K 4.0 mmol/l; Cl 99 mmol/l; HCO_3 22 mmol/l; urea 10 mmol/l; creatinine 150 mmol/l.

Serology: *Legionella* antibody negative.

Whilst in hospital the patient became confused and his serum creatine increased even further.

Aetiology and risk factors
The *Legionellaceae* are Gram-negative rods comprising at least 40 different species. They are fastidious organisms that only grow on supplemented agar containing iron, cysteine and α-ketoglutarate. *Legionella* spp. produce many extracellular enzymes, e.g. esterases, haemolysins, although the role of these in the pathogenesis of disease is uncertain. The organisms are found naturally in biofilm associated with the freshwater aquatic environment where they are believed to exist as intracellular saprophytes in protozoa. They can also colonize the biofilm of water distribution networks, e.g. hot water calorifiers or shower heads. Infection is acquired by inhalation of contaminated aerosols. The commonest species causing infection is *L. pneumophila* of which there are 14 serotypes. Serotype 1 is most commonly associated with infection. Factors predisposing to infection include smoking and immunosuppression.

Pathology
The brunt of the infection is in the lungs, which show an acute inflammatory response. *Legionella* spp. are

phagocytosed by macrophages but phagolysosome fusion is inhibited and thus the organism survives and multiplies within the macrophage until the cell is killed. *Legionella* are also phagocytosed by polymorphs and again resist cidal mechanisms. The virulence mechanisms of *L. pneumophila* are not well characterized although it does produce both a haemolysin and a protease, which may be involved in cell death. The protease can cleave IL-2 and CD4, thus inhibiting the host defences. Lipopolysaccharide from the cell wall of *L. pneumophila* may also be involved in disease pathogenesis. In the lung there are areas of interstitial inflammation and necrosis. The pathogenesis of renal failure is unclear although it may follow rhabdomyolysis. Interstitial nephritis, acute tubular necrosis, diarrhoea, and liver dysfunction may occur. Diagnosis includes culture, direct immunofluorescence, antigen detection (in the urine), serology (although the seroconversion may take up to 5 weeks after onset of the illness) and PCR.

Management

Management includes supportive measures, including ventilation if necessary and antibiotics: erythromycin plus rifampicin or ciprofloxacin. Prevention is by engineering control of water distribution systems backed by public statute.

LEIOMYOMA: A benign tumour of smooth muscle cells (see Fibroids).

LEISHMANIASIS: Infection with one of the many *Leishmania* spp.

Aetiology and risk factors

The intracellular protozoa are transmitted to humans by sandflies from other infected humans or animals. Infections are geographically separated into Old World infections (Mediterranean basin, Africa, Middle East, Indian subcontinent) and New World infections (Central and South America) (Table L1).

Pathology

The protozoa are taken up into macrophages where they replicate. The balance of control or progression within the host (the 'disease spectrum') is thought to depend on a balance between CD4 Th1 T-cells that kill infected macrophages and Th2 cells that are linked to progression, Th1 cell expansion being mainly inhibited by secretion of IL-10. The genetic makeup of the host, the size of the inoculum or the way in which the *Leishmania* antigens are presented may all be related to disease outcome by significantly altering cytokine levels and hence inhibiting or expanding different Th subsets.

There are two clinical presentations:
- visceral leishmaniasis: amastigotes infect mononuclear cells throughout the reticuloendothelial system, leading to splenic lymphoid follicles and Kupffer cells in the liver becoming enlarged, sometimes enormously. There is no Th1 response to the *Leishmania* antigens although there is a polyclonal B cell activation. Clinically the patient with visceral leishmaniasis (kala azar) may have an asymptomatic infection or present with fever, hepatosplenomegaly, weight loss, anaemia, hypergammaglobulinaemia and leucopenia. Visceral leishmaniasis is increasingly recognized in AIDS patients.
- cutaneous leishmaniasis: amastigotes infect macrophages in the skin, leading to the development of a papule. The papule may ulcerate, which is linked to a predominant Th2 response, the ulcer healing by granuloma formation when a Th1 response develops. In some cases there may be large numbers of infected skin macrophages with little cell-mediated response. In this case the nodules are disseminated over the skin in large numbers (diffuse cutaneous leishmaniasis). On the other hand, there may be few infected macrophages with a strong cell-mediated response and prominent granuloma formation in association with healed scars

Table L1 The leishmaniases – species, distribution, source and vector

Disease	Species	Distribution	Source	Vector
Visceral	*Leishmania donovani*	Indian continent	Man/dogs	*Phlebotomus*
	Leishmania infantum	Middle East, Mediterranean, Africa, S. America	Dogs	*Phlebotomus*
	Leishmania chagasi	S. America	Dogs	*Lutzomyia*
Old World cutaneous	*Leishmania major*	Middle East, Africa, Indian continent	Rodents	*Phlebotomus*
	Leishmania tropica	Mediterranean, Middle East, Indian continent	Man/dogs	*Phlebotomus*
	Leishmania infantum	Mediterranean	Dogs	*Phlebotomus*
New World cutaneous	*Leishmania mexicana*	Mexico, Central and South America	Rodents	*Lutzomyia*
	Leishmania braziliensis	S. America	Rodents	*Lutzomyia*

(leishmania recidivans). In Old World disease, in addition to the cutaneous presentation there is also a mucosal involvement which histologically has a strong mononuclear infiltrate and leads to perforation of the nasal septum and even the soft palate.

Laboratory diagnosis is by demonstration of the parasites in histological sections and treatment is with pentavalent antimony or amphotericin for cutaneous disease. Various experimental vaccines are under trial.

LEMIERR SYNDROME: Pyogenic infection of the lateral pharyngeal space caused by *Fusobacterium necrophorum*. The patient presents with a severe sore throat and cervical lymphadenopathy complicated by septicaemia, jugular thrombophlebitis and metastatic abscess in lung, bone, brain and liver.

 Necrobacillosis

LEPROSY: Infection with *Mycobacterium leprae*.

Case

A patient referred to a hospital for tropical diseases presented with skin nodules accompanied by some reddish plaques. On examination, areas of skin were anaesthetic and anhidric. Examination of motor function showed diminished strength in both hands and feet. A clinical diagnosis of leprosy was made and a biopsy taken from one of the skin lesions.

> Histopathology: granulomas and numerous acid-fast bacilli were seen in the skin biopsy (Fig. L1).

Aetiology and risk factors

Mycobacterium leprae is a slowly growing, acid-fast bacillus which has not yet been cultured on artificial medium. Leprosy is endemic in most tropical countries as well as in parts of southern Europe, e.g. Spain. An infected patient secretes large

numbers of bacilli in nasal secretions and although the exact mode of transmission is not known, it is probably via the respiratory route.

Pathology

The leprosy bacillus invades the Schwann cell surrounding the nerve axon. The disease produced is a spectrum ranging from tuberculoid, through borderline stages to lepromatous leprosy and this is probably determined by the antigenic challenge as well as certain host factors (e.g. HLA type), or environmental factors (e.g. prior exposure to other environmental mycobacteria). The classification scheme for leprosy is related to the cytology of the monocyte/macrophage and lymphocyte infiltrate and the bacterial density. Thus, in tuberculoid (TT) leprosy, there are scanty acid-fast bacilli with well-defined epithelioid granuloma surrounded by lymphocytes, associated with strong cell-mediated immunity (e.g. as judged by delayed skin testing with lepromin), whilst in lepromatous lesions (LL) there are abundant acid-fast bacilli, infiltration by foamy histiocytes and Virchow giant cells with scanty lymphocytes, associated with poor cell-mediated immunity and ineffective humoral immunity. Intermediate stages are recognized as borderline tuberculoid (BT), borderline (BB), or borderline lepromatous (BL). In tuberculoid leprosy, the skin is mainly involved, leading to depressed scars of anhidric and anaesthetic skin. In lepromatous leprosy, as well as the skin being involved, eventually becoming coarse and thick and giving rise to the 'leonine face', the nerves are also thickened. Involvement of the nerves leads to loss of the pain reflex and consequent inadvertent trauma to the limbs with resultant deformity. The nasal cartilage may eventually become destroyed. Laboratory diagnosis is by demonstration of acid-fast bacilli in either skin biopsies from the ear lobe or scrapings from the nasal mucosa.

Management

Treatment is with antibiotics, e.g. rifampicin + clofazimine + dapsone for 2–20 years. The antituberculosis vaccine gives variable but significant protection against leprosy. A specific vaccine is still experimental.

LEPTOSPIROSIS: Infection with the spirochaete, *Leptospira interrogans*.

Aetiology and risk factors

Leptospirosis is acquired indirectly from rats by contact with water contaminated with rat urine.

Pathology

The organisms enter the body via mucosal surfaces,

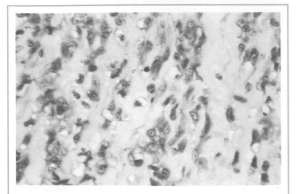

Fig. L1 A peripheral cutaneous nerve containing epithelioid granulomas and acid fast bacilli.

conjunctiva or abrasions in the skin and disseminate by the blood to all organs of the body, the liver and kidneys being most prominently affected. The illness is typically biphasic with an initial septicaemic phase which partially resolves, followed by an immunopathological phase where the leptospires have largely disappeared from the tissues and antibodies have developed. The bacteria cause tissue damage by direct-acting cytotoxic factors, the release of pro-inflammatory mediators leading to increased vascular permeability and DIC, or immunopathological mechanisms, which appear to be principally involved in the meningeal signs. There is an interstitial nephritis with neutrophils and lymphocytes. In severe cases, tubular necrosis may occur. In the liver there is a centrilobular necrosis with a predominant mononuclear cellular infiltrate. The myocardium and skeletal muscle are infiltrated with mononuclear cells and there is cellular necrosis.

In the initial phase of the illness, the patient has a headache, fever, myalgia and a peripheral leucocytosis. Renal and liver damage are evident. The renal symptoms range from mild involvement with pyuria and proteinuria to acute tubular necrosis and renal failure. The patient may be jaundiced and hepatosplenomegaly may be present. Conjunctival haemorrhages may occur and the patient may have a maculopapular or haemorrhagic skin rash. The fever and symptoms abate and recur a few days later. At this stage the hepatic and renal involvement remains or may progress, and the patient may develop signs and symptoms of meningitis and uveitis. The cellular response in the cerebrospinal fluid is principally lymphocytic. Hepatorenal failure and haemorrhages may ensue in severe cases (Weil disease*).

Laboratory diagnosis is usually by serology. The leptospires can be demonstrated in the urine by microscopy and cultured, although this is not routine. Treatment is with either penicillin or tetracycline.

LEUCOCYTE ADHESION DEFICIENCY (LAD):

An immunodeficiency disease resulting from a defect in adhesion molecules involved in attachment of neutrophils and monocytes to endothelial walls.

Patients suffer from severe bacterial infections since neither neutrophils nor monocytes can emigrate from capillaries. T-cell and NK cell-mediated cytotoxicity are also affected. The defect is in the β-chain (CD18) of the integrin C3bi receptor (CR3).

Immunodeficiency

LEUCOCYTOSIS:
An increase in total white cell count above the upper limit of normal (11×10^9/l). This may be due to an increase in neutrophils, lymphocytes, or, more rarely, other normal components of the white cell differential. The differential white cell count is performed by counting and classifying 100 white cells under the microscope.

Normal white cells
The normal white cells in peripheral blood, in order of decreasing frequency, are: (1) neutrophils, (2) lymphocytes, (3) monocytes, (4) eosinophils and (5) basophils.

Examples are shown in Fig. L2. Their numbers are best assessed by absolute rather than percentage counts. These five cell types may be classified into polymorphonuclear granulocytes, and mononuclear cells.

Granulocytes are recognized by the specific staining of their granules with Romanovsky stains (dyes which stain acid substances one colour, basic substances a different colour) as follows:
- neutrophils: indistinct neutral granules
- eosinophils: orange-brown granules
- basophils: blue-purple granules.

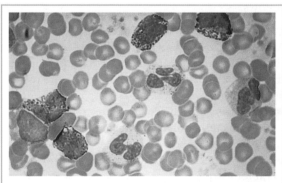

(a)

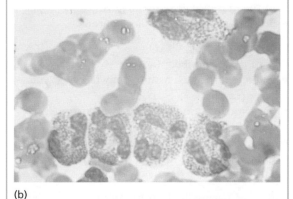

(b)

Fig. L2 (a, b) Normal white cell types in peripheral blood. (a) Neutrophils and basophils; (b) eosinophils.

The mononuclear cells of the blood are the lymphocytes and monocytes. In modern laboratories the white cell differential count is often performed by automated blood counter.

Common causes of neutrophilia (> 7.5 × 10⁹/l)
- Bacterial infection
- Tissue damage: inflammation, infarction, trauma
- Severe metabolic disorder: uraemia, acidosis
- Haemolysis and haemorrhage
- Corticosteroids: stress
- Myeloproliferative disorders*

Common causes of lymphocytosis (> 4 × 10⁹/l)
- Normal in infancy
- Viral infections: glandular fever*, influenza, rubella, hepatitis
- Some bacterial infections: whooping cough, brucella, TB
- Chronic lymphocytic leukaemia*
- Low-grade lymphocytic lymphoma* with blood spill.

Increase in other white cells that form minor components of the white cell differential count rarely results in an increase in total white cell count, but the differential count will be abnormal. Causes of increased numbers of these white cells are as follows.

Causes of monocytosis (> 1 × 10⁹/l)
Monocytes are tissue phagocytes en route to the tissues. Their numbers may be increased in any disorder associated with the death of tissues. Examples are:
- infections: particularly in the recovery phase from bacterial infection, bacterial endocarditis, tuberculosis;
- in the recovery phase from chemotherapy or radiotherapy;
- associated with malignant tumours, particularly in the presence of tissue necrosis;
- myelodysplasia, particularly chronic myelomonocytic leukaemia.

Causes of eosinophilia (> 0.5 × 10⁹/l)
- Allergic disorders: asthma, hay fever, eczema, drug reactions
- Parasitic infections: *Filaria*, *Ancylostoma*, *Ascaris*, *Toxocara*
- Hypereosinophilic syndrome
- Others: Hodgkin disease, polyarteritis nodosa, sarcoidosis

Causes of basophilia (> 0.1 × 10⁹/l)
- The myeloproliferative disorders*
- Myxoedema
- Ulcerative colitis

LEUCOPLAKIA: The term means 'white plaque' and it may be due to benign or malignant proliferation in squamous epithelium.

LEUKAEMIA: A malignant proliferation of blood-forming cells, originating in bone marrow and spilling into blood. The leukaemias are usually divided into acute and chronic varieties. Acute leukaemias are associated with an overproduction of primitive blast cells and are usually rapidly fatal without treatment. Chronic leukaemias pursue a more indolent clinical course and are associated with an excess of more mature haematological cells in bone marrow and blood.

Each of these may be further subdivided into myeloid and lymphoid types, depending on the cell lineage involved. This classification results in four major types of leukaemia: acute myeloid leukaemia*, chronic myeloid leukaemia*, acute lymphoblastic leukaemia* and chronic lymphocytic leukaemia*. Each of these may be further subclassified in various ways as described in the appropriate sections.

LI–FRAUMENI SYNDROME: An inherited syndrome due to germline mutations of the p53 gene. Patients are predisposed to various cancers including leukaemias, lymphomas, osteosarcomas and breast carcinoma.

LIPOMA: A benign tumour of fat cells (adipose tissue). Common sites are the subcutis of the trunk and extremities. Treatment is seldom required except for cosmetic reasons.

LIPOSARCOMA: A malignant tumour of adipose tissue.

Aetiology and risk factors
The aetiology is unknown. The myxoid variant of liposarcoma has been shown to be associated with a specific chromosomal translocation t(12;16).

Pathology
Liposarcomata occur in patients aged 50 years and over and rarely in the young. They usually arise within deep soft tissues, proximal extremities, or the retroperitoneum. Morphologically they are divided into well-differentiated liposarcoma, myxoid liposarcoma, round cell liposarcoma and pleomorphic liposarcoma. The characteristic diagnostic cell of liposarcoma is the lipoblast. It contains round cytoplasmic vacuoles that lead to scalloping of the nucleus.

The myxoid variant and well-differentiated type of liposarcoma have a better prognosis than the round cell and pleomorphic variants, which tend to metastasize.

Management
Surgical excision is the standard treatment.

LISTERIOSIS: An infection with *Listeria monocytogenes*.

Aetiology and risk factors
This Gram-positive bacillus is widespread in the environment and the animal kingdom and infection is acquired usually by eating contaminated food, typically sausages, coleslaw or soft cheese. The infection may also be transmitted transplacentally.

Pathology
Listeria is an intracellular pathogen and is taken up by phagocytosis into macrophages where it replicates protected from the immune system. *Listeria* causes infection in three main patient groups: pregnant females, neonates and the immunocompromised. In pregnant women, it may present as a flu-like illness with fever and myalgia. The infection may be uneventful or give rise to an infected fetus, amnionitis and premature labour. The fetus suffers a disseminated infection (granulomatosis infantiseptica) where *Listeria* forms granuloma in all the organs. The fetus may be stillborn or an infected neonate may be born. There are signs of sepsis in the neonate with a skin rash and hepatosplenomegaly. Neonates can also become infected a few days after birth, acquiring the organisms from the environment. This typically presents as a pyogenic meningitis (see Meningitis), although there may also be a high mononuclear count in the cerebrospinal fluid. Infections in the immunocompromised present either as meningitis, meningoencephalitis or septicaemia. There is peripheral neutrophilia and typical changes of a pyogenic meningitis in the cerebrospinal fluid. Laboratory diagnosis is by isolation of the organism and treatment is with ampicillin and gentamicin.

LIVER FLUKE DISEASE: Infection of the liver and biliary tract by certain helminths known as flukes.

Aetiology and risk factors
The trematodes (flukes) that cause infection are *Clonorchis*, *Fasciola* and *Opisthorchis*. *Fasciola* spp. are found in sheep-rearing areas of the UK but most infections occur in the Far East. The eggs are passed out in faeces and undergo a primary developmental stage in freshwater snails and a secondary developmental stage in fish (*Clonorchis* and *Opisthorchis* only). Infection is acquired by humans by eating raw fish (*Clonorchis* and *Opisthorchis*) or raw vegetables contaminated by the cercarial (developmental) stage.

Pathology
In the human intestine, the cercariae migrate into the bile ducts and mature into adult flukes where they lay eggs which are eventually passed out in the faeces, thus completing the cycle. The pathological changes are due mainly to mechanical irritation, leading to hyperplasia of the glandular epithelium of the bile ducts, an eosinophilic periductal infiltration, fibrosis and mechanical obstruction. Granulomas may develop in the liver parenchyma. The patient complains of mild gastrointestinal disturbances, weight loss, anorexia and fever, with pain and tenderness over the liver. There is a peripheral eosinophilia. Complications include cholangitis and cholangiocarcinoma. Laboratory diagnosis is by demonstration of the eggs in the faeces and serology. Treatment is with praziquantel (*Clonorchis* and *Opisthorchis*) and bithionol or triclabendazole (*Fasciola*).

 Schistosomiasis

LUDWIG ANGINA: A pyogenic infection of the submandibular and sublingual space, usually caused by anaerobes, that can lead to respiratory embarrassment by posterior displacement of the tongue. Treated by surgery and antibiotics.

LUNG CARCINOMA: A malignant neoplasm arising from the glandular epithelium of the bronchial tree.

Case
A 71-year-old retired clerical officer presented to the chest clinic with a 6-month history of increasing shortness of breath (SOB). He had been short of breath for many years and had been diagnosed as having emphysema 10 years previously, but the dyspnoea had become much worse recently. He also had a productive cough and over the last 2 months had noticed some flecks of blood in his sputum. He had smoked 30 cigarettes a day for the last 50 years. On further questioning, he also complained of weight loss and tiredness over the last 12 months.

Examination confirmed the weight loss. He had pallor of his conjunctiva and palpable lymph nodes were noted in the supraclavicular fossa. He also had finger clubbing. Bronchoscopy was carried out and confirmed a mass arising from the left main bronchus and biopsy was performed.

Histopathological examination: bronchial biopsies showing a poorly differentiated squamous cell carcinoma (Fig. L4).

Further staging investigations using CT scan confirmed extensive lymph node involvement in the mediastinum as well as the presence of liver metastases. The patient was treated with local radiotherapy to control his respiratory symptoms.

Haematology:
- Hb: 8 g/dl
- ESR 50.

Biochemical investigations: raised urea of 15 mmol/l.

Liver function tests were normal.

Chest radiograph: left upper lobe collapse associated with carcinoma of the bronchus (Fig. L3).

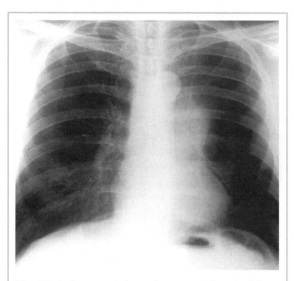

Fig. L3 Left upper lobe collapse associated with carcinoma of the bronchus. (Reproduced with permission from Curtis J, Whitehouse G. *Radiology for the MRCP*. London: Arnold, 1998)

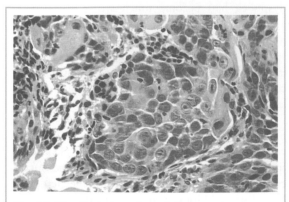

Fig. L4 Histological section of the bronchus showing a poorly differentiated squamous cell carcinoma.

Aetiology and risk factors

Risk factors include a positive family history, smoking, exposure to asbestos and exposure to radiation.

Pathology

Shortness of breath is a common presenting complaint due to obstruction to the respiratory tract. In this patient, worsening of emphysema or pneumonia could have explained his symptoms; however, haemoptysis (coughing up blood) should always be taken seriously. His long history of smoking is compatible with both the emphysema and the carcinoma. Patients with cancer can have a range of non-specific systemic symptoms including weight loss and lethargy, possibly as a result of release of tumour necrosis factor α (TNFα, also known as cachectin). Finger clubbing is often seen in patients with lung carcinoma but its aetiology is unclear. It sometimes disappears after vagotomy, implying a neural mechanism. The patient was anaemic, probably due to a combination of blood loss, malnutrition and non-specific bone marrow depression as a result of disseminated malignancy. Bone marrow involvement by metastases is another possibility. The raised blood urea indicated that his renal function was also poor; the catabolic state induced by the malignancy tends to worsen both the renal function and the symptoms of lethargy and of feeling unwell. The radiological examination demonstrated widespread, metastatic disease. The biopsy revealed a squamous cell carcinoma. The normal bronchial mucosa is glandular, so one might have expected to see an adenocarcinoma. Smoking leads to the development of squamous metaplasia of the bronchial epithelium. Further genetic damage will then produce a tumour that shows squamous differentiation. Oat cell carcinomas*, which exhibit neuroendocrine differentiation, can also occur and these tumours often secrete hormones such as parathyroid hormone (PTH) and adrenocorticotrophic hormone (ACTH). Distant metastases from a lung primary characteristically involve the liver, bone marrow and brain.

Management

This depends on the site of tumour and therefore its resectability. This man's tumour was too advanced to resect and he was therefore given palliative radiotherapy in an effort to relieve the obstruction caused by the tumour.

 Asbestosis

LUPUS ERYTHEMATOSUS: A multisystem autoimmune disorder, affecting the skin, kidneys, joints and serosal membranes, in which there is an

Table L2 Symptoms and signs of Lyme disease

Primary	Secondary
The initial sign of Lyme disease is erythema chronicum migrans: a chronic spreading redness from the site of the initial tick bite. There may be an associated fever, malaise and regional lymphadenopathy	Skin: recurrent patches of erythema. Chronic disease leads to acrodermatitis chronica atrophicans which may occur years after primary infection Joints: arthritis, arthralgia Heart: conduction disturbances Neurological: peripheral neuritis (e.g. Bell palsy), motor-sensory radiculopathy or central neurological symptoms such as meningoencephalitis Chronic symptoms are encephalopathy (personality, language, and memory changes)

array of autoantibodies, notably antinuclear antibodies.

 Systemic lupus erythematosus

LUPUS VULGARIS: A cutaneous form of tuberculosis* involving the head and neck.

LYME DISEASE: A multisystem disease caused by spirochaetes of *Borrelia* spp.

Aetiology and risk factors
Lyme disease is caused by *Borrelia burgdorferi* (principally in the USA) or *Borrelia afzelii* and *Borrelia garinii* (in Europe) and transmitted by *Ixodes* ticks. The reservoirs of infection are field voles and deer and Lyme disease is thus a zoonosis*. In the UK the disease occurs mainly in the New Forest.

Pathology
After inoculation, *Borrelia* spreads throughout the body and may avoid the host defence by means of molecular mimicry. The antigenic response to the *Borrelia* changes with time as the host recognizes new antigens expressed on the surface of the bacterium. This may explain the remitting and relapsing nature of the infection or the different clinical manifestations. In the USA, arthritis is a common sequel to infection but in Europe neurological and chronic cutaneous manifestations are more frequent. *Borrelia* can cause cell damage by a direct toxic effect, by inducing a bystander effect from the host response, and by immunopathological means, e.g. via antibodies to flagellar proteins cross-reacting to axonal proteins. Histologically the infected tissues are infiltrated with mononuclear cells and there may be vasculitis. There is a different clinical presentation at different stages of the illness, although patients may present with late disease without experiencing the early symptoms and signs (Table L2).

Laboratory diagnosis is by serology and PCR. Culture, although possible, is not routine as it has a low sensitivity. In meningeal involvement there is a lymphocytic pleocytosis, a normal glucose and elevated protein in the cerebrospinal fluid. Management is with doxycycline, amoxycillin or cefotaxime depending upon the stage of the illness.

LYMPHADENITIS: An inflammatory disorder of lymph nodes. May be secondary to infection, trauma or autoimmune disorder.

LYMPHOGRANULOMA VENEREUM: Genital infection with *Chlamydia trachomatis*.

 Chlamydial disease

LYMPHOMA: A malignant tumour arising from lymphoid cells.

 Hodgkin disease; Non-Hodgkin lymphoma

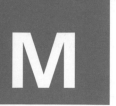

MALABSORPTION: Decreased absorption of nutrients from the gastrointestinal tract. It may be due to a primary abnormality of the intestinal mucosa, or to immune damage to the mucosa, infection, or non-specific inflammatory bowel disease.

MALARIA: A multisystem disease caused by infection with *Plasmodium* spp.

Case

A 26-year-old woman complained of an abrupt onset of chills, rigors and profuse sweating accompanied by a headache and nausea about a week after returning from a holiday in the Gambia. She had put these symptoms down to 'flu'. On examination by the GP she was noted to be pale. She was admitted to hospital with a provisional diagnosis of malaria.

Thick blood films were prepared and sent to haematology.

Haematology:
- blood smear shows intracellular protozoa characteristic of *Plasmodium falciparum* (Fig. M1).
- Hb 10 g/dl; WBC 14 000 × 10⁶/l; polymorphs 80%; Plt 120 × 10⁹/l.

Chemistry: BR 25 mmol/l; AST 100 U/l; ALT 200 U/l; APA 280 U/l; Na 120 mmol/l; K 4.8 mmol/l; HCO₃ 18 mmol/l; BU 20 mmol/l; creatinine 250 mol/l; glucose 3.0 mmol/l.

Aetiology and risk factors

There are four species of the malaria parasite that infect humans: *Plasmodium falciparum*, *Plasmodium vivax*, *Plasmodium ovale* and *Plasmodium malariae*. The parasite is transmitted by female *Anopheles* mosquitos. When the mosquito bites, sporozoites are inoculated into the bloodstream and enter hepatocytes where they undergo asexual reproduction for 1–2 weeks. In the case of *P. vivax* and *P. ovale*, the parasite can enter a dormant (hypnozoite) phase which can lead to clinical

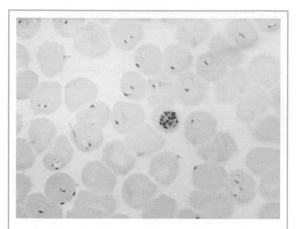

Fig. M1 Blood film stained to show malaria parasite.

relapses later in life. After asexual reproduction, the merozoites enter the bloodstream, penetrate erythrocytes and undergo schizogony (asexual reproduction). After 2 or 3 days, depending on species, the erythrocytes lyse and the released merozoites infect further red cells (Fig. M2) . The developmental cycle in the erythrocyte is synchronous, which accounts for the periodicity of the fever, all the erythrocytes being lysed at the same time, stimulating cytokines such as TNF and IL-1 which are responsible for the fever.

The parasite can undergo a sexual cycle (gametogenesis) which is completed in the mosquito when taken up in blood during a subsequent bite (Fig. M1). Malaria is restricted to tropical regions by the distribution of the vector, and local epidemiology is determined by mosquito feeding patterns and life span. Disease resistance is conferred by a variety of red cell abnormalities, notably sickle cell trait, β-thalassaemia, and G6PD deficiency, which reduce intracellular parasite survival, and this has exerted positive selection for these otherwise deleterious mutations in endemic areas.

Pathology

The liver stage of malaria is symptomless, the pathology being related purely to the blood stage. At the time of red cell rupture, the induction of inflammatory cytokines leads to the characteristic chills, fever and sweats of the 'crisis'. The principal long-term complication is anaemia, which may be life-threatening in babies and young children.

In falciparum ('malignant tertian') malaria, there are additional complications, largely consequent on adherence of the parasitized erythrocyte to vascular endothelium and sequestration within the vessel. The parasitized cell binds to ICAM-1 and CD46 as well as other endothelial receptors. Apart from

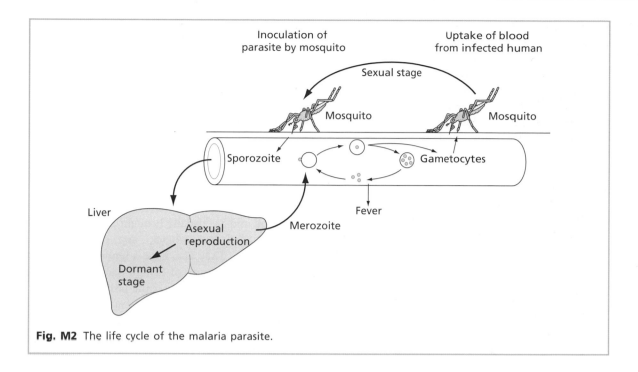

Fig. M2 The life cycle of the malaria parasite.

mechanical effects, the sequestration of the parasitized cells may lead to the release of pro-inflammatory compounds from the vascular endothelium, particularly in the brain, leading to coma which may be fatal (cerebral malaria). Histologically, the small vessels of the brain are congested with parasitized erythrocytes and there are numerous haemorrhages. Many other organs are affected, including the liver, lungs and kidneys, and there is often severe hypoglycaemia and lactic acidosis. In the lungs there is pulmonary oedema and infiltration by inflammatory cells. The patient may develop the adult respiratory distress syndrome*. Acute tubular necrosis may occur in the kidneys and the patient may develop acute renal failure, which is, however, reversible on recovery. For some reason not well understood, *P. malariae* ('quartan') malaria leads to the development of a progressive nephrotic syndrome*. Sequestration of parasitized cells in the spleen leads to gross splenomegaly. Complications include splenic rupture and hypovolaemia and secondary bacterial infection. Like several other infections, malaria causes strong immunosuppression; this may partly explain the development in malarious areas of Burkitt lymphoma*. Immunity to malaria develops slowly over 5–20 years and is easily lost on withdrawal of exposure.

Diagnosis is by examination of blood smears, which may need to be thick, since parasitaemia can be low even in severe cases. Alternatively, antigen can be detected by a dipstick test. High titres of antibody, particularly IgG, would suggest previous exposure.

Management

Management is by general supportive measures including exchange transfusion, accurate fluid balance and antimalarials such as quinine, chloroquine, primaquine or Fansidar, depending on the resistance of the parasite. In cerebral malaria, quinine is the drug of choice. Prevention is by antimalarial prophylaxis, the regimen depending upon the region to be visited and the use of mosquito netting, insect repellent and other means of reducing skin exposure. Malaria control is by reduction of malarial breeding grounds and insecticides to kill the adult mosquito. Various vaccines are currently under trial.

MALIGNANT MELANOMA: A malignant tumour of melanocytes.

Case

A 50-year-old Caucasian lady presented to the dermatology clinic with a mole on her left thigh. The mole had been present for 2 years but she had noticed a change over the last 3 months: the mole had become bigger and darker and on two occasions had bled slightly. She justified the bleeding as due to trauma. On questioning, she said she had lived in Australia for 20 years prior to settling in the UK. All her family members were fair and she and her two sisters also had ginger hair. She admitted to regular sunbathing and generally during her stay in Australia had not used sun block. There was no family history of malignancy.

On examination, the dermatologist noted the fair skin and the numerous freckles on her face, arms and legs. The lesion on her left thigh was 1 cm in diameter and jet black in colour with patchy areas of pallor at one edge. There were signs of recent bleeding. He did not find any evidence of lymphadenopathy and the rest of the systemic examination was normal. The mole was excised.

> Histopathology: Sections of the skin show a malignant melanoma in vertical growth phase. Tumour cells are seen infiltrating the epidermis with horizontal pagetoid extension as well as invading the reticular dermis (Clark level IV). The tumour measures 1.1 mm in maximum depth. A prominent lymphoid infiltrate is seen at the base with fibrosis, suggesting focal regression. The tumour is completely excised with a 1 cm margin (Figs M3, M4).

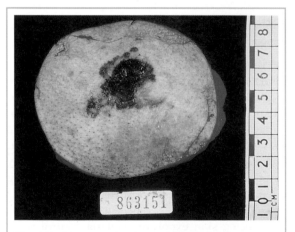

Fig. M3 Macroscopic picture of a heavily pigmented malignant melanoma.

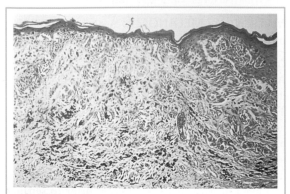

Fig. M4 Histological section showing a malignant melanoma with a junctional component. There is also an inflammatory infiltrate, indicating regression.

Aetiology and risk factors

A few cases are due to a familial predisposition. These patients have the dysplastic naevus syndrome and develop multiple atypical naevi with an almost 100% risk of melanoma during their lifetime. Most cases are sporadic secondary to skin damage due to excessive sunbathing.

Pathology

Most people have benign naevi and since they can be present anywhere on the body, most people are unaware of all the moles they carry. Malignant melanomas are most common on the extremities and trunk and are usually brought to attention due to colour (dark brown/black), size, or a change in these features. They also have a tendency to bleed, which is not a feature of benign naevi. Due to the intense media publicity over the last 5 years, many more people are aware of these features and hence are more vigilant. The classical melanoma victim is a fair-skinned, ginger-haired person with numerous freckles, the lack of skin pigmentation making them susceptible to the damaging effects of UV radiation from the sun.

The neoplastic melanocytes may invade upwards to involve the epidermis and may also spread horizontally, both in the epidermis and upper dermis. They may remain in this state for a long time. It is at the stage of vertical growth that they become dangerous. At this stage, the cells acquire the ability to invade downward, usually in the form of a nodular proliferation. It has been shown that the depth of invasion and, in particular, the size (thickness) are strong prognostic factors, tumours below 0.75 mm in thickness having a better prognosis than larger lesions. This lady had a lesion 1.1 mm in thickness, which is a bad prognostic feature. It is important that the lesion is completely excised with a wide margin as melanoma cells do have a tendency to invade horizontally and on histopathological examination this may be underestimated.

Metastases generally occur first in regional lymph nodes, and in this case the lymph nodes in the groin would have to be examined with care. Some centres also perform lymphangiography to check for metastatic disease in these regional nodes at the time of diagnosis.

Management

This comprises adequate surgical excision. If patients have metastatic disease, chemotherapy, either single agent or combination, may be tried; however, results have been disappointing in terms of survival with any form of treatment once metastases have occurred.

 Naevus

MALIGNANT MESOTHELIOMA: A malignant tumour arising from either the parietal or serosal pleural lining.

Case

A 62-year-old carpenter presented to his medical practitioner with a 2-month history of dyspnoea. This had been getting worse over 6 months but over the last 2, he had found it increasingly difficult to climb up to his first floor flat. There were no lifts in the building. He was otherwise well and gave no significant previous medical history.

On examination, the left lung fields were dull to percussion with reduced breath sounds. A clinical diagnosis of pleural effusion was made and he was referred to hospital. There were no other physical findings of note.

Chest radiograph findings: pleural effusion with deviation of the mediastinum.
Haematological examination: a mild, normochromic, normocytic anaemia of 10 g/l. ESR: 35 mm/h.

Biochemical investigations were all normal.

A chest drain was introduced through the intercostal space and 4.5 litres of blood-stained fluid was removed. Some of the fluid was sent for cytological examination.

Cytological examination: pleomorphic tumour cells, positive for cytokeratin but negative for carcinoembryonic antigen (CEA). Features are suggestive of mesothelioma (Fig. M5).

Further direct questioning revealed that the patient had helped with refurbishment of a building 25 years previously and had handled asbestos

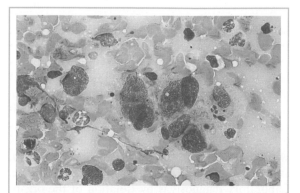

Fig. M5 Pleural fluid with pleomorphic tumour cells.

MRI: a pleural effusion is present together with solid masses on the chest wall and the mediastinal aspect of the pleural cavity.
Abdominal ultrasound: normal.
Pleural biopsy: pleomorphic tumour cells invading the pleura. The tumour cells are positive for cytokeratin including C56 but negative for CEA, AUA1 antigen and mucin. Electron microscopy of the tumour cells shows long slender microvilli on the cell surface. Features are of malignant mesothelioma (Fig. M6).

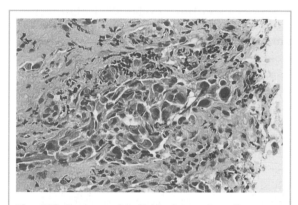

Fig. M6 Groups and individual tumour cells infiltrating the pleura. An inflammatory cell response is also present.

containing partition boards. This job had lasted 6 months and he had no other known contact with asbestos.

A pleural biopsy was also carried out and the patient had staging investigations including MRI of the chest and abdominal ultrasound.

The pleural effusion was re-drained and tetracycline was introduced into the cavity to create a pleurodesis. Chemotherapy and radiotherapy were not felt appropriate.

Aetiology and risk factors

There is an increased incidence of mesothelioma in those exposed to asbestos. A large proportion of mesotheliomas arising in people working in the shipping industry has been due to asbestos exposure. Lifetime risk is about 10% after heavy exposure. There is a long latent period of 25–40 years. Unlike lung carcinoma, smoking is not an important risk factor.

Pathology

SOB is a common presenting symptom for both cardiac and respiratory diseases and the differential diagnosis is wide. It includes cardiac failure, myocardial infarction, asthma, chronic bronchitis and emphysema, and tuberculosis, to list just a few. In this case, tumour within the pleural cavity had led to accumulation of an exudate – a pleural effusion. By restricting lung expansion, this had caused respiratory failure. The patient's symptoms had come on very quickly and would have been consistent with either rapid onset cardiac failure or respiratory failure.

Clinical examination revealed a large pleural effusion and this was drained to relieve symptoms and to try and establish a diagnosis. The fluid was sent for cytological diagnosis and this revealed the features of malignancy, i.e. pleomorphism, increased n:c (nuclear:cytoplasmic) ratio, mitoses (Fig. M6). It can be very difficult to differentiate between mesothelial cells and metastatic carcinoma. Carcinoma cells tend to mould around each other and may contain acidic or neutral mucins. They may also express antigens such as CEA, which are not generally seen on mesothelial cells. Hence, special stains looking for mucins or these antigens may be helpful. In practice, it is not safe to rely entirely on one marker and a panel of special stains is used, whose positive and negative results should permit a correct diagnosis. Electron microscopy is used infrequently now due to the availability of immunohistochemistry but it can be very useful in some instances and in the differentiation of mesothelioma and adenocarcinoma, it may be the best diagnostic tool. Mesothelioma may be localized to an area in the pleural cavity or may spread through it to involve the entire lining and even extend to the contralateral chest wall. It rarely invades directly through the diaphragm to involve the liver. Extension into the mediastinum (MRI scan) may cause symptoms due to obstruction of nerves or major vessels.

Management

In this patient, the tumour was already extensive and apart from symptomatic relief, chemotherapy and radiotherapy were felt to be inappropriate.

MARFAN SYNDROME: A disorder of connective tissue, which leads to defects in the skeleton, cardiovascular system and eyes.

Aetiology and risk factors

The majority of cases have a familial predisposition and the inheritance is of autosomal dominant type. Molecular studies suggest that the locus for Marfan syndrome resides on 15q21.1. Immunohistochemical studies have suggested that the basic defect lies in the fibrillin protein and mutations in the fibrillin gene have been identified in some patients with sporadic disease.

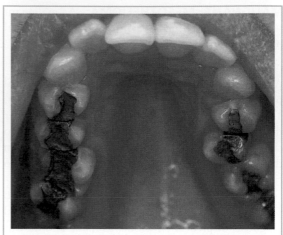

Fig. M7 Patient with Marfan syndrome with a high arched palate. (Reproduced from Browse NL. *An Introduction to the Symptoms and Signs of Surgical Disease*, 3rd edn. London: Arnold, 1997)

Pathology

The patients are usually very tall with long extremities and tapering fingers and toes and a high arched palate (Fig. M7). The ligaments of the joints of the hands and feet are lax and patients are able to hyperextend the wrists. Spinal deformities such as kyphosis and scoliosis may also be present. The chest may be abnormal with a pigeon-breast deformity.

Cardiovascular problems are the most dangerous and include mitral valve prolapse, dilatation of the aortic root with aortic regurgitation, and aortic dissection as a result of cystic medial necrosis. Mitral valve prolapse is more common but less dangerous than the aortic disease. Aortic dissection can result in sudden haemorrhage, shock and death. Ocular changes take the form of lens dislocation.

Management

Management is symptomatic and usually required for the skeletal and cardiac manifestations.

MASTOIDITIS: Infection of the mastoid bone, frequently associated with otitis media*. The mastoid air cells are lined with respiratory epithelium and become hyperaemic and oedematous. Pus may accumulate in the air cells and cause pressure necrosis, leading to abscess formation. Complications include brain abscess and septic thrombosis of the adjacent lateral sinus. The patient presents with signs of otitis media complaining of pain, swelling and tenderness over the mastoid bone. Laboratory diagnosis is by isolation of the organism and management is with appropriate antibiotics.

MEASLES: See Exanthema.

MEDULLARY SPONGE KIDNEY: A disorder of unknown aetiology in which there is cystic dilatation of the collecting ducts within the medulla, usually diagnosed in adults as an incidental finding and due to renal calcification, hematuria or urinary calculi.

MEGALOBLASTIC ANAEMIA: Macrocytic anaemia associated with a series of characteristic morphological appearances in blood and bone marrow, collectively known as megaloblastic change. Besides oval macrocytes, neutrophils with hypersegmented nuclei (neutrophil right shift) are found in the blood (see Fig. P10, p. 201). In the marrow there is delay in nuclear maturation with erythroid precursors having larger nuclei than expected for the degree of cytoplasmic maturation, as judged by haemoglobin content. Because of defective manufacture of nucleic acids, many of the nuclei have a lacy appearance (Fig. M8). Megaloblastic change also affects the white cell series with the formation of giant metamyelocytes.

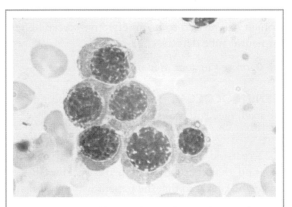

Fig. M8 Megaloblasts. The nuclei are larger than normal for the degree of red cell maturation (judged by pinkness of cytoplasm) and the nuclear chromatin has a lacy appearance.

Megaloblastic anaemia is most commonly due to vitamin B12 (pernicious anaemia*) or folic acid deficiency, which are required for nucleic acid manufacture. It may also be caused by drugs that interfere with nucleic acid manufacture, particularly cytotoxic agents such as cytosine, hydroxyurea and azathioprine. Megaloblastic change may also be found in some cases of myelodysplasia and acute leukaemia.

MELANOMA: See Malignant melanoma.

MELANOSIS COLI: Presence of melanin pigment within macrophages in the colonic mucosa. Often the aetiology is unknown but it is linked to the use of purgatives

MELENY GANGRENE: Spreading necrotic infection of the skin and subcutaneous tissues.

 Necrotizing fasciitis

MELIOIDOSIS: An infection with the Gram-negative bacillus *Burkholderia pseudomallei*.

Aetiology and risk factors
Melioidosis is endemic in parts of Asia and northern Australia. The organism is found in the soil and surface water and infection is acquired following minor abrasions, although airborne transmission also occurs.

Pathology
Infection may be asymptomatic but with waning immunity it may reactivate years after the initial colonization. The organism has lipopolysaccharide in the cell wall and produces a number of extracellular hydrolytic enzymes. Clinically, the patient may present with widespread abscesses (see Glanders) throughout the body, particularly evident in the skin or lungs, which can be pyogenic with neutrophils or granulomatous, depending on the length of infection and the host reaction. The patient may also be septicaemic with fever, elevated acute phase proteins, neutrophilia, evidence of DIC* and liver and renal failure (see Endotoxic shock). Alternatively, the patient may present with a more indolent picture of low-grade fever, weight loss, night sweats and pulmonary cavities and the suspicion is often of tuberculosis. In children parotid abscesses are particularly common. Laboratory diagnosis is by isolation of the organism and treatment is with ceftazidime.

MEN SYNDROME: Multiple endocrine neoplasia (MEN) or multiple endocrine adenomatosis (MEA) syndromes are a rare, inherited group of multiple endocrine neoplasms.
At least three types of MEN syndromes have been identified:
- MEN type I. The glands affected are the parathyroid, pancreatic islets, anterior pituitary, adrenal cortex and thyroid (follicular cells).
There is an increased incidence of peptic ulceration in these patients as a result of the increased gastrin from pancreatic islet neoplasms.
- MEN type IIa (Sipple syndrome). The glands affected are the thyroid (medullary cells) and

adrenal medulla. There is no increased incidence of peptic ulceration in these patients.

- MEN type IIb. The glands affected are the thyroid (medullary cells), adrenal cortex and parathyroids. In addition, this subgroup of patients with MEN type II have mucocutaneous neuromas, marfanoid habitus and pigmentation. This syndrome is sometimes referred to as MEN type III.

MENINGIOMA: A benign neoplasm arising from the arachnoid cells of the leptomeninges lining the external surfaces of the brain and the spinal cord.

Meningiomas are usually solitary, grow slowly and present with localizing symptoms and signs caused by compression of the underlying nervous tissue. They can produce convulsions or a vague syndrome of headache, giddiness, vomiting and psychic changes. They account for around 15% of all intracranial tumours and show a slight predilection for females. The commonest sites for development of meningiomas are the olfactory groove, tuberculum sellae, parasagittal region, cerebellopontine angle and spinal canal. Macroscopically, they are well-circumscribed, solid nodules, usually attached to the overlying dura mater. Microscopically they show several different appearances, named according to the dominant histological pattern: syncytial, fibroblastic, transitional, psammomatous, secretory or papillary (Fig. M9).

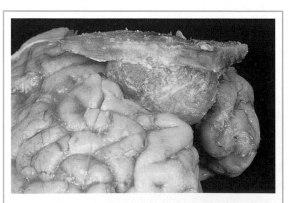

Fig. M9 Macroscopic appearance of meningioma arising from dura and compressing the underlying brain.

Rarely, meningiomas with histological features of malignancy can arise. These tend to invade the brain tissue, can metastasize, and are associated with a bad prognosis. Cytogenetic studies have demonstrated loss of the long arm of chromosome 22 in meningiomas, suggesting the presence of a tumour suppressor gene at this location. Treatment consists of surgical removal, irradiation being used only for non-operable tumours.

 Neurofibromatosis

MENINGOCELE: A sac-like structure containing meninges and cerebrospinal fluid, caused by herniation of meninges through a defect in the skull or vertebral body.

Meningoceles are caused by incomplete closure of the neural tube during fetal development, most commonly affecting the lower lumbar vertebrae or the skull. The mildest form is called spina bifida where there is a defect in the posterior part of lumbar vertebrae but no herniation. In more severe forms the meningocele contains neural tissue as well as the meninges and is called a myelomeningocele or an encephalocele, depending on the type of neural tissue. The cause of this developmental defect is not known; however, strong evidence suggests a link with folate deficiency. Daily folate supplements are recommended to pregnant women to reduce the risk. Neural tube defects often lead to an increase in the concentration of alpha-fetoprotein in amniotic fluid and maternal serum, and determination of alpha-fetoprotein in pregnant women has proved to be an effective screening test for neural tube defects.

 Germ cell tumour; Hepatocellular carcinoma

MENINGOCOCCAL MENINGITIS: Infection of the meninges with *Neisseria meningitidis*.

Case

A 22-year-old man was complaining of a headache and said that the light hurt his eyes. His GP was called and observed that the patient was pyrexial and disorientated and that he had a stiff neck. A provisional diagnosis of meningococcal meningitis was made. He gave the patient an injection of benzylpenicillin and arranged for his admission to hospital. On admission to hospital it was noted that the patient had developed a petechial rash that did not blanch on pressure and that he was hypotensive. Blood was taken for culture and a full blood count. As there was no evidence of papilloedema, a lumbar puncture was

Haematology: Hb 13 g/dl; WBC 18 000 × 10⁶/l; polymorphs 80%; Plt 120 × 10⁹/l.
Fibrinogen: 1 g/l.
Microbiology: CSF WBC 1000/cm³; polymorphs >90%; RBC 0–2/cm³; protein 0.6 g/l; glucose 2.0 mmol/l with a blood glucose of 5.3 mmol/l.

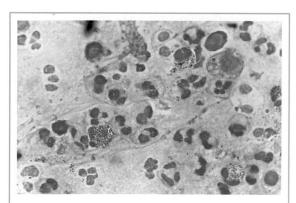

Fig. M10 Gram stain of CSF showing intracellular Gram-negative cocci.

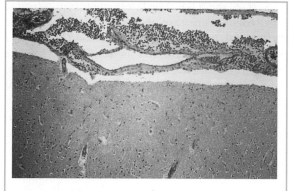

Fig. M11 Inflammation of the arachnoid membrane in meningitis.

performed. Benzylpenicillin was continued whilst awaiting the results of microbiology

Gram-negative intracellular diplococci were seen (Fig. M10). *Neisseria meningitidis* was grown from blood and CSF culture.

Aetiology and risk factors

Neisseria meningitidis is a fragile Gram-negative diplococcus that readily dies under adverse environmental conditions such as drying and low temperatures. It is spread by droplet infection and colonizes the nasopharynx. Many individuals who acquire the organism may remain asymptomatic but can act as sources of infection. The organism has a polysaccharide capsule which can be used to differentiate strains into serotypes, e.g. A, B, C, W135 and Y. Type A commonly causes epidemics in sub-Saharan Africa, whilst serotypes B and C are common in the UK. The polysaccharide of type B is similar to a neuraminic acid found in the CNS (and the capsule of *E. coli* K1) and is therefore poorly immunogenic, as it is perceived by the host to be 'self'. The capsule of types A and C form the basis for the current vaccine. Transmission is facilitated by overcrowding and readily occurs under poor social circumstances. Predisposing factors for disease include complement deficiencies. The organism also has outer-membrane proteins which can be used to further subdivide the strains, e.g. strain B15.PI 16, pili which are important for the attachment to non-ciliated nasopharyngeal epithelium, and a polysaccharide capsule which is antiphagocytic. Neisserial infections are relatively common in patients with complement deficiencies of C6–C9 (membrane attack complex), indicating the important role of these components in protection against these organisms.

Pathology

The attached bacteria penetrate the mucosal barrier and the capillaries in the submucosa where they are spread by the bloodstream to the capillaries of the choroid plexus. Meningococci bind to the endothelium of the capillaries and penetrate to the subarachnoid space where they are protected by the relative immunological deficiencies of this compartment (low complement and immunoglobulin levels). An acute inflammatory reaction is produced (Fig. M11) with neutrophil recruitment, pus formation, cytokine release, and the disruption of the blood–brain barrier by breakdown of the normally tight junctions of the capillary endothelium. Vascular damage ensues with oedema and fibrin deposition leading to haemorrhage and infarction.

Endotoxin (cell wall lipopolysaccharide, LPS), which is released from the meningococci, is responsible for the local vascular damage as well as the systemic vascular collapse (endotoxic shock*) that may occur in some patients. LPS activates the complement cascade, activates the coagulation cascade leading to disseminated intravascular coagulation and stimulates the production of IL-1,

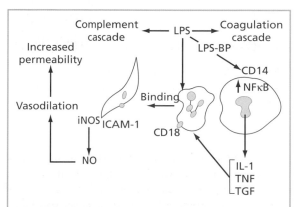

Fig. M12 Diagram of the action of LPS in endotoxic shock.

IL-8, IL-6 and TNF. The latter stimulates inducible nitric oxide synthetase (iNOS) production from the endothelial cells forming nitric oxide. This is a powerful vasodilator and is responsible for the hypotension associated with shock (Fig. M12). Complications include haemorrhage in the adrenal gland (Waterhouse–Friderichsen syndrome*).

Laboratory diagnosis is by isolation of the organism from blood or CSF, or detection using PCR or antigen detection assays.

Management
Management includes antibiotics (usually benzylpenicillin) and systemic support if shock is present. The disease is notifiable.

MENINGOENCEPHALITIS: Inflammation of both the brain and meninges.

 Encephalitis

METASTASIS: Spread of a neoplasm from the primary site to a distant site via blood vessels, lymphatics or body cavities, generally considered to be the hallmark of malignancy.

MICROANGIOPATHIC HAEMOLYTIC ANAEMIA (MAHA): Destruction of red cells associated with the deposition of fibrin in small blood vessels. The fibrin strands act like wire cheese cutters, slicing up red cells. Fragmented cells and helmet-shaped cells may be seen on the blood film along with the general effects of a haemolytic anaemia* such as reduced haemoglobin level, increased reticulocyte count and raised bilirubin levels.

Causes of fibrin deposition in the circulation, and hence of MAHA, are disseminated intravascular coagulation*, disseminated malignancy, vasculitis*, malignant hypertension, thrombotic thrombocytopenic purpura* and glomerulonephritis. Very rarely, giant cavernous haemangiomas* may cause MAHA and consumption thrombocytopenia.

MICROSPORIDIOSIS: Infection with the obligate intracellular protozoan pathogens *Enterocytozoon bieneusi, Encephalitozoon intestinalis, Encephalitozoon hellum, Encephalitozoon cuniculi, Pleistophora* sp. and *Nosema* sp. The microsporidia are widespread in the animal kingdom but the source of human infection is generally unknown. The majority of infections have been reported in AIDS patients. Infection in immunocompetent individuals appears to be asymptomatic but is recognized from seroepidemiological studies. *Enterocytozoon bieneusi* infects the enterocytes, causing a chronic diarrhoea; the bile duct epithelium, causing a cholangitis; and the nasal mucosa, causing polyps. *Encephalitozoon intestinalis* also infects the enterocytes, causing chronic diarrhoea. *Encephalitozoon hellum* infects the cornea, causing keratoconjunctivitis. *Encephalitozoon* species infect the macrophage and may cause disseminated infection, e.g. kidneys, liver. *Pleistophora* spp. have been associated with myositis. Laboratory diagnosis is by histology. For most infections there is no effective treatment, although *Encephalitozoon intestinalis* does respond to albendazole.

MIKULICZ SYNDROME: The combination of inflammation of salivary and lacrimal glands, seen mainly in Sjögren disease*, but also in association with leukaemia, lymphomas and sarcoidosis.

MILLER–FISHER SYNDROME: A peripheral neuropathy affecting the cranial nerves.

 Guillain–Barré syndrome

MIXED CONNECTIVE TISSUE DISEASE(S): A syndrome displaying features of several rheumatic diseases, e.g. SLE (arthritis, rash, antinuclear antibodies); scleroderma (Raynaud phenomenon) and polymyositis (muscle pain and weakness). Treatment is with steroids.

MOLLUSCUM CONTAGIOSUM: Viral infection of the skin presenting with small umbilicated papules widely distributed over the body and face and occurring commonly in AIDS patients. Specific treatment (cryotherapy or curettage) may be required.

MONOCLONAL GAMMOPATHY OF UNDETERMINED SIGNIFICANCE (MGUS): Paraproteins are sometimes found in the blood in patients with no evidence of B-cell malignancy. These are particularly common in the elderly and their importance lies in the fact that they may be confused with the more serious myeloma*. These benign monoclonal proteins are generally of low concentration (<20 g/l for an IgG) and the other immunoglobulins are not depressed as in myeloma. The patient does not have bone pain, hypercalcaemia, or renal impairment. Over a period of observation the concentration of a benign paraprotein does not rise.

MUCOCELE: A mucus-filled cyst usually formed secondary to obstruction of secretory ducts of an organ such as the salivary gland or gallbladder.

MUCORMYCOSIS: An infection with a zygo-mycete fungus (e.g. *Mucor*) which particularly affects the paranasal sinuses (rhinocerebral mucor-mycosis). The fungus is found in rotting vegetables and the route of infection is principally inhalation of spores, although invasive gastrointestinal and skin disease may also occur. Predisposing factors for rhinocerebral disease include diabetic ketoaci-dosis. The fungus proliferates at the point of entry and invades the adjacent tissue, particularly the vasculature, leading to thrombosis and tissue necro-sis. The patient presents with a fever, facial pain and oedema. There may be proptosis because the fungus invades the structures behind the eye. It may also invade the brain tissue and carries a high mortality. Laboratory diagnosis is by isolation of the fungus and treatment is a combination of surgery and amphotericin. A similar illness can develop with *Aspergillus*.

MULTIPLE SCLEROSIS: A chronic demyelinating disease of the nervous system characterized by recurrent attacks with predilection for the spinal cord, the optic nerves and the brain.

Case

A 35-year-old female presented with loss of vision in her left eye. Within the last year her appetite had diminished and she had lost 5 kg in weight, she had attacks of insomnia and she felt tired and depressed. Her past medical history was unremark-able but she remembered an episode of tingling sensation in her left leg 3 years ago, which had lasted for a few weeks and had gradually disap-peared.

On examination her vital signs were normal. Neurological examination revealed partial loss of vision in her left eye. Ophthalmoscopy showed an inflamed optic nerve head (papillitis). The right eye was normal. Both legs were hyper-reflexic, with increased muscle tone.

Examination of CSF by lumbar puncture showed 7 cells/ml, normal protein concentration (0.43 g/l) but increased IgG concentration (0.12 g/l).
An MRI scan revealed multiple foci of demyelination in both cerebral lobes as well as the left optic nerve.

In this case the presence of a long history, relaps-ing remitting symptoms, evidence for involvement of multiple parts of the nervous system, plus the CSF and imaging findings strongly suggested a diagnosis of multiple sclerosis.

Aetiology and risk factors

The cause of multiple sclerosis is unknown. The disease is thought to develop as a result of an autoimmune reaction against the myelin basic protein, the main constituent of the myelin sheath of nerve cells. It is a relatively common disease in northern countries, the prevalence reaching 1 per 1000 persons in Europe and the USA. Females are affected twice as much as males. Other risk factors include a family history and certain MHC antigens, e.g. DR2, B7.

Pathology

The main pathological feature of multiple sclerosis is focal or patchy destruction of myelin sheaths with relative preservation of the axons in the central nervous system (Fig. M13). Loss of myelin leads to significantly diminished transmission of signals by the nerves. The presentation of multiple sclerosis is very variable depending on the site and the extent of nerve cell involvement.

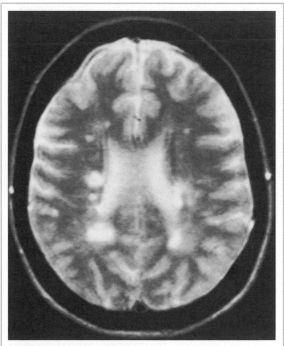

Fig. M13 MRI scan showing lesions in the periventricular white matter of both hemispheres. (Reproduced with permission from Curtis J, Whitehouse G. *Radiology for the MRCP*. London: Arnold, 1998)

Approximately 40% of multiple sclerosis patients develop optic neuritis usually affecting only one eye and causing total or partial visual loss. Other common findings include involvement of the

M

spinal cord leading to upper motor neuron dysfunction with weakness and spasticity in the involved areas and loss of joint position and vibration senses. Involvement of the cerebellum causes impairment in cerebellar functions. Generalized involvement of the cerebral hemispheres can lead to depression, by far the commonest emotional symptom of multiple sclerosis. Characteristically, the disease has a relapsing and remitting clinical course with eventual neurological deterioration in some of the patients.

CSF examination usually reveals a normal or mildly increased cell and protein content but the proportion of the IgG compared to total protein is characteristically increased. On electrophoresis a restricted number of bands are observed, suggesting that the IgG content is oligoclonal. It is thought that the immunoglobulin is secreted by the B-cells in the central nervous system.

On postmortem examination of the central nervous system, the involved areas of the white matter generally show multiple well-circumscribed areas of grey discoloration representing 'plaques' of demyelination (Fig. M14). Microscopically, in

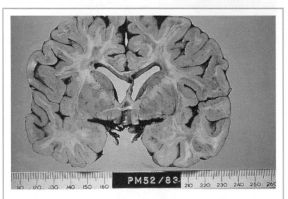

Fig. M14 Macroscopic appearance of multiple sclerosis brain showing loss of white matter in the temporal and parietal lobes.

active plaques, loss of myelin can be demonstrated using special stains. By contrast, axonal processes are relatively well preserved. Additionally, focal accumulation of lymphocytes and macrophages, particularly around vessels, is observed. These include both helper and cytotoxic T-cell subsets and antigen-presenting cells and are thought to account for the cellular immune response observed in these patients against the myelin basic protein. In inactive plaques, the demyelination persists but the inflammatory response subsides and instead an astrocytic proliferation is seen. Although it is thought that there is limited potential for remyelination in

affected areas, most of the plaques remain unmyelinated.

The disease follows a chronic course with episodes of relapses and partial remissions. The cellular basis of remissions is unclear as potential for remyelination is thought to be limited. After 10 years, approximately 50% of the patients become disabled. Occasionally the disease can follow a rapid course with rapid neurological deterioration.

A variant of multiple sclerosis (also called neuromyelitis optica or Devic disease), characterized by bilateral optic neuritis and spinal cord involvement, is seen in Asians. Other demyelinating diseases include acute disseminated encephalomyelitis and central pontine myelinolysis.

Management
No effective treatment of multiple sclerosis is known, but interferon-β has been shown to reduce relapse rates in severe cases. Steroids can be helpful during acute flare-ups, otherwise treatment is directed to relieve the symptoms.

MUMPS: Infection with the mumps virus.

Aetiology and risk factors
Mumps occurs mainly in children and may affect many organs, but most obviously the parotid glands. Transmission requires close contact and is by the respiratory route or direct contact.

Pathology
The initial infection is of the upper respiratory tract followed by a viraemia, following which the virus can localize in many organs, e.g. parotid, pancreas, testes, ovary, meninges. In the infected glandular tissues there is a periductal infiltration of lymphocytes with tissue oedema and cell necrosis within the duct systems of the gland, which may also be infiltrated with neutrophils. With orchitis*, if oedema is severe, there may be pressure necrosis of germinal epithelium, leading to sterility. Clinically the patient has a temperature and complains of pain over the angle of the jaw with obvious swelling of the parotid and sublingual glands. The mouth is dry and swallowing may be difficult. Alternatively, the patient may present with meningitis (with or without preceding parotitis), the mumps virus being one of the commonest causes of viral meningitis*.

Complications include orchitis or oophoritis which may develop in a small proportion of patients about a week after the parotid swelling is evident. There is recurrence of the fever with a swollen and oedematous scrotum and pain in the testis (orchitis) or abdomen (oophoritis). Although atrophy can occur, sterility is unusual. There may also be some degree of pancreatitis or myocarditis. An early-onset encephalitis associated with neuronal cell death and a late-onset demyelinating post-infectious encephalitis may also occur. The mumps virus may possibly be causally related to endocardial fibroelastosis. Laboratory diagnosis is by serology or virus isolation (from saliva or cerebrospinal fluid). There may be a peripheral leucopenia or leucocytosis and if pancreatitis occurs there will be an elevated serum amylase. Management is symptomatic and prevention is by vaccination as part of the live measles, mumps, rubella (MMR) vaccine.

MYASTHENIA GRAVIS: A disorder of neuromuscular transmission characterized by weakness and fatiguability of voluntary muscles.

Aetiology and risk factors

The aetiology is unknown but there is experimental evidence for infectious agents playing a role in induction. Although it can occur at any age, it affects mainly young women, where there is usually accompanying thymic hyperplasia with medullary germinal centres, and middle-aged men, in which the MG is sometimes associated with a thymoma of mixed epithelial and lymphocyte type. Overall, about 10% of the patients have a thymoma. Women are twice as likely to get MG as men. It usually presents with weakness in the external ocular muscles (ocular myasthenia) or facial and pharyngeal muscles, and progresses to more generalized muscle weakness. The disease may progress rapidly or slowly over many years. HLA-A1, B8 and DR3 are associated with the early onset disease in women, whilst B7 and DR2 are associated with the middle-aged male disease. A neonatal form of the disease occurs in one in eight babies born to mothers with MG but resolves over a few weeks, suggesting that the IgG acetylcholine receptor (ACR) antibodies (see below) are causative. D-Penicillamine therapy may also induce MG but this resolves on removal of the drug. It is often associated with other autoimmune diseases including thyrotoxicosis, diabetes mellitus, rheumatoid arthritis and SLE.

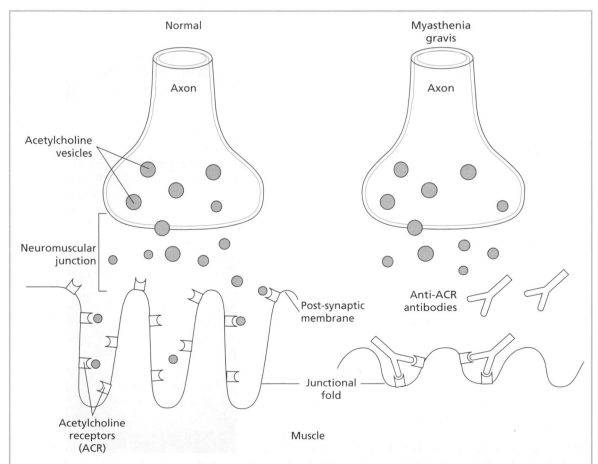

Fig. M15 Note the antibodies blocking/modulating the acetylcholine receptor (ACR), reduction in number of receptors, and the flattening of the junctional folds.

Pathology

The histopathology of the muscle shows scattered lymphocytic aggregates with a widening of the synaptic cleft at neuromuscular junctions. There is evidence of damage to the post-synaptic membrane. MG patients in most cases (90%) have autoantibodies to the ACR and this antibody is itself pathogenic. It binds to and destroys (via complement) the ACR and prevents neuromuscular transmission (Fig. M15) – an example of type II hypersensitivity.

Autoantibodies to thyroglobulin and thyroid microsomes are found in 40% of patients and about 60% have antibodies to skeletal muscles and thymic epithelial cells. These are, however, not pathogenic and probably result from muscle damage or cross-reacting thymic antigens.

Management

Although the severity of the disease does not correlate directly with antibody levels, reduction in autoantibody production is highly effective in reversing symptoms. This is achieved through immunosuppression with azathioprine and prednisolone and for more severe cases, plasmapheresis (plasma exchange) combined with immunosuppression. Thymectomy is also effective, probably because it removes some of the anti-ACR antibodies (plasma cells synthesizing these antibodies are normally present in the thymus) and also a source of antigen. Anticholinesterase drugs are also used as long-term therapy.

MYCETOMA: A chronic infection of subcutaneous tissue, muscle and bone caused by a number of different fungi or bacteria (actinomycetes).

Aetiology and risk factors

Some of the organisms causing mycetoma are shown in Table M1. The organisms are found in the soil and on vegetation. Infection occurs after minor trauma. Mycetoma is endemic in tropical areas, e.g. Africa, India and the Middle East.

Table M1 Organisms causing mycetoma

Fungus	Actinomycete
Madurella mycetomatis	Actinomyces madurae
Madurella grisea	Nocardia brasiliensis
Pseudallescheria boydii	Streptomyces somaliensis

Pathology

After inoculation, the organism spreads along the fascial planes, invading skin, muscle and bone. There is a fibrotic and mixed cellular reaction to the micro-colonies of the organism which are surrounded by a hyaline material produced by the host (Splendore–Hoeppli phenomenon) with a neutrophilic infiltration around the granules further surrounded by epithelioid and giant cells (pyogranuloma). The disease presents with an indurated area of the skin, usually the lower limb (Madura foot) but it can also occur on any part of the body following trauma. Eventually sinuses develop, discharging characteristic and diagnostically useful coloured granules (red, black, yellow). The sinuses heal, only for new ones to develop. As the micro-organism invades the surrounding structures, the bone and muscle are destroyed. Laboratory diagnosis is by histology and isolation of the organism. If the disease is caused by an actinomycete, treatment is with streptomycin and sulphonamides; if by a fungus, some may respond to azoles although surgery may also be necessary.

MYCOBACTERIOSIS: Infection with mycobacterial species other than *Mycobacterium tuberculosis* (see Tuberculosis) or *Mycobacterium leprae* (see Leprosy).

Aetiology and risk factors

Mycobacterial species and the diseases they cause are shown in Table M2. These mycobacterial

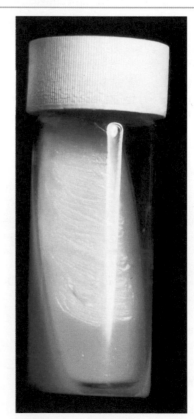

Fig. M16 Atypical mycobacterium growing on Lowenstein–Jensen medium.

Table M2 Species of mycobacteria, source and resultant disease

Species	Source	Disease
M. bovis BCG	Vaccine	Focal or disseminated disease in immunocompromised patients receiving the vaccine or following immunotherapy with BCG
M. kansasii	Water supplies	Pulmonary or disseminated disease
M. xenopi	Water, endoscope washer/disinfectors	Pulmonary, soft tissue, joint disease in immunocompetent individuals and disseminated disease in AIDS patients
M. ulcerans	Soil	Buruli ulcer
M. marinum	Water: swimming pools, fish tanks. Fish pathogen	Superficial granulomatous lesion of skin. Bursitis, tenosynovitis associated with T-cell anergy
M. malmoense	Water, soil	Pulmonary disease and lymphadenitis in immunocompetent individuals and disseminated disease in AIDS patients
M. chelonei/fortuitum	Water, endoscope washer/disinfectors	Soft-tissue infection (injection abscess) and lymphadenitis
M. scrofulaceum	Water	Cervical adenitis
M. paratuberculosis	Water	May be causally linked to Crohn disease
M. haemophilum	Water, soil	Soft-tissue infections, lymphadenitis and disseminated disease principally in immunocompromised individuals
M. avium/intracellulare	Water supplies	Disseminated disease characteristically in AIDS patients. Lymphadenitis, tenosynovitis and pulmonary disease (in women) occurs in immunocompetent individuals

species are environmental saprophytes, found in soil or water. Some may be present in the biofilm found in endoscope-washer/disinfectors. Mostly they are opportunist pathogens causing soft tissue, joint, pulmonary or disseminated disease. Some affect principally immunocompromised patients, particularly AIDS patients (e.g. *Mycobacterium avium*), where they frequently cause disseminated disease, whereas others cause local infection following trauma (e.g. *Mycobacterium chelonei*).

Pathology

Like *M. tuberculosis* and *M. leprae*, they are intracellular pathogens overcoming host defences by preventing phagolysosome fusion or inhibiting acidification of the phagolysosome. Other virulence factors of the mycobacteria include the cell wall glycolipids and catalase. *Mycobacterium ulcerans* produces a lipid cytotoxin and causes Buruli ulcer*, an ulcerating skin lesion found in Africa and Australia. Histologically, the host response of mycobacterial disease is granuloma formation. Laboratory diagnosis is by isolation from appropriate specimens. Management is by various combinations of antibiotics and antimycobacterial agents.

MYCOSIS FUNGOIDES: A low-grade T-cell lymphoma of the skin characterized by infiltration of the epidermis by atypical lymphocytes with cerebriform nuclei. At first, only the skin is involved, but after many years the tumour may become aggressive and involve local lymph nodes and other organs. Occasionally leukaemic dissemination occurs – the so-called Sézary syndrome*.

MYELODYSPLASIA: Potentially premalignant clonal haematological disorders, characterized by dysplastic changes in blood and bone marrow and cytopaenias.

MYELOFIBROSIS: Increase in reticulin and collagen in the marrow cavity. Sometimes this may be a local reactive phenomenon to infection, trauma or local tumour, but it is usually due to

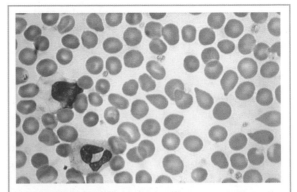

Fig. M17 Blood film in myelofibrosis showing teardrop poikilocytosis.

M

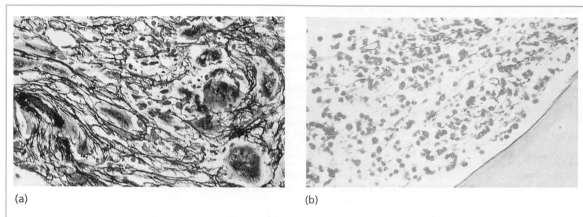

Fig. M18 (a, b) Bone marrow trephine biopsy which has been sectioned and stained by a silver impregnation method demonstrating reticulin. This is increased in myelofibrosis (a) compared with a normal marrow biopsy (b).

primary myelofibrosis, a myeloproliferative disorder*

Pathology

Approximately 25% of cases have a history of another myeloproliferative disorder, particularly polycythaemia* rubra vera or essential thrombocythaemia*, which may burn out as myelofibrosis. All the general features of the myeloproliferative disorders may be present. Massive splenomegaly is common and may be an incidental finding on abdominal examination. Splenic infarcts may occur, causing pleuritic pain in the left hypochondrium, sometimes associated with a rub.

The blood shows a leucoerythroblastic anaemia with pear-shaped red cells – teardrop poikilocytes (Fig. M17).

The white cell and platelet counts may be high, normal or low. In the bone marrow there is an overgrowth of the reticulin framework within which the haemopoietic cells live. This may eventually turn to fibrous tissue, preventing the normal aspiration of bone marrow samples (dry tap) and necessitating a trephine bone marrow biopsy for diagnosis (Fig. M18).

Management

Regular red cell transfusions are often required. Patients with bulky or painful spleens may benefit from splenectomy, particularly when red cell transfusion requirements are high. The excessive cellular proliferation may lead to folate deficiency and folate supplementation may help maintain the haemoglobin level.

MYELOMA: A marrow-based malignant proliferation of plasma cells that frequently secrete a

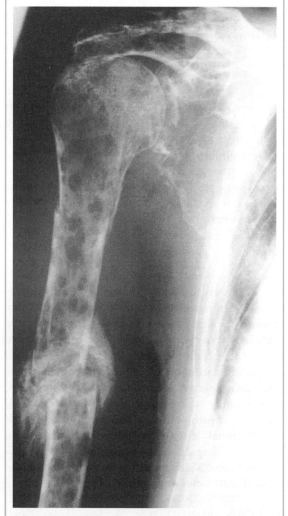

Fig. M19 Radiograph of humerus showing two fractures, one recent and one old with multiple lytic areas in a patient with myeloma.

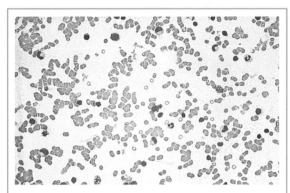

Fig. M20 Blood film showing rouleaux formation. Increased amounts of gammaglobulin in the plasma allows the red cells to adhere to each other along their short axis. The appearance is similar to piles of coins gently tipped over to form long branching chains.

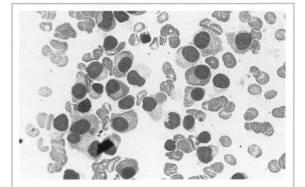

Fig. M21 Bone marrow aspirate in myeloma showing plasma cells with multiple nuclei.

monoclonal antibody and cytokines that stimulate osteoclasts. Because of its various effects on blood, bone and kidney, myeloma may present to almost any clinical speciality.

Case

A 70-year-old man complained of backache. This initially responded to non-steroidal anti-inflammatory agents but become more intractable as the weeks passed. Eventually things come to a head when he fell downstairs in his house for the second time in a month and was admitted to the A&E department as an emergency. On examination he appeared pale and was confused and incontinent of urine. His right humerus was obviously fractured. Firm pressure on the sternum with the flat of the hand produced pain.

Radiography of the right arm demonstrated a fracture of the humerus with some callus formation (Fig. M19). The rest of the humerus showed multiple lytic bone deposits and he was detained in the radiology department so that x-rays could be taken of his skull, chest, spine and pelvis. These all demonstrated multiple lytic bone deposits.

His plasma electrolytes showed a reduced sodium of 131 (135–145 mmol/l), normal potassium, elevated urea and creatinine. Bone chemistry results confirmed that he was hypercalcaemic with a serum calcium of 3.26 (2.25–2.55 mmol/l), but normal phosphate and alkaline phosphatase. Total protein was elevated, which was due to an increased globulin. The serum albumin concentration was reduced. His blood count showed a normocytic anaemia with normal white cell and platelet counts. The blood film showed blue background protein staining and heavy rouleaux formation (Fig. M20).

The ESR was greatly increased at >140 mm/h. Plasma viscosity was modestly increased 2.1 (1.5–1.75 cp). A bone marrow aspirate was performed, which showed 30% plasma cells (normally less than 5%) of nucleated cells with many binucleate and abnormal plasma cells (see Fig. M21). Scrum electrophoresis was performed which showed a monoclonal band in the gamma region, with reduction in the remainder of the gammaglobulin levels.

Immunoglobulin measurement showed the IgG concentration to be elevated threefold over normal whilst the levels of the other immunoglobulins were reduced. Bence Jones protein was detected in urine as free kappa chains of immunoglobulin.

Aetiology and risk factors

As in other haemopoietic malignancies, cytogenetic abnormalities are sometimes found in the myeloma cells. However, these are not characteristic of the disease and their causation is uncertain. An increased incidence of myeloma has been found in agricultural workers, perhaps related to exposure to farm animals or pesticides. Recently, evidence for herpesvirus type 8 infection (the virus that causes Kaposi sarcoma*) has been found in the bone marrow stroma from patients with multiple myeloma, though whether this is the cause of the disease remains controversial.

Pathology

Hyponatraemia is commonly found in the presence of large concentrations of paraprotein. This is due to the protein molecules occupying much of the plasma volume and contributing to the plasma oncotic pressure.

Renal impairment is common in myeloma. This may be due to plasma hyperviscosity, as discussed below, or dehydration due to hypercalcaemia.

Sometimes the increased calcium in the urine interferes with tubular function (nephrocalcinosis) or may even result in urinary stones. Renal tract infections, like other infections, are common in myeloma. Sometimes abnormal immunoglobulin molecules may be precipitated in the tissues as amyloid.

The malignant plasma cells secrete cytokines (osteoclast activating factors, OAF) which stimulate the bone osteoclasts to resorb bone. This causes hypercalcaemia and dehydration with osteoporosis, lytic bone lesions and pathological fractures as seen in this case. Unlike most other causes of hypercalcaemia, myeloma usually shows normal alkaline phosphatase levels.

Malignant plasma cells infiltrate the bone marrow, disrupting normal blood cell production and resulting in anaemia (sometimes macrocytic), neutropenia and thrombocytopenia.

Many of the clinical manifestations of myeloma result from the production of a monoclonal paraprotein. This is an antibody sometimes manufactured by the malignant plasma cells. If this is a large molecule such as IgM, it may cause the plasma to be abnormally thick and viscous. This results in a syndrome of confusion, oedema, purpura and renal impairment – plasma hyperviscosity. On the blood film, the abnormally high protein concentration may impart a blue tinge to the staining so that a diagnosis of myeloma may be suspected without even putting the film under the microscope. The paraprotein reduces the normal electrical charge on red cells that keeps them apart, so that they tend to clump together in rouleaux, looking like piles of coins gently tipped over (Fig. M20). The ratio of volume to surface area of the red cells is thus changed and they tend to sediment faster through the plasma when the blood sample is allowed to stand, resulting in a high erythrocyte sedimentation rate.

A useful diagnostic test in myeloma is the bone marrow aspirate. Plasma cells are present in normal marrow but number less than 5% of all nucleated cells. If there are more than 20% plasma cells in the marrow, the diagnosis is almost always myeloma, particularly if abnormal and multinucleate cells are common.

The paraprotein consists of single type and class of antibody molecule produced by a single clone of plasma cells. Electrophoresis of normal serum usually shows a broad band in the gammaglobulin region (Fig. M22), reflecting the diversity of antibodies made against many different antigens. The paraprotein forms a single tight band in the gammaglobulin region, an M (for monoclonal)

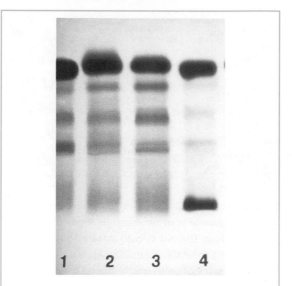

Fig. M22 Protein electrophoresis of three controls and a patient with myeloma. There is a monoclonal paraprotein in the gamma region at the bottom of the patient's track, which contrasts with the diffuse gammaglobulin bands in the normal patients.

band. Other antibody production is suppressed, contributing to the immunodeficiency found in this disease.

Malignant plasma cells may fail to make a complete immunoglobulin molecule and only make part of it. Commonly light chains are manufactured and released from the plasma cells and these are small enough to pass through the glomerulus and appear as Bence Jones protein (BJP) in the urine. Classically this protein precipitates when the urine is heated (like most urinary proteins) but, unlike other urinary proteins, the BJP re-dissolves when the urine is heated further. In modern laboratories BJP is usually detected by sensitive immunological techniques rather than heating. BJP may form casts in the renal tubules, another cause of impaired renal function in myeloma.

Management

Hypercalcaemia, if present, is managed by vigorous hydration, and steroid and bisphosphonate administration. Supportive treatment, such as red cell transfusion, antibiotics and platelet transfusion, are given as in any case of marrow failure. Chemotherapeutic treatment may consist of single-agent oral alkylating drugs such as melphalan or combination chemotherapy regimens such as VAD (vincristine, Adriamycin and dexamethasone). Younger patients may benefit from stem cell autografts, particularly if the response to initial chemotherapy has been good and the ability to selectively purify the stem cells in the graft is locally available. Radiotherapy effectively treats painful lytic lesions and the services of an orthopaedic surgeon may be required for the fixation of pathological fractures.

MYELOPROLIFERATIVE DISORDERS:

A group of neoplastic disorders of the bone marrow resulting in the overproduction of relatively normal blood and bone marrow cells. Four haematological diseases are classified as myeloproliferative disorders (Table M3).

Table M3 The myeloproliferative disorders

Disease	Major proliferating cell type
Polycythaemia* rubra vera	Red cell precursors
Essential (primary) thrombocythaemia*	Platelet precursors
Myelofibrosis*	Marrow reticulin framework
Chronic myeloid (granulocytic) leukaemia* (may also be classified as a chronic leukaemia)	Myeloid precursors

The divisions between the four myeloproliferative disorders are not absolute and many patients may have intermediate disorders with features of more than one, e.g. some cases of polycythaemia rubra vera may have very high platelet counts as well as a high haemoglobin; some cases of essential thrombocythaemia may have inaspirable marrow due to marrow fibrosis.

Common features of the myeloproliferative disorders

- Extramedullary haemopoiesis: the presence of developing myeloid and erythroid cells in tissues other than the bone marrow, particularly in spleen and liver. This haemopoiesis may result in mature red and white cells being released into the blood, or it may not (ineffective haemopoiesis). Extramedullary haemopoiesis may be regarded as metastasis* of bone marrow to other tissues.
- Marrow hyperplasia: the bone marrow has a higher density of cells than normal, which can be seen on biopsy, and may extend further down the long bones than usual, replacing white (fatty) marrow.
- Increased marrow reticulin: this is most noticeable in myelofibrosis*, when the increase in the reticulin framework on which the bone marrow

cells live is so thickened as to form fibrous tissue and prevent aspiration of marrow.
- Platelet dysfunction: particularly found in essential thrombocythaemia, but also in the other myeloproliferative disorders. The platelets may clump when they should not, leading to thrombosis, or not clump when they should, leading to bleeding.
- Hyperuricaemia: due to increased nucleic acid turnover, particularly if cytotoxic agents are used in treatment; may lead to gout.
- Clonality: all the cells of the disease can be demonstrated to have arisen from one parent cell.
- Predisposition to transform to acute leukaemia: This is high in chronic myeloid leukaemia, when more than 90% of cases will undergo blast transformation, and lower in the other myeloproliferative disorders.
- Basophilia: the myeloproliferative disorders are the commonest cause of an increased basophil count.

MYOCARDIAL INFARCTION:

Coagulative necrosis of the myocardium secondary to ischaemia.

Case

A 58-year-old man was admitted with severe, blunt, centrally located chest pain extending to his left arm and difficulty in breathing. The pain had started suddenly when he was having his breakfast and had become gradually unbearable within the last 3 hours. It was constant and did not change with movement or breathing. He had been well until that morning though he had noticed that he had started getting very tired after climbing stairs or walking uphill within the last year. He had been overweight all his life and had smoked 20 cigarettes a day for the last 40 years. His father had died of heart disease at the age of 65.

On physical examination his pulse rate was 122 beats/min, the respiration rate was 28/min, the blood pressure 150/95 mmHg. On auscultation his heart beat was regular though occasional extra beats were heard. His lung sounds were normal. There was no epigastric sensitivity. No other physical signs were present.

Blood chemistry showed increased creatine levels at the time of admission and increased aspartate aminotransferase and lactic dehydrogenase levels were detected next day.

Blood count showed a mild leucocytosis and increased ESR. An ECG showed characteristic changes of acute full thickness anterior wall infarction. Chest radiograph was normal. A radionuclide assay showed anterior wall myocardial hypoperfusion.

The patient was administered analgesic to control pain and anxiety and thrombolytic agents to help restore the coronary artery patency and β-adrenoreceptor antagonists to control tachycardia and arrhythmia.

Aetiology and risk factors

Myocardial infarction is almost always caused by atherosclerotic occlusion of the coronary arteries. Rarely, congenital abnormalities or vasculitis could be responsible.

Therefore risk factors associated with myocardial infarction are the same as those associated with the development of atherosclerosis. These include male sex, old age, family history, smoking, hypertension, hypercholesterolaemia, lack of physical activity and obesity.

Pathology

The cardinal symptom of myocardial infarction is chest pain which is characteristically severe, dull, constricting and continuous. The pain is a result of severe myocardial ischaemia and necrosis. A past history of angina as described in this patient suggests the presence of long-standing ischaemic heart disease. Patients suffering from myocardial infarction often feel breathless because of pain, although the respiratory capacity is not usually affected. The critical pathological event in myocardial infarction is an acute reduction in myocardial perfusion. Myocardial infarction takes two clinico-pathological patterns:
- transmural infarction,
- subendocardial infarction.

In transmural infarction the underlying event is occlusion of one of the coronary arteries by a sudden change in an atheromatous plaque, usually fissuring or ulceration of the plaque leading to platelet activation and thrombosis in the coronary artery lumen. In some cases, coronary artery spasm also contributes to the occlusion. This event is almost always limited to a single coronary artery and myocardial infarction is seen in the zone perfused by the particular coronary artery. The infarction involves the full thickness of the myocardium. In about 50% of cases the left anterior descending coronary artery is blocked and the infarction, as described in this case, is seen in the anterior wall of the left ventricle and anterior part of the interventricular septum. In other cases, either the right coronary artery or the left circumflex coronary artery is involved, leading to posterior wall or lateral wall infarctions, respectively. By contrast, in subendocardial infarction the area of necrosis is limited to the inner third of the myocardium. The necrosis usually shows patchy distribution and may encircle the whole of the inner myocardium. The subendocardial myocardium is very vulnerable to any reduction in blood flow. There is usually multivessel disease involving several arteries but no plaque fissuring or ulceration with thrombosis is seen.

Macroscopically, the area of damaged myocardium is not usually identifiable within the first 12 hours. After 12 hours the infarction can be identified as a pale zone. Histologically the first visible sign of infarction is wavy fibres. Microscopically identifiable coagulation necrosis appears 10–12 hours after the infarction and becomes established by 48 hours. There is usually interstitial infiltration by neutrophils, which leads to lysis of the necrotic tissue. This is followed by a reparative response. First, macrophages phagocytose the necrotic debris and inflammatory granulation tissue replaces the necrotic area. Eventually a scar tissue, predominantly composed of collagen fibres, is formed at the zone of the infarction. The whole process from infarction to scarring takes around 2 months (Fig. M23).

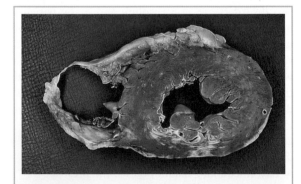

Fig. M23 Macroscopic appearance of heart after massive myocardial infarction involving the posterior wall of the left ventricle.

During the acute phase of myocardial infarction a number of enzymes are released into the circulation from the dying myocytes. Serial determination of plasma levels of these enzymes, in particular creatine kinase, aspartate aminotransferase and lactic dehydrogenase, is very helpful in the diagnosis and monitoring of myocardial infarction.

Although some patients suffering from acute myocardial infarction recover without problems, the majority develop complications secondary to the damage inflicted to the myocardium. The most

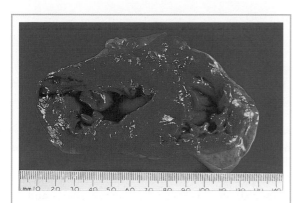

Fig. M24 Myocardial rupture in the lateral wall of the left ventricle following myocardial infarction.

Table M4 Infectious agents causing myocarditis

Viruses	Bacteria	Parasites
Coxsackie	*Strep. pyogenes*	*Trypanosoma* spp.
Influenza	*C. diphtheriae*	*Trichinella spiralis*
Echovirus	*Staph. aureus*	*Toxoplasma gondii*
Adenovirus	*M. pneumoniae*	
Mumps virus	*Ch. psittaci*	
Rabies virus	*Rickettsia rickettsii*	
CMV	*Borrelia burgdorferi*	
Rubella virus		

common complication is the development of arrhythmias, which are the main cause of sudden cardiac death in myocardial infarction. Other complications include cardiogenic shock, left ventricular aneurysm, cardiac rupture (Fig. M24), pericarditis and mural thrombus formation.

Management
The treatment is directed towards control of pain and arrhythmias, and thrombolytic measures where indicated.

MYOCARDITIS: Inflammation of the cardiac muscle (myocardium), usually as a result of an infectious process.

The clinical presentation of myocarditis is variable. In some patients the disease can be completely asymptomatic, in others arrhythmias, congestive heart failure, and even sudden cardiac death can occur. Physical examination can be normal or there may be changes in heart sounds and rhythm disturbances.

Aetiology and risk factors
Myocarditis can be seen in any age group; however, infants, pregnant women and immunosuppressed patients are more vulnerable. Myocarditis is caused most commonly by infectious agents (see Table M4). Other causes include hypersensitivity*, toxins (e.g. alcohol) and systemic diseases (e.g. rheumatoid arthritis*).

Pathology
Morphologically the ventricles are usually enlarged and the myocardium shows small areas of haemorrhage. Microscopically in viral myocarditis, the myocardium is infiltrated by inflammatory cells, which are predominantly lymphocytes. The myocytes adjacent to the myocardial infiltrate show focal areas of necrosis. In most cases the myocarditis is self-limited and resolves without complications. However, a proportion of the cases are thought to progress to develop dilated cardiomyopathy*. With viral myocarditis, replication of virus occurs in the myocytes (Coxsackievirus) or vascular endothelium (CMV). There is infiltration of the myocardium with inflammatory cells (mainly lymphocytes and macrophages) and necrosis of the myocytes, probably caused by a combination of direct cytolysis by the virus and the presence of autoreactive cytolytic T-cells, which also kill uninfected myocytes. Anti-myocardial antibodies can also be detected and may contribute to pathogenesis. Laboratory diagnosis is by histology of endocardial biopsy specimens, by isolation or detection of the causative infectious agent, by serology or by PCR.

Management
Treatment is usually limited to bed rest and control of complications such as arrhythmia and heart failure.

 Cardiomyopathy; Chagas disease; Lyme disease; Rheumatic fever

MYOSITIS: Inflammation of muscle. It may be due to infections (e.g. gas gangrene, Coxsackievirus) or part of a larger syndrome such as polymyositis* or dermatomyositis.

MYXOEDEMA: The syndrome of lethargy, weight gain, hair loss, low BMR, and localized oedema, due to deficiency of thyroid hormones. It is the commonest manifestation of hypothyroidism*, but the latter may also be due to Hashimoto disease*, iodine deficiency, or secondary to pituitary disease.

N

NAEVUS: Mole, a congenital benign skin lesion most often developing as a result of growth of melanocytes in the dermoepidermal junction, dermis or both.

 Malignant melanoma

NASOPHARYNGEAL CARCINOMA: A malignant tumour arising from the epithelial lining of the nasopharynx. It is rare in the West but endemic in southern China, SE Asia and the Mediterranean basin. EBV infection is thought to be critical in the development of the tumour.

 Burkitt lymphoma

NECROBACILLOSIS: A disease, usually of the head and neck, with tissue necrosis and abscess formation caused by *Fusobacterium necrophorum*.

 Lemierr syndrome

NECROSIS: Death of cells in a tissue or organ in a living individual. Necrosis is invariably due to some external factor (e.g. heat, toxins, anoxia), in contrast to apoptosis*, the 'planned suicide' mechanism used in tissue modelling.

NECROTIZING FASCIITIS: Infection of the subcutaneous tissues, typically with *Streptococcus pyogenes*.

Case

A patient was admitted to hospital with an area of spreading erythema on the arm following a minor injury. Over a short period of time his temperature rose and he became hypotensive, confused and tachycardic. The skin became a dusky purple colour, bullae had developed on the arm, and the area of inflammation had spread proximally and was very painful. A diagnosis of necrotizing fasciitis was made and a surgical opinion sought. The patient was started on antibiotics and wide surgical debridement of the necrotic tissue performed. Tissue specimens and blood cultures were sent to the laboratory.

Haematology: Hb 14 g/dl; WBC 17 000 × 10⁶/l; polymorphs 80%; Plt 120 × 10⁹/l.
Chemistry: CPK 250 U/l.
Microbiology: *Streptococcus pyogenes* isolated from the blood and tissue cultures.

Aetiology and risk factors

β-Haemolytic Gram-positive streptococci can be differentiated by the cell wall carbohydrate into Lancefield groups, A, B, C, G, etc. Lancefield group A is also called *Streptococcus pyogenes* and is responsible for a variety of different diseases as shown in Table N1.

Table N1 Lancefield groups and associated diseases

Lancefield group	Organism	Associated diseases
Lancefield Group A	*Strep. pyogenes*	Impetigo, pharyngitis, wound infection, erysipelas, necrotizing fasciitis, septicaemia, scarlet fever, toxic shock, rheumatic fever, glomerulonephritis, chorea
Lancefield B	*Strep. agalactiae*	Neonatal meningitis and septicaemia
Lancefield C	*Strep. zooepidemicus, Strep. equisimilis*	Pharyngitis and wound infections
Lancefield G	*Strep. equisimilis, Strep. canis*	Pharyngitis and wound infections

Note that the same Lancefield group carbohydrate can be found in separate species, and conversely different Lancefield carbohydrates may be found in the same species.

Strep. pyogenes can be further subdivided into Griffith types based upon antigenic differences in cell wall proteins (M, T, R). The organism is found as a commensal in the nasopharynx of a small proportion of individuals. It is transmitted by either droplet infection or contact. *Strep. pyogenes* adheres to fibronectin, which is expressed on the surface of epithelial cells in the pharynx, by lipoteichoic acid, found in the cell wall of the organism. The organism avoids the host defences by possessing a hyaluronic acid capsule and expressing M proteins on the surface of the bacterium. Both components are antiphagocytic. M proteins bind fibrin and a protein that inhibits the complement cascade, thus preventing opsonization. The large number of different M proteins that exist in different strains also means that repeated infections can occur with different Griffith types.

Pathology

The presence of the organism in the tissues stimulates an acute inflammation with recruitment of polymorphs to the site of infection. Superficial infections may remain relatively localized but if inoculated into deep tissue the organism may spread rapidly through the tissues, destroying them. In necrotizing fasciitis the organism spreads through the subcutaneous tissues, causing a vasculitis of the superficial blood vessels supplying the skin and leading to necrosis of the skin above the infection. The organism produces a number of extracellular enzymes such as hyaluronidase, lipase, DNase, streptolysin, streptokinase, which facilitate spread of the organism through the tissues (Fig. N1). Some strains also produce streptococcal pyrogenic exotoxins (speA, B and C) responsible for toxic shock and scarlet fever. These toxins are superantigens and stimulate the excessive release of pro-inflammatory cytokines from T-cells, macrophages, and monocytes.

Diagnosis is clinical and laboratory confirmation is by isolation of the organism. Evidence of a recent infection is supported by serology – the antistreptolysin O (ASO) and anti DNase titre.

Management

Management is by wide surgical debridement and benzylpenicillin.

 Glomerulonephritis; Rheumatic fever; Scarlet fever; Toxic shock syndrome

NEOPLASIA; NEOPLASM: Literally means 'new growth'. A neoplasm, by definition, demonstrates uncontrolled growth and is clonal – both features differentiate neoplasia from hyperplasia. Neoplasms may be benign or malignant.

NEPHRITIS: Inflammation of the kidney.

 Glomerulonephritis; Pyelonephritis

NEPHROTIC SYNDROME: A syndrome characterized by excessive proteinuria (>3.5 g/24 h), hypo-

N

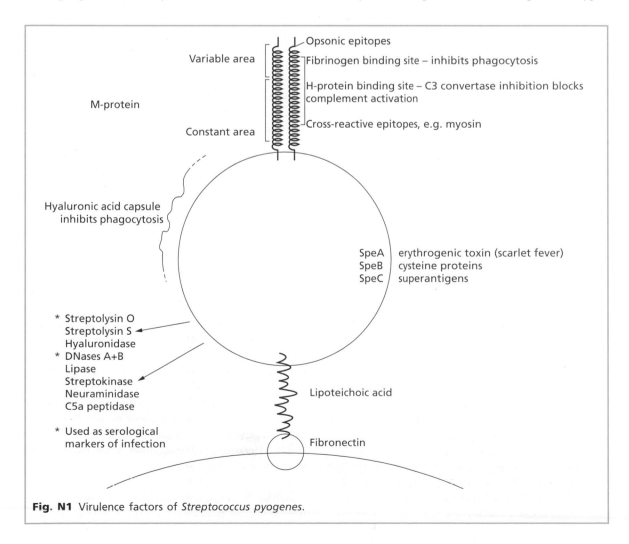

Fig. N1 Virulence factors of *Streptococcus pyogenes*.

albuminaemia and oedema. Hypercholesterolaemia is frequently also present.

Aetiology and risk factors

Any condition that causes increased glomerular capillary permeability (primary or secondary) to proteins will give rise to the nephrotic syndrome. The prognosis depends on the underlying cause. Examples of such conditions are as follows:

- primary glomerular disease: minimal change, membranous, mesangial proliferative and focal glomerulonephritis;
- secondary glomerular disease: diabetes, Alport syndrome, drugs, toxins, systemic lupus erythematosus, amyloidosis, renal vein thrombosis and multiple myeloma.

Pathology

In nephrotic patients the mechanism for the large amounts of proteinuria is complex. However, it occurs partially as a result of damage that occurs to the glomerular basement membrane allowing the passage of large protein molecules. This results in urinary excretion of albumin, reducing the osmotic pressure which maintains fluid within the blood vessels. With the loss of osmotic pressure, sodium and water escape into the extravascular compartments, resulting in a reduction in plasma volume. As a consequence the renin-angiotensin–aldosterone system is activated (secondary hyperaldosteronism), resulting in oedema. Due to the loss of other proteins apart from albumin, e.g. immunoglobulins and complement factors, there is increased susceptibility to infection. However, there is an increase in high molecular weight proteins such as fibrinogen, apolipoproteins and α2-microglobulin, resulting in elevated levels of fibrinogen, cholesterol and triglycerides. The increased fibrinogen makes nephrotic patients prone to thrombosis.

The presence of nephrotic syndrome is established by measuring 24-hour urinary protein concentration, serum albumin, creatinine, urea and creatinine clearance. Serum protein electrophoresis shows a reduced albumin and an increase in α- and β-globulin fractions.

Management

Management mainly lies in treatment of the underlying cause, where identifiable, and managing the consequences of the protein loss (high protein diet, antibiotics, anticoagulants, etc.).

NEUROBLASTOMA: A solid malignant tumour arising from primitive neuroepithelial cells, often located in the adrenal medulla or other paravertebral sympathetic ganglia.

Neuroblastoma is one of the commonest malignant tumours of childhood. The patients usually present with an abdominal mass, fever and weight loss. The tumour size is variable but can be as large as 1000 g. Histologically, the tumour is composed of small blue round cells similar to embryonic neuroepithelial cells. The tumour cells form solid nests or may form rosettes around a central fibrillary area. Some tumours contain mature ganglion cells between the primitive elements. Neuroblastomas metastasize early and extensively into liver, lung and bones. The prognosis depends on various factors, including the stage on presentation, DNA ploidy, the presence or absence of specific chromosomal deletions or amplifications, and histological grade. The treatment of neuroblastoma depends on the stage, and includes surgical excision, multi-agent chemotherapy, and bone marrow therapy.

NEUROFIBROMATOSIS: An inherited autosomal dominant disease characterized by development of multiple neurofibromas and sometimes other neurogenic tumours.

At least two distinct subtypes are recognized; neurofibromatosis-1 (von Recklinghausen disease) and neurofibromatosis-2. The more common of the two, neurofibromatosis-1, is characterized by the presence of multiple cutaneous and internal neurofibromas (Fig. N2), numerous irregular pigmented skin lesions with brownish coffee colour (so-called *café au lait* spots) and iris hamartomas* (Lisch nodules). These patients also have increased risk of developing meningiomas*, optic gliomas and phaeochromocytomas*. The gene (*NF-1*) involved has been mapped to chromosome 17 and codes for neurofibromin, a putative tumour suppressor gene. The much less frequent neurofibromatosis-2 is characterized by the presence of bilateral acoustic schwannomas and sometimes multiple meningiomas. The affected gene has been mapped to chromosome 22 and is also thought to be a tumour suppressor gene.

The clinical presentation shows a wide range due to variable gene expression and various locations of the tumours. The diagnosis can be made with some confidence in the presence of multiple nerve tumours and *café au lait* spots. Histologically, the neurofibromas seen in neurofibromatosis-1 are of plexiform subtype and may show malignant change in a small percentage of patients.

There is no treatment other than excision of symptomatic tumours.

NEUROPATHY: Non-neoplastic diseases of peripheral nerves secondary to various factors includ-

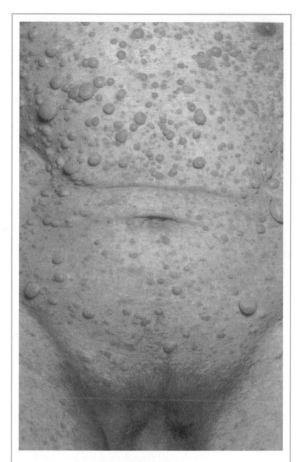

Fig. N2 A patient with neurofibromatosis. Numerous nodules are seen on the skin. (Reproduced from Browse NL. *An Introduction to the Symptoms and Signs of Surgical Disease*, 3rd edn. London: Arnold, 1997)

ing inflammation, infection, toxins, metabolic alterations and genetic diseases.

NEUROSYPHILIS: Infection of the central nervous system by *Treponema pallidum*.

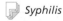 *Syphilis*

NEUTROPENIA: A reduction in the neutrophil count below the lower limit of the normal range $(2.0 \times 10^9/l)$. The neutrophil granulocyte is the major cellular defence against bacterial infection. Below a count of $1 \times 10^9/l$ a risk of bacterial infection exists. Below 0.5 this risk is marked and if in hospital the patient will usually be isolated.

Neutropenia may be found as an isolated problem, or associated with a reduction in red cells or platelets. When other cells are reduced the most likely cause is bone marrow infiltration, such as an

acute leukaemia* or other malignancy, or some cause of general marrow impairment, such as aplastic anaemia*.

Isolated neutropenia may be found as an idiosyncratic drug reaction, in myelodysplasia and autoimmune diseases*. Some normal Black and Middle East individuals run a persistently low neutrophil count in the blood but appear to have normal defences against infection. In this benign racial neutropenia it is likely that many of the neutrophils are held in the marginating pool in the tissues rather than in the circulation.

In the rare condition cyclical neutropenia there is defective physiological control of neutrophil production so that numbers in the blood fall very low before the bone marrow is stimulated into normal myelopoiesis, restoring the neutrophil count to normal. The bone marrow then switches off, allowing the neutrophil count to drop again, repeating the cycle.

 Agranulocytosis; Bone marrow failure

NOCARDIASIS: Infection caused by *Nocardia* spp. The organisms are found in the environment and may be opportunist pathogens in immunocompromised patients, e.g. renal transplant recipients. *Nocardia* can give rise to both focal and disseminated disease. The main route of entry for immunocompromised patients is probably via the lungs, leading to pulmonary disease, or by disseminating to, e.g. the brain. Clinically the patient can present with an acute pneumonia, chronic pulmonary disease (resembling tuberculosis) or focal signs of an abscess. Laboratory diagnosis is by isolation of the organism and treatment is with sulphonamides, amikacin or tetracyclines.

NON-GONOCOCCAL (NON-SPECIFIC) URETHRITIS: Genital infection principally caused by *Chlamydia trachomatis*.

 Chlamydial disease

NON-HODGKIN LYMPHOMA: A malignant tumour arising from B- or T-lymphocytes.

Case

A 53-year-old woman was seen in the outpatient department complaining of swelling in her neck. She was first seen by her GP a year ago complaining of sore throat and swelling in the neck and had received a course of antibiotics for upper respiratory infection after which the swelling had partially subsided. However, the size of the neck lump had gradually increased in the last 6 months and she

N

was referred by her GP to the haematology outpatients. She had no other complaints and was physically fit. Her past medical history and family history were unremarkable.

On physical examination she appeared well. Her vital signs were normal. She had palpable lymph nodes on both sides of her neck, axilla and groins measuring between 0.5 and 4 cm in diameter. The liver and spleen were not palpable. Neurological examination was normal. The routine hematological and blood chemical values and urine analysis were normal.

FNA of one of the cervical lymph nodes showed a monotonous infiltrate of small to medium-sized lymphocytes consistent with a low-grade lymphoma (Fig. N3).

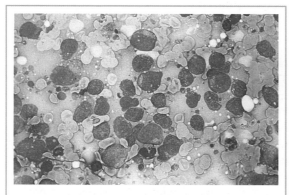

Fig. N3 FNA of the lymph node showing monotonous infiltrate of small to medium-sized lymphocytes.

One of the cervical lymph nodes was biopsied to confirm the cytological findings.

Histological examination of the cervical lymph node biopsy showed that the normal structures of the lymph node were replaced by a tumour composed of medium to small size lymphocytes. The tumour cells were forming follicular structures, which showed a back-to-back arrangement. Immunohistochemistry showed that the tumour cells were B-lymphocytes expressing bcl2 protein and showing light chain restriction. A diagnosis of low-grade non-Hodgkin lymphoma, follicle centre subtype (follicular lymphoma) was made (Fig. N4).

In the light of the diagnosis, a number of additional tests were performed to establish the extent of disease (staging).

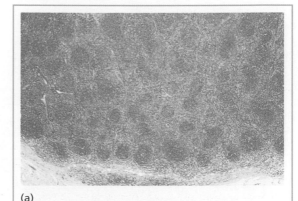

(a)

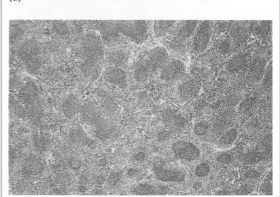

(b)

Fig. N4 (a) Histology of follicular lymphoma showing bare follicles arranged in a back-to-back pattern. (b) Same lymph node immunostained for bcl2 protein, which is expressed by the neoplastic follicles.

A chest radiograph was normal. CT scan of the abdomen showed enlargement of para-aortic lymph nodes.
A bone marrow trephine biopsy showed a normocellular bone marrow with paratrabecular aggregates of small lymphocytes consistent with lymphoma involvement.

Staging showed that the patient had stage 4 disease with bone marrow involvement and she was treated with chemotherapy.

Aetiology and risk factors

In the majority of cases the aetiology of non-Hodgkin lymphoma is not known. However, there are a number of risk factors and diseases associated with different subsets of non-Hodgkin lymphomas. These include immunodeficiency states, chronic inflammatory states (particularly autoimmune disorders), drugs (in particular cancer chemotherapeutics), environmental factors such as ionizing radiation, and viruses such as EBV in Burkitt lymphoma*.

The majority of non-Hodgkin lymphomas occur after the age of 40; however, every age group can be effected. There is a slight male to female predominance and a higher incidence in whites than blacks.

Pathology

Approximately two-thirds of non-Hodgkin lymphomas present with persistent painless enlargement of the lymph nodes as observed in this case. In low-grade lymphomas the patient usually feels well and no other symptoms may be present. However, occasionally, systemic symptoms such as fever, night sweats and weight loss or symptoms due to involvement of extranodal sites can be present.

On physical examination the patient usually has generalized lymphadenopathy and enlargement of spleen and liver may be detected if these organs are also involved.

As a number of other diseases such as infections, autoimmune diseases or other neoplasms can cause generalized lymphadenopathy, examination of the lymph node with FNA and followed by biopsy is essential to establish the diagnosis.

Accurate classification of lymphomas is critical as clinical features, treatment and prognosis depend on the lymphoma subtype. This area has been subject to intense debate and controversy for many years. In Europe a scheme called the Revised European–American Lymphoma (REAL) classification is currently being used. This sets forth the diagnostic features of lymphomas that are widely recognized and diagnosable by contemporary techniques. For practical purposes, over 85% of non-Hodgkin lymphomas derive from B-lymphocytes and thus are called B-cell lymphomas. Most B-cell lymphomas arising in the lymph nodes fall into two main categories: follicle-centre (follicular) lymphomas and diffuse large-cell lymphomas. Follicular lymphomas, as observed in the above case, are composed of medium to small size neoplastic B-cells which efface the normal lymph node architecture and form neoplastic follicles. In most cases the neoplastic B-cells express the anti-apoptotic bcl2 protein as a result of the t(14;18) chromosomal translocation which juxtaposes the *bcl2* gene to the transcriptionally active immunoglobulin heavy chain gene. This is thought to be the critical though not the sole abnormality in lymphomagenesis. As bcl2 expression is absent in normal follicle centres, immunohistochemical demonstration of bcl2 in tumour cells as described in this case is a very helpful tool in the establishment of the diagnosis of lymphoma. These tumours are considered to be cytologically low grade and follow an indolent clinical course over many years. They respond poorly to conventional therapies and most patients die of the disease within 10 years.

By contrast, the diffuse large-cell lymphomas are composed of large neoplastic lymphocytes with high-grade cytology and follow an aggressive clinical course. If untreated, most patients die of the disease within a few months. However, most cases of large-cell lymphoma respond dramatically to therapy, around 30–40% of patients being eventually cured of the disease.

Management

The treatment of malignant lymphoma is influenced by many factors including histological subtype, site and stage of disease. Treatment options include:

- observation (some low-grade lymphomas);
- surgery (some extranodal lymphomas);
- chemotherapy;
- radiotherapy;
- salvage therapeutic approaches;
- biological therapeutic approaches.

 Burkitt lymphoma; Chronic lymphocytic leukaemia; Hodgkin disease

NOSOCOMIAL INFECTION: Also called hospital-acquired infection.

 Hospital-acquired infection

O

OAT CELL CARCINOMA: A malignant epithelial tumour of the lung composed of clusters of small cells showing features of neuroendocrine differentiation.

Oat cell carcinoma, also known as small cell carcinoma, accounts for around 25% of all malignant tumours of the lung. The tumour is almost always associated with a history of smoking and is thought to arise from the bronchial epithelium. Histologically, the tumour is composed of clusters of small cells with dark irregular nuclei and no or very little cytoplasm (Fig. O1).

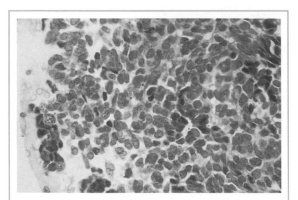

Fig. O1 Histological section of oat cell carcinoma (small cell carcinoma) showing small dark blue cells with smudging artefact.

Generally no glandular or squamous cell differentiation is seen; however, neuroendocrine features can be identified in tumour cells by electron microscopy and immunohistochemistry. The diagnosis is usually established by a biopsy performed under bronchoscopy. The tumour is usually widely spread locally and sometimes systemically at the time of diagnosis. Occasionally oat cell carcinoma can secrete ectopic hormones, in particular ADH and ACTH. The treatment of choice for oat cell carcinoma is chemotherapy. Despite initial dramatic responses and symptomatic relief, the prognosis remains dismal.

Hormone-secreting tumours; Lung carcinoma; Paraneoplastic syndromes

OBESITY: Usually defined as a body mass index >30. The body mass index (BMI) is calculated from the formula: $BMI = weight\ (kg)/height^2\ (m)$. Obese individuals have an increased mortality from diabetes mellitus, heart disease, cerebrovascular disease and chest infections.

Pathology

Two types of obesity are recognized, childhood-onset and adult-onset obesity. In the former, obesity results from an increase in number of fat cells, whilst in the latter it is due to hypertrophy of the existing cells. Obesity is a consequence of excess calorie intake, this excess being converted to fat and stored in the adipose tissue which is distributed in internal organs. Obesity can arise from certain pathological conditions such as Cushing syndrome*, hypothyroidism* or hypothalamic disease.

Table O1 shows some conditions associated with obesity and their pathogenesis.

Table O1 Conditions associated with obesity

Condition	Pathogenesis
Hypoventilation syndrome (Pickwickian syndrome)	Excessive fat accumulation in chest wall resulting in alveolar hypoventilation
Osteoarthritis	Increase in body weight on weight-bearing joints
Diabetes mellitus	Increased insulin release and resistance
Gallstones	Increased synthesis of cholesterol and lipoproteins
Hypertension	Increased adrenal corticosteroids
Atherosclerosis	Increased cholesterol and lipoproteins, diabetes mellitus and hypertension
Myocardial infarction	Ischaemic heart disease from atherosclerosis
Stroke	Ischaemic heart and cerebral disease from atherosclerosis

Management

Management is usually difficult but involves the use of advice, exercise, dieting (low calorie), drugs (fenfluramine) and gastric restriction surgery. Very severe obesity is associated with a high morbidity.

OCCUPATIONAL LUNG DISEASE: See pneumoconiosis.

OEDEMA: A collection of tissue fluid in the inter-cellular spaces of the body secondary to changes in hydrostatic or oncotic pressures.

 Ascites; Heart failure

OESOPHAGEAL CARCINOMA: A malignant epithelial tumour of the oesophagus arising from the native squamous epithelium or from metaplastic gastric mucosa.

Aetiology and risk factors
The aetiology of oesophageal carcinoma is not known but there are several well defined risk factors. These include alcohol, smoking, dietary factors including deficiencies in vitamins and essential metals, and long-standing oesophageal irritation. Men are affected several-fold more often than women.

Pathology
The cardinal presenting symptom of oesophageal carcinoma is difficulty in swallowing (dysphagia) due to obstruction of the oesophageal lumen by the tumour mass. Bleeding may occur, especially when the tumour is ulcerated. Diagnosis is usually established by endoscopic examination of the oesophagus and histological examination of the endoscopic biopsy. Macroscopically, tumour is seen either as an exophytic mass or as a diffusely infiltrative lesion with deep ulceration (Fig. O2). Histologically, most tumours are moderately to well-differentiated squamous cell carcinomas. These usually start as *in situ* carcinoma and develop into invasive cancer. Increasingly, invasive adenocarcinomas are also being diagnosed in the oesophagus. These start as glandular dysplasia in Barrett oesophagus* and eventually develop into invasive adenocarcinomas. Oesophageal carcinomas remain clinically silent till late in the disease. Usually extensive local spread and distant metastasis has occurred by the time of diagnosis. The prognosis for superficial cancers is good as they can be completely removed by surgical resection. However, little can be done for deeper invasive tumours.

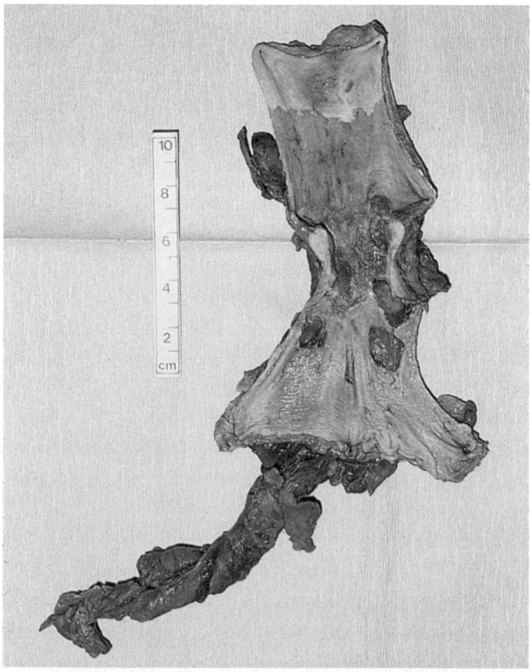

Management
Primary management is surgical but radiotherapy or chemotherapy may be needed to prevent recurrence or treat systemic disease.

 Barrett oesophagus

ONCHOCERCIASIS: See Filariasis.

ONCHRONOSIS: See Alkaptonuria.

ONYCHOMYCOSIS: Infection of the nails with a fungus (dermatophyte, *Fusarium*, *Candida*, *Scytalidium* or *Scopulariopsis*). The nails become discoloured, hypertrophic soft and friable.

Ringworm

OPPORTUNISTIC INFECTION: A generic term meaning an infection by an organism normally of relatively low pathogenicity occurring in an immunocompromised host.

ORCHITIS: Acute or chronic inflammation of the testis, usually secondary to an infectious process.

In most instances the orchitis develops secondary to an epididymal infection. Common bacterial urinary tract infections can spread to the testis in this way. Specific inflammations such as gonorrhoea* and tuberculosis* may also cause orchitis by extension of epididymitis into the testis. On the other hand, both congenital and acquired syphilis* tend to directly involve the testis. Orchitis may also be a consequence of systemic viral infections, in particular mumps infection in postpubertal males. In this case the involvement of the testis is usually unilateral and patchy, rarely causing infertility.

The presenting symptom is usually testicular enlargement associated with pain. The morphology

Fig. O2 Macroscopic appearance of oesophageal cancer involving the middle part of the oesophagus.

of orchitis depends on the infecting agent and the stage of the infection. Initially there is usually an interstitial inflammatory infiltrate containing neutrophils as well as lymphocytes and macrophages. The inflammation then extends into the tubules and suppurative necrosis and microabscess formation can be seen. Healing may lead to extensive fibrosis. In tuberculosis* the histological changes mimic the features of tuberculous infection elsewhere.

Treatment is directed against the offending agent.

OROYA FEVER: A rare infection caused by *Bartonella bacilliformis* and geographically restricted to the northern Andes. It is transmitted by the sandfly. The micro-organism parasitizes the erythrocyte and causes an acute haemolytic anaemia. The patient presents with a fever, a low haemoglobin and splenomegaly. Laboratory diagnosis is by microscopy of a blood film and treatment is with chloramphenicol.

OSLER–WEBER–RENDU DISEASE: A rare autosomal dominant disorder characterized by the presence of numerous small vascular ectasias (telangiectases) in the skin or mucous membranes. Also known as hereditary haemorrhagic telangiectasia*.

OSTEITIS DEFORMANS: A chronic disease of bone characterized by periods of osteoblastic and osteoclastic activity resulting in irregular bone formation.

 Paget disease of bone

OSTEOARTHRITIS: A degenerative disease of the joints characterized by destruction of articular cartilage, usually leading to disability.

Case

A 72-year-old man was admitted complaining of long-standing pain in the right knee joint. The symptoms had started 5 years ago. Initially they were intermittent with discomfort in the right knee joint which was brought about by activity and disappeared with rest. The pain had become worse in the last 3 years and limited the patient's movements considerably. Since that time he had been receiving physiotherapy to maintain joint function and using analgesics to control the pain. The movement of the joint was now very limited and he had difficulty in walking. There was also pain associated with movement in the left knee joint, though much less severe. He had no other diseases and his past medical history was unremarkable.

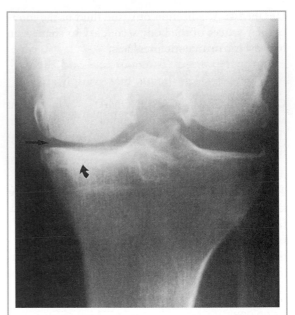

Fig. O3 Radiograph of the knee showing joint space (straight arrow), osteophyte formation and sclerosis (curved arrow). (Reproduced with permission from Lisle DA. *Imaging for Students*. London: Arnold, 1996)

On examination the right knee joint was painful when moved and the movement capacity was very limited. There was wasting in associated muscle groups. Other physical signs were unremarkable.

Peripheral blood count, ESR and blood chemistry were within normal limits.

Radiographs of the right knee showed loss of joint space, formation of osteophytes and subchondral sclerosis (Fig. O3).

As the pain persisted despite medical treatment and the movement of the joint was severely limited, a right knee-joint replacement was performed.

The histopathological examination of the joint removed during surgery showed loss of articular cartilage, thickened subchondral bone and cystic change in the subchondral bone. Osteophytes were present at the periphery. No inflammatory reaction was present.

Aetiology and risk factors

Osteoarthritis is one of the commonest diseases affecting the elderly, most of the population above the age of 65 having at least one joint involved. The aetiology of osteoarthritis is unclear. Either an abnormality in the articular cartilage or changes in the joint stresses is considered to be the initiating event.

In the majority of the cases no reasons for development of osteoarthritis is apparent (so-called primary osteoarthritis) and a change in cartilage secondary to ageing has been suggested. In a small percentage of cases a preceding condition is associated with the development of the disease (so-called secondary arthritis). These include repeated trauma, metabolic diseases such as haemochromatosis, inflammatory conditions such as septic arthritis or rheumatoid arthritis, developmental abnormalities and systemic diseases such as diabetes. The anatomical distribution of the diseases differs between men and women, the hip joint being more often involved in men, in contrast to the knees and hands in women.

Pathology
The underlying event in osteoarthritis is the destruction of the articular cartilage and underlying (subchondral) bone. The first changes seen in the articular cartilage are chondrocyte proliferation in clusters and biochemical changes in the matrix. This is followed by fibrillation and fragmentation of the cartilage. Eventually the cartilage is lost and subchondral bone forms the articular surface. Microfractures on the bone surface allow synovial fluid into the subchondral bone and lead to cyst formation. Attempts in regeneration result in sclerosis and development of bony outgrowths (osteophytes) as observed in this case. Occasionally fragments of cartilage or bone separate and fall into the joint space, forming so-called loose bodies. Unlike rheumatoid arthritis*, no significant inflammatory reaction is seen in osteoarthritis.

Osteoarthritis has a slow but progressive course, eventually leading to disability in many patients.

Management
Treatment is aimed at relieving symptoms with simple analgesia and maintaining or improving joint functions with exercises and physiotherapy.

 Ankylosing spondylitis; Rheumatoid arthritis

OSTEOMALACIA: Defective mineralization of bone occurring in the adult. There are associated structural and metabolic abnormalities.

Aetiology and risk factors
Osteomalacia is a disorder resulting from failure of bone mineralization (low calcium and low phosphate) and defective osteoblast function in adults. The causes of osteomalacia as a result of low calcium include a lack of adequate sunlight, postgastrectomy, abnormal vitamin D metabolism, malabsorption syndromes, chronic renal disease and anticonvulsant therapy. The causes of osteomalacia

as a result of low phosphate include those hereditary and acquired conditions associated with a renal tubular phosphate loss, such as Fanconi anaemia*, cystinosis, Wilson disease*, lead nephropathy and cadmium nephropathy. Osteomalacia as a result of defective osteoblast function is seen in relation to aluminium retention and high-dose treatment with diphosphonates in patients with Paget disease.

Pathology
In osteomalacia, as a result of defective mineralization, there is uncalcified osteoid. The consequence is softening of the bone with an increase in osteoblasts, resulting in soft bones, weakness, bowing deformity of the long bones and incomplete fractures. Osteomalacia causes significant bone pain. However, unlike rickets there are very few skeletal deformities seen in adults.

Blood/urine tests reveal a normal or low serum calcium, normal or low serum phosphate (subsequently elevated as a result of increase in PTH), normal or raised serum alkaline phosphatase, increase in PTH levels and normal or low levels of 25(OH)D.

Bone histology reveals evidence of osteomalacia or hyperparathyroidism.

Management
Osteomalacia is best treated using oral calcitriol or alfacalcidol and phosphate supplements. Caution must be taken in phosphate replacement because of the risk of metastatic calcification.

OSTEOMYELITIS: Infection of bone.

Case
A young child was feverish and off his food. He complained of pain in the leg and was unwilling to walk. The thigh was hot, swollen and tender to palpation. A provisional diagnosis of osteomyelitis was made and the patient admitted to hospital. A blood culture and full blood count was taken and a radiograph performed.

> Haematology: Hb 11 g/dl; WBC 15 000 × 10⁶/l; polymorphs 80%; ESR 40 mm/h.
> Microbiology: *Staphylococcus aureus* isolated from the blood cultures (Fig. O4).
> Radiology: The radiograph showed elevation of the periosteum of the femur.

Aetiology and risk factors
Most cases are caused by *Staphylococcus aureus* although other organisms can also cause infection (Table O2).

O

Table O2 Causes of osteomyelitis

Infants	Group B streptococcus, *E coli*	Subperiosteal abscess common
Children	*Staph. aureus*	Frequently follows minor trauma. Occurs in the metaphysis of long bones
Adults	*Staph. aureus, E. coli*	Commonly occurs in vertebrae as well as the diaphysis of long bones
Any age	*Salmonella* Dimorphic fungi, e.g. *Coccidioides, Histoplasma* as part of systemic disease *Brucella* sp. *M. tuberculosis*	Associated with sickle cell disease

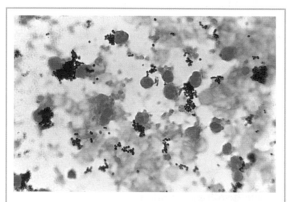

Fig. O4 Gram stain of blood cultures showing Gram-positive cocci in clusters.

Staph. aureus is a Gram-positive coccus that is differentiated from all the other staphylococci by producing coagulase, an enzyme that converts fibrinogen to fibrin and is a virulence characteristic (Fig. O5). *Staph. aureus* is associated with a wide range of diseases as follows:

- impetigo and boils
- wound infections
- abscess
- septicaemia
- pneumonia (secondary to influenza or in patients with cystic fibrosis)
- osteomyelitis and arthritis
- endocarditis (in IVDU)
- meningitis(following surgery or trauma)

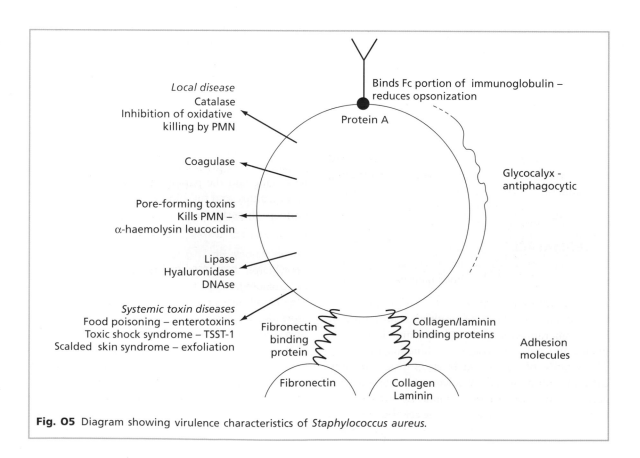

Fig. O5 Diagram showing virulence characteristics of *Staphylococcus aureus*.

- scalded skin syndrome
- food poisoning
- toxic shock syndrome.

The virulence characteristics of *Staph. aureus* are shown in Fig. O5.

Pathology

Staph. aureus may spread to the bones either following trauma or via the bloodstream. The organism localizes to the metaphysis of the long bones because of the presence there of large venous sinusoids which lead to sluggish blood flow. The organism produces an acute inflammation and oedema, which reduces the blood flow to the periosteum, leading to necrosis of bone. There is infiltration with neutrophils and a local acidosis compromising the host defences. The infection can spread through the bone leading to a raised periosteum, which further diminishes the blood supply and leads to further bony necrosis. The organism grows in the necrotic tissue as a microcolony surrounded by a glycocalyx where it is relatively protected from the host defences, predisposing to chronic infection. Laboratory diagnosis is by isolation of the organism from the blood or a specimen of bone.

Management

Management is with appropriate antibiotics, usually flucloxacillin with or without Fucidin for *Staph. aureus* infections. Surgery may be required but usually not in children.

OSTEOPOROSIS: A generalized term defining a reduction in bone mass associated with a decrease in structural strength of the bone.

Aetiology and risk factors

A large number of clinical states can be associated with osteoporosis; the most important ones are:
- ageing
- postmenopausal hormonal changes
- reduced physical activity
- endocrine disorders (hyperparathyroidism*, hyperthyroidism*, diabetes*)
- neoplasia (plasma cell myeloma*, carcinomatosis)
- gastrointestinal diseases (malnutrition, malabsorption, vitamin C and D deficiencies)
- rheumatic diseases
- drugs.

The pathogenesis of osteoporosis is complex and depends on the underlying cause. In the osteoporosis of ageing, decreased osteoblastic activity and growth factor secretion and decreased physical activity are thought to contribute. In post-

menopausal osteoporosis, decreased serum oestrogen levels are believed to be the main cause.

Pathology

The clinical features depend on the bones involved. The most common symptoms are pain in the back and deformity of the spine due to collapse of vertebral bodies. Fractures of long bones, in particular in the hip, humerus and wrists, can also occur. Osteoporosis can be difficult to diagnose until complications develop. Radiological changes can be demonstrated only after substantial bone loss and blood biochemistry is not generally helpful. Histologically in osteoporotic bone the cortex and trabeculae are thin and the trabeculae have lost their interconnections and may show microfractures.

Management

Treatment depends on the underlying cause and includes preventive measures such as increased exercise, calcium supplements and oestrogen replacement therapy and treatment of complications.

 Osteomalacia

OTITIS EXTERNA: Acute inflammation of the external auditory meatus and pinna, which can be caused by a number of different micro-organisms, particularly *Aspergillus* sp. and *Pseudomonas aeruginosa*. Moist conditions predispose to infection and otitis externa may be a particular problem in deep-sea diving bells. Severe invasive disease may also occur, especially with *Ps. aeruginosa*, where the organism invades the underlying structures, such as bone and cartilage, producing 'malignant' otitis externa. The condition presents with pain, erythema and swelling of the tissues. Complications of malignant otitis externa include mastoiditis and brain abscess. Laboratory diagnosis is by isolation of the responsible organism and management is with local cleansing, topical antibiotics, or, if invasive disease is present, parenteral antibiotics.

OTITIS MEDIA: Acute inflammation of the middle ear caused mainly by respiratory viruses, *Streptococcus pneumoniae*, *Haemophilus influenzae* and *Moraxella catarrhalis*. The infection occurs principally in children. The middle ear is lined by ciliated mucus-secreting respiratory epithelial cells and communicates with the posterior nasopharynx by the eustachian tube. The eustachian tube allows drainage of secretions from the middle ear and ensures equalization of pressure inside and outside the middle ear. If the eustachian tube becomes blocked, secretions will accumulate and an infection may follow. The patient presents with fever, pain in the ear and possibly a discharge. There may be tinnitus and vertigo. On examination the tympanic membrane appears bulging and erythematous. Complications include mastoiditis, brain abscess, rupture of the tympanum, chronic effusion (glue ear) and hearing loss. Management of the acute episode relies on empirical antibiotics to cover the known pathogens (ampicillin, co-amoxiclav), although tympanocentesis and isolation of the pathogen may occasionally be required. Chronic infection unresponsive to medical management may require the placement of tympanostomy tubes.

OVARIAN CANCER: A malignant tumour of the ovary arising most commonly from the surface epithelium but also occasionally from the germ cells. Most present as cystic masses and are discussed under a separate entry (see Ovarian cyst).

 Ovarian cyst; Teratoma

OVARIAN CYST: Cystic dilatation of the ovaries secondary to physiological processes, neoplastic or non-neoplastic diseases.

Broadly, ovarian cysts can be classified into two groups: non-neoplastic and neoplastic (Table O3).

Table O3 Ovarian cysts

Category	Histological type and characteristics
Non-neoplastic cysts Follicular cyst	Physiological. Usually incidental finding during palpation or ultrasonography. Often multiple and less than 2 cm in diameter. Occasionally larger ones can arise as a result of iatrogenic ovarian stimulation. They contain clear fluid and are lined by granulosa cells
Luteal cyst	Physiological. These are cystically dilated corpora lutea, usually secondary to haemorrhage after ovulation. They are lined by luteinized granulosa cells giving a yellow colour to the cyst wall
Polycystic ovaries	See Polycystic ovary*
Endometriotic cyst	See Endometriosis*
Neoplastic cysts Serous tumours	These arise from the surface epithelium. Around 70% are benign, the rest being either of borderline malignancy or frankly malignant. Serous cystic tumours can be very large and bilateral. The cysts characteristically contain clear, serous liquid. In benign serous cysts, the wall is lined by a single layer, tubal-type, columnar epithelium. In borderline and malignant tumours the epithelium forms multiple layers and papillary projections
Mucinous tumours	These also arise from the surface epithelium and have benign, borderline and malignant varieties. They are lined by mucinous type epithelium and the cysts contain mucin. When the borderline or malignant mucinous tumours spread to the peritoneal cavity they form numerous small tumours containing mucin and scanty tumour cells. This pattern of spread is called 'pseudomyxoma peritonei' and may have serious consequences for the patient
Endometrioid tumours	These are thought to arise from the surface epithelium. The majority are malignant and are composed of glands resembling endometrium
Germ cell tumours	The majority of germ cell tumours arising in the ovary are benign mature teratomas*. Characteristically these are cystic tumours containing sebaceous material and hair. The cyst is usually lined by squamous epithelium and underlying skin appendages mimicking normal skin. For this reason these are also called 'dermoid cysts'. Occasionally other tissues such as bone, thyroid, respiratory epithelium or brain can be seen. Rarely, immature teratomas containing primitive epithelial or mesenchymal elements can arise. These may behave aggressively and have overall poor prognosis

O

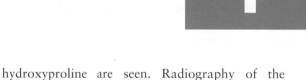

PAGET DISEASE OF BONE: Also known as osteitis deformans; a bony disorder seen in the UK in about 10% of the elderly. It affects about 1% of the population of men above 50 years of age in Western Europe and the United States. The condition is usually asymptomatic and men are more commonly affected.

Aetiology and risk factors
The aetiology of this disease is unknown but there are some suggestions that a virus infection may be implicated.

Pathology
Clinical features of Paget disease are pain in the affected bone, bony deformities (bowing of the tibia and femur) and fractures (spine). Biochemically, serum calcium, phosphorus and parathyroid hormones are normal. Increased levels of serum alkaline phosphatase (bony origin) and urine hydroxyproline are seen. Radiography of the affected bones shows a mixture of osteolytic and osteosclerotic changes (Fig. P1).

One or more bones may be involved. The more commonly affected bones include the pelvis, skull, spine scapula, femur, tibia, humerus and mandible. The disease process starts with an irregular increase in osteoclastic resorption of bone followed by an osteoblastic reaction, laying down new bone, which is highly vascular. This process usually maintains the total bone volume. Finally, there is a sclerotic phase in which the osteoblastic exceeds the osteoclastic activity, resulting in marked thickening of the bony trabeculae and cortex. High-output cardiac failure is a major complication and there is an increased risk (2–5%) of involved bones becoming malignant (osteogenic sarcoma).

Management
Paget disease is treated with diphosphonates and calcitonin.

PAGET DISEASE OF BREAST: Involvement of the epidermis of the nipple and surrounding skin of breast by ductal breast carcinoma*, clinically resembling eczema. There is almost always an underlying *in situ* ductal carcinoma (see also Fig. B9, p. 41).

PANCOAST TUMOUR: Apical lung cancer which invades the cervical sympathetic chain to produce ipsilateral Horner syndrome (ptosis, miosis, anhidrosis and enophthalmos). It may also invade the axillary plexus.

PANCREATIC CARCINOMA: A malignant epithelial tumour of the pancreas, arising from ducts or acini of the exocrine pancreas.

Aetiology and risk factors
Pancreatic carcinoma is one of the most frequent cancers in the West. The aetiology is not known, but a history of smoking and excess alcohol consumption are important risk factors. The oncogene K-*ras* has been shown to be mutated in most pancreatic carcinomas and the tumour suppressor gene, *p53*, is affected in the majority of cases.

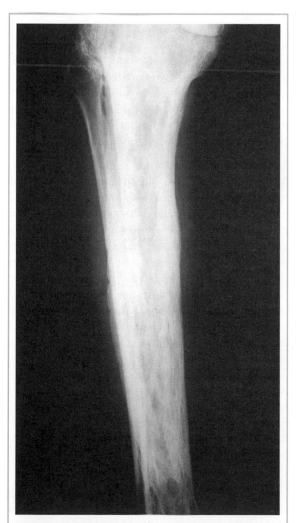

Fig. P1 Radiograph of leg showing increased density of bone in tibia.

Pathology

Most pancreatic carcinomas produce clinical symptoms and signs only late in the disease when the cancer has spread beyond the pancreas. Abdominal pain is the main symptom when the tumour involves main nerve trunks in the lesions. The majority of the tumours arise in the head of the pancreas and these often cause jaundice by blocking the common bile duct. Other symptoms and signs include weight loss, anorexia and generalized weakness. If the pancreas is diffusely infiltrated, diabetes may develop due to loss of endocrine pancreas. With tumours of the body or tail of the pancreas, laboratory tests are often normal, but with cancers of the head of the pancreas, serum bilirubin and alkaline phosphatase, and prothrombin time, are raised, and urobilinogen absent from urine and stools.

The diagnosis is reached by imaging and biopsy of the lesion by a percutaneous trucut biopsy. Histologically most cancers are moderately differentiated adenocarcinomas of pancreatic duct origin. The tumour stroma shows dense desmoplastic reaction and perineural invasion is usually present. Locally, pancreatic carcinoma infiltrates the retroperitoneal space and adjacent organs such as the duodenum, stomach, adrenals and kidneys as well as regional lymph nodes, nerve trunks and large vessels. Distant metastasis is predominantly seen in the liver, lungs and bones. As most cases are diagnosed late, the prognosis is very poor. Only in 10% of cases can successful curative surgery be performed.

Management

Management consists of surgery to resect small tumours or to relieve bile-duct obstruction.

PANCREATITIS: Acute or chronic inflammation of the pancreas.

Case

A 43-year-old woman presented to the casualty department with a history of severe abdominal pain radiating to her back. The pain had started the night before and gradually worsened. She had developed nausea and vomiting within the last 6 hours. She had a history of vague abdominal discomfort in the right upper quadrant for the last year; otherwise her past medical history and family history were unremarkable.

On examination she was febrile with a temperature of 38.7°C. Her pulse was 120 beats/min, blood pressure was 90/50 mmHg, respiratory rate was 25/min. Her skin was dry and skin turgor was increased. On palpation there was sharp abdominal tenderness limited to the epigastric region. Her liver and gallbladder were not palpable and the right upper quadrant was relatively free of pain. On auscultation the intestinal sounds were diminished.

A plain film of the abdomen showed localized ileus involving the jejunum (sentinel loop). Ultrasonographic examination of the abdomen and abdominal CT scan showed oedema and enlargement of the pancreas as well as multiple small stones in the gallbladder but no evidence of a perforated viscus.

> Blood count and chemistry: Hb 13.5 g/l; Hct 41%; ESR 40 mm/h; WBC 1.8×10^9/l; serum amylase: 2000 units/l.
> Liver and kidney function tests were within normal limits.

The presence of characteristic symptoms and signs and increased serum amylase strongly suggested a diagnosis of acute pancreatitis secondary to cholelithiasis in this case. The patient was treated medically with analgesics to control the pain and i.v. fluids to maintain intravascular volume. The symptoms subsided and the patient recovered within the next 5 days. An elective cholecystectomy was performed at a later date.

Aetiology and risk factors

Acute pancreatitis is caused by the release of pancreatic digestive enzymes into the interstitial tissue, usually secondary to obstruction of the pancreatic duct. In the great majority of cases it is associated with either biliary tract disease (in particular cholelithiasis) or alcoholism. In cholelithiasis it is thought that the blockage of the ampulla of Vater by gallstones leads to the ductal obstruction. In the case of alcoholic pancreatitis, increased viscosity of pancreatic secretion is thought to cause impaction of secretions within the ductules leading to obstruction. Alcohol can also damage acinar cells by direct toxicity. Other less common risk factors for the development of pancreatitis include drugs, viral infections, abdominal surgery, metabolic disorders such as hyperlipidaemia and hypercalcaemia. In about 10% of cases no precipitating factors can be identified.

Pathology

Most of the clinical features of acute pancreatitis can be attributed to the release of digestive enzymes of the pancreatic acini into surrounding tissues and the systemic circulation. Proteolytic and lipolytic digestion of the pancreatic and peripancreatic

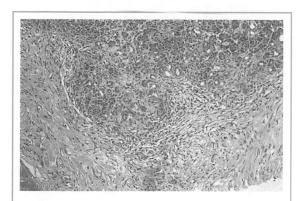

Fig. P2 Histological section of pancreas showing fibrosis and a mixed inflammatory infiltrate.

tissues leads to destruction of pancreatic acini and necrosis of intra- and peripancreatic fat. Involvement of blood vessels causes interstitial haemorrhage. An inflammatory infiltrate composed mainly of neutrophils soon accumulates (Fig. P2).

Features of an acute abdomen with severe abdominal pain and ileus develop as a consequence of involvement of the peritoneum, the mesentery, the omentum and the abdominal wall. Ascites containing digested tissue components and pancreatic enzymes such as amylase may accumulate. Measurement of amylase in the ascites may be helpful in the diagnosis of acute pancreatitis. Other local complications include formation of a pancreatic abscess secondary to liquefaction of pancreatic tissue and formation of pseudocysts.

Release of pancreatic enzymes into the systemic circulation results in increased blood levels of amylase and lipase. Measurement of these enzymes in the serum, though not entirely specific for acute pancreatitis, provides a very useful diagnostic tool. Increased levels of serum amylase activity can be detected between 2 and 12 hours of onset of the attack. If there are no further complications the levels will return to normal within 3–5 days. The magnitude of the rise of serum amylase activity does not correlate with the severity of the disease, and about 15–20% of patients with acute pancreatitis will have normal levels. Systemic complications of acute pancreatitis include hypovolemic shock secondary to fluid loss and release of vasodilator inflammatory mediators, pleural effusions, adult respiratory distress syndrome and acute tubular necrosis. An important biochemical complication is that of hypocalcaemia; this is as a combined result of reduced parathormone levels, loss into necrotic fat and low albumin.

Repeated attacks of acute pancreatitis, usually secondary to alcoholism or biliary tract disease, can lead to the development of chronic pancreatitis. Clinically the patients suffer from abdominal pain and weight loss. Symptoms related to destruction of pancreatic tissue are often observed. These include steatorrhoea, malabsorption and weight loss secondary to loss of exocrine pancreas, and diabetes secondary to loss of endocrine pancreas. Morphologically, the pancreas becomes fibrotic with loss of pancreatic acini and obliteration of pancreatic ducts. The remaining ducts become enlarged and contain inspissated secretions, which may be calcified and can be detected on radiographs.

Management

In most patients with acute pancreatitis the disease is self-limiting and supportive therapy to control pain and correct fluid balance is sufficient. If malabsorption is present in chronic pancreatitis, pancreatic enzyme replacement therapy is administered.

PANNICULITIS: Inflammation of the subcutaneous fatty tissue.

PAPILLOMA: A benign tumour of the epithelium, morphologically characterized by finger-like projections in a fibrovascular stroma. Papillomas most commonly arise from the skin, oral mucosa or urothelium.

PARACOCCIDIODOMYCOSIS: Or South American blastomycosis, an infection with the dimorphic fungus *Paracoccidioides brasiliensis*.

Aetiology and risk factors

The infection is endemic in South America and the natural habitat of the fungus is unknown although it may be the soil. The infection is probably acquired by the respiratory route.

Pathology

Once in the lungs, the conidia germinate as yeasts and invoke a granulomatous response. With progression of disease there is mediastinal lymphadenopathy and ultimately there may be fibrosis of the lungs and airways, leading to respiratory problems. Disseminated disease can involve the adrenals (leading to Addison disease*), skin, central nervous system and liver. Clinically the patient may remain asymptomatic or develop acute or chronic disease. With waning immunity, disease may reactivate in an asymptomatic individual. Disease can be either acute or chronic.

Acute disease presents with involvement of superficial lymph nodes and hepatosplenomegaly, and may have mucocutaneous involvement or disease of the gastrointestinal tract. Pulmonary involvement is uncommon. The patient is pyrexial with weight loss, mucocutaneous ulceration or symptoms of malabsorption. There may be a peripheral eosinophilia and a low serum albumin, leading to oedema.

In chronic disease, the main organ affected is the lungs, though other systems such as the larynx, trachea or skin may often be involved. Uncommonly abdominal organs and bones are affected. The presentation is indolent with productive cough, dyspnoea and weight loss. Oropharyngeal and respiratory mucosal ulcers are common, causing dysphagia and hoarseness, and with fibrosis they may lead to stenosis.

Laboratory diagnosis is by histology, serology and isolation of the fungus. Treatment is with amphotericin or azoles. It may also be treated with sulphonamides.

PARAGONIMIASIS: Infection with the lung fluke *Paragonimus* sp., acquired by eating raw crustaceans infected with the cercariae. After ingestion, the cercariae pass through the peritoneal cavity and diaphragm and enter the lungs where they encyst, mature and produce ova. The ova are expectorated or swallowed and passed out in the faeces into the environment where they hatch and infect freshwater snails. They undergo a developmental stage in the snails before infecting crustaceans, thus completing the life cycle. The encysted flukes cause an acute inflammation in the lungs producing abscesses, tissue necrosis and granuloma. There is peripheral eosinophilia and eosinophils can be found in the sputum. Clinically the patients have an initial allergic reaction with fever and urticaria. Chronic infection presents with a productive cough with reddish sputum, chest pain and dyspnoea. Symptoms may arise from lesions in other organs, e.g. brain. Laboratory diagnosis is by demonstration of the characteristic ova in sputum or faeces and serology. Treatment is with praziquantel.

PARANEOPLASTIC SYNDROMES: Symptoms and signs seen in cancer patients which cannot be explained by the direct effects of the primary tumour or its metastases.

A variety of pathogenetic mechanisms can cause paraneoplastic syndromes and in some instances no cause is apparent. Clinically the paraneoplastic syndrome may be the presenting symptom of a malignancy and in some instances can be life-threatening. Ectopic hormone secretion by the tumour is the most frequent cause of paraneoplastic syndrome and is discussed under a separate entry

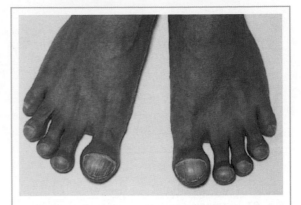

Fig. P3 Clubbing of the toes in a patient with cancer. (Reproduced from Browse NL. *An Introduction to the Symptoms and Signs of Surgical Disease*, 3rd edn. London: Arnold, 1997)

Table P1 Paraneoplastic syndromes

Ectopic hormone secretion*	
Skin disorders	Acanthosis nigricans*, dermatomyositis*
Neurological disorders	Myasthenia
Haematological disorders	Venous thrombosis, non-bacterial thrombotic endocarditis
Renal disorders	Glomerulonephritis*
Bone and soft tissue	Clubbing (Fig. P3); hypertrophic osteoarthropathy
Metabolic	Hypercalcaemia*

(see ectopic hormone secretion). Others are shown in Table P1.

PARAPROTEIN: A localized band of immunoglobulin usually detected in the gamma region of serum protein electrophoresis (see Fig. M22, p. 174). The antibody molecules in the band are all identical, being the product of a single clone of plasma cells.

A paraprotein is sometimes an incidental finding in otherwise healthy individuals, when it is known as monoclonal gammopathy of undetermined significance*. It is also a feature of malignant B-cell lymphoproliferative disorders such as myeloma* and Waldenström disease*.

PARATHYROID ADENOMA: A benign tumour of the parathyroid gland acini, often producing excess quantities of parathyroid hormone.

 Hyperparathyroidism

PARKINSON DISEASE: A disease affecting the extrapyramidal system, particularly the basal ganglia of the central nervous system, and characterized by rigidity and abnormal involuntary movements.

Case

A 75-year-old man presented with shakiness of both hands. The symptoms had started 2 years ago and had worsened during the last 6 months. His physical activity was reduced, he no longer played golf and he felt old and tired. His past medical history was unremarkable and he was not taking any drugs. His physical examination was normal. On neurological examination there was effacement of both nasolabial folds (masked face). There was resting tremor with a 'pill rolling' pattern in both hands. He had rigidity, slowness of movement (bradykinesis), difficulty in starting movement and postural instability. There was no loss of sensory functions or intellectual capacity.

In the presence of classical clinical findings, the patient was diagnosed as having idiopathic Parkinson disease and was put on dopamine replacement therapy. He responded very well to dopamine and remains well.

Aetiology and risk factors

The cause of Parkinson disease is not known. Genetic factors are not thought to be important. Certain drugs such as methyl-phenyl-tetrahydropyridine can cause a similar clinical syndrome, as can brain injury (e.g. in boxers). The disease usually presents after 50 years of age and affects approximately 1% of the population above the age of 80. Males and females are affected equally.

Pathology

The motor disturbances seen in Parkinson disease are thought to be the result of loss of dopaminergic neurons in the nigrostriatal system. This system is important in regulating signals from the thalamus to the motor cortex. Postmortem examination of the brain stem shows loss of pigmentation in the substantia nigra and nucleus ceruleus (Fig. P4).

Microscopically there is loss of neurons and reactive gliosis in these areas. Some of the neurons contain round, eosinophilic, intracytoplasmic inclusions called Lewy bodies (Fig. P5) These are composed of neurofilament material and are believed to be the result of neuronal injury.

The features found in the substantia nigra are associated with reduction in striatal dopamine levels, and the severity of symptoms appears to be directly proportional to the dopamine loss. Around 10% of cases of idiopathic Parkinson disease are complicated by dementia – so-called Lewy body dementia – similar to Alzheimer disease*. The neuronal damage is irreversible and the disease usually progresses, albeit slowly, rendering a proportion of the patients severely disabled.

Management

In earlier stages of the disease the patients may respond to selegiline, a MAO-B inhibitor. In later stages dopamine replacement is the cornerstone of therapy. The dopamine precursor L-dopa, which can cross the blood–brain barrier, is administered in combination with carbidopa which controls the systemic side-effects. There are experimental attempts to control the disease with surgery or transplantation of fetal brain tissue.

 Alzheimer disease

PAROXYSMAL NOCTURNAL HAEMOGLOBINURIA (PNH): Acquired loss of cell membrane proteins on haemopoietic cells which protect against damage by complement. Without these

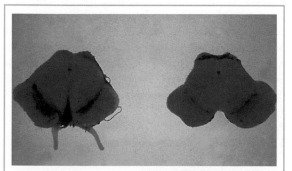

Fig. P4 Macroscopic appearance of brain stem showing loss of pigmentation in substantia nigra (right) compared to the normal brain stem (left).

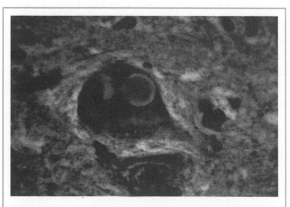

Fig. P5 Histological section showing Lewy body.

defences the cell membranes are under constant attack from miniature enzymatic explosions. This results in destruction of red cells, white cells and platelets. Bone marrow stem cells may also be affected, causing aplastic anaemia*.

Aetiology and risk factors

PNH is a clonal disorder due to a defect of a gene on the X chromosome which codes for a transmembrane protein anchor glyceryl phosphatidyl inositol (GPI). Without GPI, a variety of other proteins cannot maintain their attachment to the cell membrane, particularly the complement inactivating proteins DAF (decay-accelerating factor – CD55) and MIRL (membrane inhibitor of reactive lysis – CD59).

Pathology

The intermittent haemolysis of red cells is intravascular and the released haemoglobin appears in the urine, often most noticeable in the concentrated early morning specimen. Anaemia due to haemolysis may be exacerbated by iron deficiency due to chronic urinary blood loss. Some of the voided haemoglobin is phagocytosed by renal tubular cells. These are later shed into the urine and detection of a positive urinary haemosiderin provides a useful way of confirming intravascular haemolysis.

Perhaps because of the chronic release of tissue thromboplastin from damaged blood and bone marrow cells, patients with PNH are at risk from thrombosis. This may be in unusual sites such as the portal or hepatic veins. PNH is thus a rare cause of acquired thrombophilia*.

The classic diagnostic test for PNH is the Ham acid serum haemolysis test (Fig. P6). Because complement-mediated haemolysis particularly occurs in an acid medium, hydrochloric acid is added to the patient's red cells, with some fresh complement. The patient's red cells will haemolyse but normal control red cells will not. Many patients have had their anaemia corrected by transfusion with normal red cells before the diagnosis of PNH is entertained, so the Ham test will be negative. The diagnosis may then be made by detecting the absence of particular antigens from the patient's cell surface (Fig. P7).

Besides acquired aplastic anaemia, patients with PNH may also develop acute myeloid leukaemia*. A clone of PNH red cells may be found in a variety of haematological malignancies.

Management

This involves the correction of anaemia by red cell transfusion, treatment of thrombosis* by anticoag-

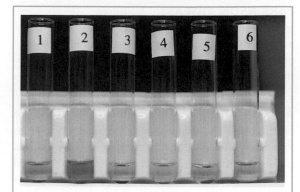

Fig. P6 Hams acidified serum haemolysis test. Haemolysis is visible in tube 2 when acid, patient red cells and fresh complement are all present. The other tubes are all controls, lacking these three essential components. Tube 1, fresh normal serum + patient red cells; tube 2, fresh normal serum + patient red cells + hydrochloric acid; tube 3, heat-inactivated normal serum + patient red cells + hydrochloric acid; tube 4, fresh normal serum + normal red cells; tube 5, fresh normal serum + normal red cells + hydrochloric acid; tube 6, heat-inactivated normal serum + normal red cells + hydrochloric acid.

ulation, and correction of iron deficiency by iron supplementation. Bone marrow transplantation is a curative treatment available for the minority of younger patients with an HLA-matched donor available.

PASTEURELLOSIS: Infection with *Pasteurella* spp., mainly *Pasteurella multocida*, which can range from a localized skin infection to disseminated disease. *Pasteurella* are normal flora in the oropharynx of animals; however, they can also cause animal disease. Human infection frequently follows animal bites. Clinically, the patient may present with signs of an acute inflammatory reaction (cellulitis) at the site of the bite and regional lymphadenopathy. Systemic disease may also occur with meningitis, arthritis, endocarditis, osteomyelitis or septicaemia. Diagnosis is by isolation of the organism and treatment with penicillin.

PATERSON–KELLY/PLUMMER–VINSON SYNDROME: See Iron-deficiency anaemia.

PELIOSIS HEPATIS: Cystic disease of the liver caused by *Bartonella henselae*.

 Bacillary angiomatosis

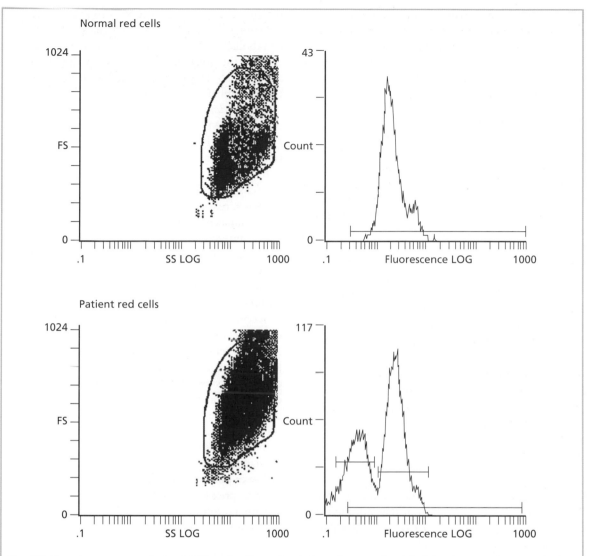

Fig. P7 Flow cytometry analysis of PNH red cells. Red cells have been stained for the CD59 antigen. Each dot on the scatter plot from the flow cytometer (left-hand graph) represents a red cell. The vertical axis (FS, forward light scatter) represents cell size and the horizontal axis (side scatter) cell granularity. The operator has drawn a line around the population of red cells for analysis. The right-hand histogram shows an analysis of cell intensity of staining for CD59 (fluorescence) on the horizontal axis and numbers of cells showing that degree of staining (count) on the vertical axis. In the patient's test, there are two populations of red cells, one of which lacks CD59 antigen.

PELVIC INFLAMMATORY DISEASE: Ascending infection of the endometrium and fallopian tubes caused by *Neisseria gonorrhoeae*, *Chlamydia trachomatis* or endogenous vaginal microflora.

Case

A 17-year-old sex-worker presented with a history of 1 week's abdominal pain and vaginal discharge following her period. The pain was described as a dull ache and occurred on both sides of the lower abdomen. She gave a history of having her appendix removed some years previously. On examina-

tion there was no guarding and the abdomen was soft with normal bowel sounds. On pelvic exami-

Microbiology: MSU negative; pregnancy test negative. Smear showed numerous pus cells. Culture for *N. gonorrhoeae* negative. LCR for *Chlamydia* positive.
Haematology: Hb 12.7; WBC 12 000 × 10⁶/l; polymorphs 70%.
Chemistry: C-reactive protein 60 mg/l.

nation, the adnexa were tender to palpation. A provisional diagnosis of pelvic inflammatory disease (PID) was made and a pregnancy test was performed, an MSU sent, and a cervical smear taken. Specimens were also taken for *Neisseria* and *Chlamydia*.

Aetiology and risk factors

The two most important causes of PID are *Chlamydia trachomatis* and *Neisseria gonorrhoeae*. The genus *Chlamydia* is an obligate intracellular pathogen and consists of at least three species, one of which, *Chlamydia trachomatis* serovar D–K, is associated with genital and neonatal infections (see Chlamydial disease). *Neisseria gonorrhoeae* is a fastidious Gram-negative diplococcus (see Gonorrhoea) that causes gonorrhoea*, septicaemia, arthritis and occasionally, endocarditis.

Infection rates for chlamydia range from 25 to 40% in Europe and in many cases chlamydial salpingitis may be asymptomatic. However, up to 55% of patients with clinically overt PID have evidence of chlamydial infection. An important sequela of chlamydial PID is infertility, which can be as high as 13% following a first attack, rising to 75% after a second attack. Also, ectopic pregnancy occurs 10 times more frequently following chlamydial salpingitis. The organisms are transmitted by sexual contact.

Pathology

Cervical infection with *Neisseria* or *Chlamydia* may lead to an ascending infection of the endometrium, fallopian tubes, ovaries or peritoneum. A chlamydia-induced perihepatitis may also occur, associated with pain in the right upper quadrant of the abdomen and fibrous adhesions between the liver capsule and the adnexa. Cervical infection with either of the two primary causes of PID results in damage to the endocervix, which may allow both the initial pathogen and endogenous bacteria to ascend into the upper genital tract. In addition, there is extension of the border of columnar epithelium which may allow further bacterial adhesion.

Only some strains of *N. gonorrhoeae* are prone to cause PID. The organism attaches to non-ciliated epithelial cells by pili and outer-membrane proteins (see Gonorrhoea). The organism is taken up into a phagosome and eventually penetrates the subepithelial tissues where it induces an acute inflammatory reaction with sloughing of the damaged epithelium. The lipopolysaccharide of *N. gonorrhoeae* induces TNF production which may be responsible for the destruction of ciliated epithelium in the fallopian tubes, thereby nullifying one of the host defences. In addition, gonococci can induce production of C5a

which recruits more neutrophils to the area, further damaging host cells by the release of oxygen metabolites. Activation of phospholipase A2 may activate the prostaglandin cascade with the production of leukotrienes and PGE, which contribute to the inflammatory response.

Chlamydia attach to epithelial cells of the genital tract by OMPs and are taken up into vacuoles. Fusion with lysosomes is inhibited and the infectious elementary bodies change to reticulate bodies and the organism divides. The replicative form condenses into infectious particles again and the cell lyses, releasing the elementary bodies to reinfect other adjacent cells or another individual during sexual intercourse. The initial cellular response to chlamydia is with neutrophils but, in established infections, plasma cells dominate. Production of TNF, IFN-γ and IL-1 may also be involved in the pathogenesis of PID. INF-γ induces MHC II expression on the epithelial cells which may have the effect of either down-regulating the immune response, allowing endogenous organisms to invade, or activating B- and T-cells that will act against the cells expressing the MHC II and thereby destroy the epithelial lining. The immune response to chlamydial antigens, particularly the 60 kDa heat shock protein antigen, may be responsible for the scarring associated with tubal adhesions.

Diagnosis is by clinical exclusion of other causes of lower abdominal pain in a woman, particularly ectopic pregnancy and appendicitis. There is no specific laboratory test for PID although specimens for both *Chlamydia* and *Neisseria* should be taken.

Management

Management includes the use of appropriate antibiotics, e.g. tetracycline, metronidazole. A vaccine using one of the OMP antigens is currently under trial.

PEMPHIGUS; PEMPHIGOID: Autoimmune bullous diseases of the skin characterized by blister formation secondary to suprabasal (pemphigus) or subepidermal (pemphigoid) separation of the epidermis from the underlying skin.

 Bullous skin disease

PENICILLIOSIS: Infection with the fungus *Penicillium* spp., usually occurring in immunocompromised patients. *Pencillium marneffei* is particularly common in AIDS patients and is acquired in SE Asia, causing a disseminated disease similar to histoplasmosis.

 Histoplasmosis

PEPTIC ULCER: An inflammatory lesion of the gastrointestinal tract where an area of the mucosa and usually underlying submucosa have been lost secondary to digestion by acid and digestive enzymes.

Case

A 34-year-old man presented with a long-standing history of episodic epigastric pain. The pain occurred intermittently during the day when the stomach was empty. He was occasionally woken with pain during the night. The symptoms were usually relieved by eating or by antacids. He remembered a 3-day episode 6 months ago when the pain was associated with black coloured sticky stools. His past medical history was otherwise unremarkable. On examination his vital signs were normal. There was mild epigastric sensitivity on palpation.

His blood count was normal. An ELISA test detected serum IgG antibodies to *Helicobacter pylori*. Gastroduodenal endoscopy showed features of gastritis in the gastric antrum and an ulcer measuring 2 cm in diameter was seen in the first part of the duodenum. Biopsies of the gastric and duodenal mucosa were obtained.

> Histological examination of the gastric biopsy showed active chronic gastritis with *H. pylori* (Fig. P8). The duodenal mucosa showed severely inflamed small intestinal mucosa with regenerative features representing the ulcer edge, but no malignancy.

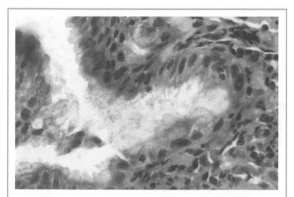

Fig. P8 Histological section of stomach showing numerous small bacteria in the surface mucus layer.

He was diagnosed as having a duodenal peptic ulcer. He received histamine H2-receptor antagonists to control the acute disease and *H. pylori*

eradication therapy was administered. He responded well to treatment and the symptoms subsided. A repeat endoscopy at 6 months showed that the duodenal ulcer was healed and the *H. pylori* infection was eradicated.

Aetiology and risk factors

Peptic ulcers are caused by an imbalance between the protective mechanisms of the mucosa and damaging forces of digestive enzymes and acid. The most important risk factor for development of peptic ulcer is *H. pylori* infection of the gastric antrum, which affects over 90% of patients suffering from duodenal ulcers and over 70% of those suffering from gastric ulcers. How *H. pylori*-associated antral gastritis leads to duodenal ulcer is not known, but an inflammatory response against the *H. pylori* is thought to play a role. Other risk factors include non-steroidal anti-inflammatory drugs, steroids, cigarette smoking and diseases associated with abnormal gastric acid secretion. It is estimated that around 10% of the population develop peptic ulcers at least once during their lifetime. The male-to-female ratio is 2:1.

Pathology

The cardinal symptom of peptic ulceration, pain, is a result of irritation of mucosal nerves exposed to gastric acid and enzymes. Food or antacids neutralize the acid and thus control the pain. The majority of peptic ulcers are seen in the first part of the duodenum and some in the gastric antrum. The oesophageal mucosa can be affected in those

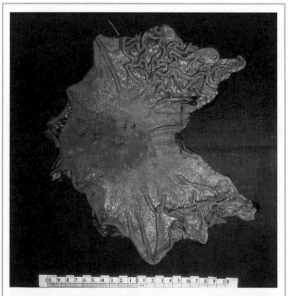

Fig. P9 Macroscopic appearance of a gastric ulcer located in the lesser curve.

patients with gastro-oesophageal reflux or Barrett oesophagus*. Rarely a Meckel diverticulum containing ectopic gastric tissue can cause peptic ulceration in the adjacent intestinal mucosa. Macroscopically, all peptic ulcers have round punched-out craters in the mucosa measuring 1–4 cm in diameter (Fig. P9).

Microscopically, the mucosal lining is absent at the centre of the ulcer crater and usually ulceration extends into the muscularis propria. The ulcer base is covered with necrotic debris and beneath this, inflammatory granulation tissue and extensive fibrosis are seen. At the edges the mucosal epithelium shows regenerative features.

The gastric mucosa in duodenal ulceration almost invariably shows *H. pylori*-associated gastritis as observed in this patient. Peptic ulcer is a chronic, relapsing and remitting disease and if untreated can cause a number of complications. The most common complication is bleeding from an ulcer, possibly as a result of peptic injury to one of the large vessels. The history of dark stools suggests an episode of bleeding in this patient. Other common complications are perforation of the ulcer and strictures secondary to extensive fibrosis.

Management

Management is directed towards eradicating the predisposing factors, most importantly the *H. pylori* infection, by antibacterial treatment and control of acid secretion by histamine H2-receptor antagonists in the acute phase. Occasionally surgery may be necessary for disease unresponsive to medical treatment or if complications have developed.

 Zollinger–Ellison syndrome

PERICARDITIS: Inflammation of the pericardial sac.

Aetiology and risk factors

Pericarditis is either of infectious aetiology, or associated with some other medical or surgical condition, e.g. rheumatoid arthritis*, post-cardiac surgery, or idiopathic. Infectious pericarditis is most commonly viral, but other microbial agents can be responsible (see Table P2).

Pathology

Following a viral infection, inflammation of the mesothelial cells lining the pericardial sac occurs with the accumulation of a serofibrinous effusion. A purulent effusion with large numbers of neutrophils is seen with a bacterial pericarditis. In tuberculous pericarditis there is the characteristic granuloma formation in the pericardium, which becomes lined by a thick fibrinous exudate. The pericardium becomes infiltrated with lymphocytes and monocytes. In the later stages of infection, adhesions occur between the opposing layers of the pericardium obliterating the sac. The accumulation of an effusion or blood secondary to metastatic disease leads to tamponade, whilst inflammatory adhesions cause constrictive pericarditis, which interferes with the ventricular stroke volume and cardiac output. Patients may present with chest pain and tachycardia, frequently accompanied by fever and myalgia attributed to the underlying systemic infection. On examination, a pericardial friction rub may be heard and ST elevation may be seen on the ECG; the accumulation of an effusion may be seen using echocardiography. Laboratory diagnosis of infection relies on histology, isolation of the causative agent (either from the pericardial sac in cases of bacterial or fungal disease or more usually from faeces or throat washings in the case of viral causes) or detection of a serological response to the infecting agent.

Management

Management depends upon the cause. There is no specific treatment for viral pericarditis; bacterial, fungal and parasitic diseases require the appropriate antimicrobial agent. Surgery may be necessary to relieve tamponade.

PERIODONTITIS: Inflammation of the gums (gingivitis) and the deep periodontal tissue (periodontitis).

Table P2 Agents responsible for pericarditis

Viruses	Bacteria	Fungi	Parasites
Coxsackie A, B	*Strep. pneumoniae*	*Histoplasma capsulatum*	*Toxoplasma gondii*
Adenovirus	*Staph. aureus*	*Coccidioides immitis*	*Entamoeba histolytica*
Influenza virus	*Mycobacterium tuberculosis*		
Mumps virus	*Mycoplasma pneumoniae*		
ECHO	*Haemophilus influenzae* *Neisseria meningitidis* and *N. gonorrhoeae*		

Aetiology and risk factors

Periodontitis is probably the commonest infection world wide. It results from an interaction between a complex microflora, including *Bacteroides*, *Fusobacterium*, *Actinobacillus*, *Eikenella*, *Porphyromonas*, *Prevotella* and *Treponema* species; environmental factors such as smoking, and host factors such as oral hygiene, HLA type and associated disease, e.g. diabetes.

Pathology

Initially there is a local acute inflammatory response with infiltration by neutrophils and elevated levels of pro-inflammatory cytokines in the gingival crevicular fluid. IL-1 may be particularly relevant to periodontal disease as it is associated with bone resorption and may be involved in alveolar bone loss. Following neutrophil infiltration there is a T-cell and plasma cell infiltrate with peripheral activation of T-cells. The gingival neutrophils, and B- and CD4 T-cells may be involved in tissue damage rather than being protective. The bacteria in the plaque produce immunomodulatory factors (e.g. porins) that may temporarily inhibit host defences. These porins are B-cell mitogens and can induce polyclonal B-cell activation. There is destruction of connective tissue mediated by proteinases and the rate of progression of periodontal disease may be linked to the proteinase/inhibitor ratio. Along with tissue destruction there is the development of periodontal pockets and loosening of teeth. Some metabolic products of the anaerobic bacteria can inhibit fibroblast function and therefore impair healing. Diagnosis is clinical and treatment is by descaling, improved oral hygiene and giving up smoking. Periodontal pockets may be treated surgically.

PERITONITIS: Infection in the peritoneal cavity which can be caused by several different bacteria, usually following a perforation of a viscus.

PERNICIOUS ANAEMIA: Vitamin B12-deficient, macrocytic, megaloblastic anaemia due to an autoimmune attack against the gastric parietal cells which results in lack of intrinsic factor. The name of this disorder is unfortunate, as it is easily and cheaply treated by quarterly B12 injections.

Case

A 68-year-old housewife was referred to the endocrine clinic with a 6-month history of lassitude and depression. She also gave a 2-month history of tingling in her toes at night. Twenty years before she had a thyroidectomy for thyrotoxicosis. Her sister had also received treatment for 'thyroid trouble'. On examination she was a pale lady with blue eyes, 'blue rinse' hair, and vitiligo on both arms. Her mouth was normal. Examination was otherwise normal except for absent vibration sense below both knees. A blood count was performed:

WBC 3.0×10^9/l
RBC 0.39×10^{12}/l; Hb 8.8 g/dl; Hct (ratio) 0.277
MCV 116 fl; MCH 36.0 pg
MCHC 32.0 g/dl; RDW 12.8 %
Plt 138×10^9/l.

Blood film examination showed oval macrocytes and hypersegmented neutrophils (Fig. P10). Urea and electrolytes were normal, liver function showed a minor increase in unconjugated bilirubin. Prompted by the macrocytic anaemia, serum B12 and red cell folate levels were measured. Serum B12 was reduced at 60 ng/l (normal 150–900). Red cell folate was in the low-normal range.

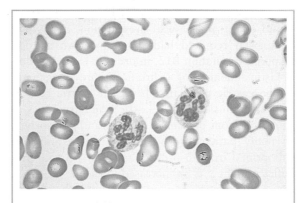

Fig. P10 Blood film in pernicious anaemia showing oval macrocytes and hypersegmented neutrophils.

Daily intramuscular vitamin B12 injections were started. The reticulocyte count rose, closely followed by the haemoglobin level. A Schilling vitamin B12 absorption test was performed. This showed 2% absorption in the part I test, which was corrected to 15% by addition of intrinsic factor in the part II test. This demonstrated that the B12 deficiency was due to lack of intrinsic factor, the commonest cause of which is pernicious anaemia.

Autoantibodies to gastric parietal cells and intrinsic factor were found in the serum. Although 20% of women over 60 may have parietal cell antibodies, few normal women have intrinsic factor antibodies and their presence helps to confirm pernicious anaemia.

P

Aetiology and risk factors

Other autoimmune disorders may be associated with pernicious anaemia, and this lady has had previous autoimmune thyroid disease and vitiligo, an autoimmune attack against the melanocytes of the skin. Pernicious anaemia is commonest in blue-eyed, blonde northern European races. Like most autoimmune disorders, it is commoner in women.

Pathology

Because many of the oval macrocytes characteristic of the disorder die before they leave the bone marrow (ineffective erythropoiesis), there is in effect a haemolytic element to the anaemia, which may cause a tinge of jaundice. Vitamin B12 and folic acid are needed for all rapidly dividing cells of the body, including the lining of the gastrointestinal tract, so that some patients with megaloblastic anaemia may suffer mild diarrhoea and sore mouths. Deficiency in the bone marrow results in modest leucopenia and thrombocytopenia as well as the classic macrocytic anaemia. Bone marrow examination to prove megaloblastic erythropoiesis was not performed in this case in view of the classic blood count and clinical presentation, but would have been required had she not shown a good response to vitamin B12, in order to exclude sideroblastic anaemia* or a chronic erythroleukaemia.

The gastric parietal cells secrete gastric acid as well as intrinsic factor. Gastric acid is required to split iron from protein so that it can be absorbed, so many patients with pernicious anaemia have suboptimal iron absorption and may become iron deficient. There is an increased incidence of gastric carcinoma in pernicious anaemia so this should also be borne in mind as a cause of occult blood loss and iron-deficiency anaemia* in cases of pernicious anaemia.

Though autoantibodies to gastric parietal cells and intrinsic factor are found in the great majority of patients, the actual damage to the gastric mucosa is thought to be largely T-cell mediated.

Normal vitamin B12 absorption Liver, red meat and fish are the principal dietary sources of vitamin B12. In the stomach, intrinsic factor, secreted by the gastric parietal cells, couples to the B12 and carries it to the terminal ileum. Here the B12 is transferred into the intestinal mucosa.

Vitamin B12 absorption can be investigated by means of the Schilling test. A 'flushing' dose of ordinary vitamin B12 is given by intramuscular injection. An oral dose of radioactive B12 is then given. If it can be absorbed, it will, but being super-fluous to requirements it is excreted in the urine. A 24-hour urine collection should therefore contain at least 10% of the swallowed radioactivity. If the result of this investigation is normal, the B12 deficiency is due to lack of intake, such as may be found in vegans. If absorption is reduced, then the part II Schilling test is performed. The procedure is the same as part I except that radioactive B12 and intrinsic factor are given by mouth. The purpose of the part II test is to determine whether the malabsorption found in part I is due to lack of intrinsic factor or to a defective terminal ileum. Lack of intrinsic factor may be due to pernicious anaemia or gastrectomy. Disorders of the terminal ileum that may affect B12 absorption include Crohn disease* and surgical resection.

Neurological damage in B12 deficiency Vitamin B12 is required for maintenance of nerve function and its deficiency from any cause may result in neurological damage. The classic neurological problem is subacute combined degeneration of the spinal cord, but peripheral neuropathy, dementia and optic atrophy may also be found. Careful neurological testing, as in the case described above, may reveal minor neurological abnormalities in cases of B12 deficiency prior to their clinical presentation. Rarely, such neurological damage may be present in the absence of anaemia, but macrocytosis will almost always be present. Because such neurological problems take months or years to recover, it is important to recognize and treat B12 deficiency as early as possible in the course of the disease. Hydroxocobalamin, the usual form of B12 to be used therapeutically, is cheap and overdose does no harm.

Administration of folic acid may worsen the neurological problems of B12 deficiency, so treatment of a macrocytic megaloblastic anaemia should be with both B12 and folic acid until the results of B12 and red cell folate assays are known.

PEUTZ–JEGHER SYNDROME: A rare autosomal dominant familial syndrome characterized by multiple polyps along the gastrointestinal tract and increased pigmentation in face, lips, hands and genitalia (Fig. P11).

PHAEOCHROMOCYTOMA: A tumour arising from the sympathetic nervous system giving rise to an overproduction of adrenal medullary hormones (catecholamines).

Case

A 30-year-old male had been attending the hypertension clinic for the last 2 years. His medical history revealed that he had suffered from several episodes of hypertension, weight loss, headache and

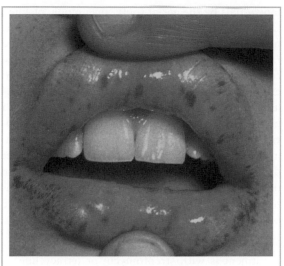

Fig. P11 Patient with Peutz–Jegher syndrome showing circumoral pigmented naevi. (Reproduced from Browse NL. *An Introduction to the Symptoms and Signs of Surgical Disease*, 3rd edn. London: Arnold, 1997)

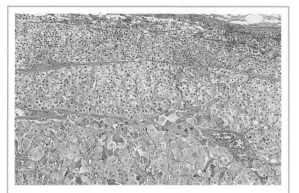

Fig. P12 Histology of phaeochromocytoma. The normal adrenal cortex is seen at the top, the large dark staining cells of the phaeochromocytoma are seen at the bottom of the picture.

occasional palpitations. On clinical examination, he had tachycardia, a bounding pulse and a fine tremor. On this occasion his blood pressure was 130/100 mmHg.

A number of biochemical blood tests were requested, including serum electrolytes, urea, creatinine, and glucose:

Serum: sodium 138 mmol/l; potassium 3.8 mmol/l;
Urea 5.7 mmol/l;
Creatinine 90 mmol/l;
Glucose 7.5 mmol/l.

Urinary 24-hour cortisol and catecholamine excretion was measured on three occasions. His cortisol excretion was normal but he had elevated catecholamines.

A tentative diagnosis of phaeochromocytoma was made. He had a CT scan, which confirmed a left adrenal mass.

Aetiology and risk factors

Phaeochromocytomas are a very rare cause of hypertension in the UK (<0.1%). About 90% of tumours are adrenal in origin, the remaining 10% arising from the sympathetic ganglia. Ten per cent of phaeochromocytomas are multiple and 10% are malignant. Phaeochromocytoma is also a component of the multiple endocrine neoplasia (MEN) syndrome. A small proportion of patients (5%) give a positive family history. A variety of drugs can precipitate a hypertensive attack in individuals with a phaeochromocytoma, including tricyclic anti-depressants, antidopaminergic agents, metoclopramide and naloxone.

Pathology

Phaeochromocytomas are usually well circumscribed tumours, varying in size (Fig. P12). Electron microscopy of the tumour shows the presence of membrane-bound neurosecretory granules in the cytoplasm containing neuron-specific enolase, chromogranin and catecholamines. The clinical features described in this patient resulted from increased catecholamine secretion. This causes peripheral vasoconstriction (α-receptor mediated) and increased cardiac output (β-receptor mediated). Hypertension is the most common presentation; this can be episodic, episodes of hypertension being precipitated by drugs, bending, increased abdominal pressure and meals. The other clinical signs and symptoms seen in this patient, such as palpitations, headaches and tremors, were the result of increased sympathetic activity. The serum glucose level is elevated (hyperglycaemia) as a result of impaired glucose tolerance from the insulin antagonistic action of catecholamines. The diagnosis is suspected when a 24-hour urine is screened for catecholamines. In some centres, failure to suppress plasma catecholamine with clonidine is used to support the diagnosis.

Management

When the diagnosis has been made, the tumour is localized prior to surgery by using either a CT scan, adrenal vein catheterization, or MIBG (radiolabelled metaiodobenzylguanidine) scan. The tumour is then removed surgically after a sympathetic blockade (beta-blockade). Patients are usually started on alpha-blockers before using beta-blockers.

PHAEOHYPHOMYCOSIS: A general term denoting infections with brown pigmented (i.e. dematiaceous) moulds, commonly found in soil and causing skin, eye, sinus, subcutaneous or disseminated disease, usually in compromised individuals.

PINTA: A non-venereal treponemal disease of the skin caused by *Treponema carateum*.

 Treponematosis

PITYRIASIS VERSICOLOR: A superficial infection of the skin with *Malassezia furfur* (*Pityrosporum obiculare*, *Pityrosporum ovale*), which is a commensal on the skin. Common triggers for disease are overexposure to sunlight and immunosuppression. The patient complains of hypo-(or hyper-)pigmented scaling areas on the arms or trunk. Other infections associated with these yeasts are a folliculitis and seborrhoeic dermatitis, which occurs commonly in AIDS patients. The patient complains of pruritus and scaling of the upper trunk and a greasy skin. Laboratory diagnosis is by demonstration of the fungus in skin scrapings and treatment is with topical selenium or azoles.

PLAGUE: Infection with the Gram-negative bacillus *Yersinia pestis*.

Aetiology and risk factors
Plague is an infection of historical significance as it was probably the cause of The Black Death, which killed about a quarter of the European population in the fourteenth century (a good account of a modern outbreak occurs in *La Peste* by Albert Camus). It is caused by *Yersinia pestis* and is a potential agent of biological warfare. The organism is endemic in rats, where it causes epizootic infections and is transmitted by the flea to humans (and other rats).

Pathology
Virulence factors of *Y. pestis* are carried on plasmids and cause lysis by disrupting cell signalling. *Yersinia* is taken up by neutrophils and macrophages, but resists intracellular killing, spreading by the lymphatics to the regional lymph nodes, where the organism multiplies. Haemorrhagic necrosis of the lymph node occurs, which becomes infiltrated by neutrophils and contains abundant micro-organisms (bubonic plague). Septicaemia occurs and the organisms can then spread to any organ, particularly the lung, from which the organism can be transmitted to other

individuals by the aerial route (pneumonic plague). Clinically the commonest presentation is bubonic plague with the patient complaining of fever and rapidly developing painful swollen lymph nodes – called buboes (usually in the groin or axillae) – and endotoxic shock*. The infection may spread to the lungs and the patient becomes dyspnoeic, with a productive cough and haemoptysis. There is peripheral leucocytosis. There may be evidence of disseminated intravascular coagulation* and of liver damage with elevated transaminases. Death can occur within a day or two. Laboratory diagnosis is by microscopy of an aspirate from a bubo, culture of the organism and serology.

Management
Treatment is with streptomycin or tetracycline. A vaccine is available and the disease is notifiable.

PLASMACYTOMA: A localized tumour of malignant plasma cells which may, rarely, present without evidence of the generalized bone disorder multiple myeloma*, for example with a pathological fracture. Local radiotherapy may be curative in this situation, but regular follow-up with paraprotein measurement is important, as about a third of these patients eventually develop multiple myeloma.

PLEURISY: Inflammation of the pleura.

PNEUMOCOCCAL PNEUMONIA: Acute inflammation in the lungs caused by *Streptococcus pneumoniae*.

Case
A 27-year-old homeless male presented to casualty with rigors and a productive cough with blood-stained sputum. He also complained of a sharp pain on the right side of his chest, which was worsened during breathing. He had a high temperature and was tachypnoeic. On examination he had signs of consolidation on the right side of the chest with decreased movement of the chest. Auscultation revealed crepitations with the presence of a pleural rub and bronchial breath sounds over the right lower lobe.

Haematology: Hb 13 g/dl; WBC 27 000 × 10⁶/l; polymorphs 80%.
Radiology: lobar consolidation in right lower lobe.
Chemistry: Po_2 8.5 kPa; Pco_2 5.5 kPa; pH 7.4; HCO_3 23 mmol/l.
Microbiology: *Strep. pneumoniae* isolated from the sputum and blood culture.

A diagnosis of community-acquired pneumonia was made. Blood gases were measured and specimens sent for a full blood count, blood and sputum culture.

Aetiology and risk factors

Strep. pneumoniae is a Gram-positive 'viridans' streptococcus (i.e. only causing partial haemolysis of blood when grown on blood agar). It is the commonest cause of community-acquired pneumonia. Risk factors for disease include splenectomy and alcoholism. The organism is transmitted by droplet infection and can cause a wide variety of infections as follows:

- pneumonia
- otitis media
- sinusitis
- meningitis
- septicaemia
- endocarditis
- arthritis
- empyema
- peritonitis.

Pathology

The organism gains entry to the lower respiratory tract, particularly if the normal host defences such as the mucociliary escalator and the alveolar macrophages are compromised by virtue of a preceding viral infection, poor cough reflex, or excess alcohol intake. Once in the lungs, the organism induces an acute inflammatory response in the alveoli which therefore fill with fluid and pus cells, compromising gas exchange and resulting in a low P_{O_2} (Figs P13, P14).

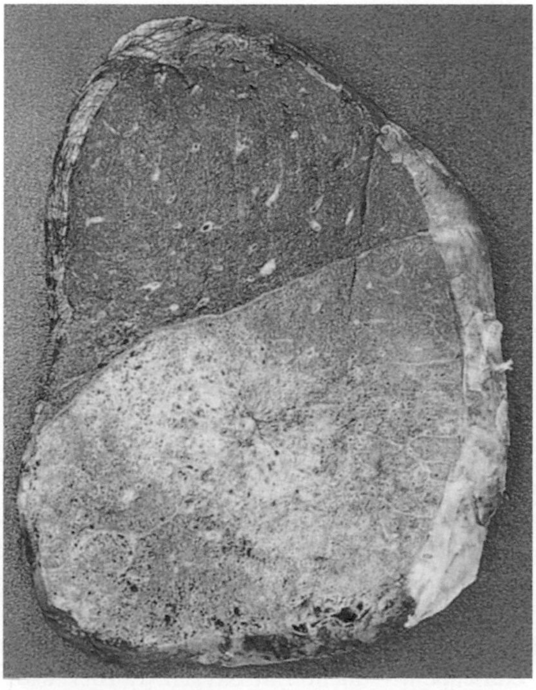

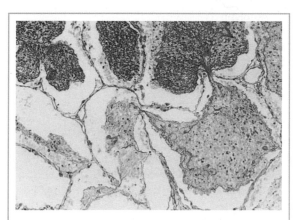

Fig. P14 Microscopic section of lung showing acute inflammatory exudate within alveoli.

The P_{CO_2} is usually normal unless respiratory failure occurs. The cell wall of the pneumococcus contains a teichoic acid (incorporating choline) and this combines with C-reactive protein, an acute phase protein, which activates the alternative complement pathway, leading to a chemotactic signal (C5a) for the accumulation of the neutrophils. Cell wall components of the pneumococcus stimulate the production of pro-inflammatory cytokines (TNF, IL-1 IL-8) from monocyte/macrophages and endothelial cells which, in turn, up-regulate endothelial receptor molecules ICAM-1 and ELAM, allowing the polymorphs to escape into the alveoli. *Strep. pneumoniae* avoids phagocytosis because it possesses a polysaccharide capsule which is antiphagocytic. In addition to the polysaccharide capsule, the pneumococcus expresses a number of choline-binding protein antigens on the cell wall, such as an amidase (autolysin) and PspA (pneumococcal surface adhesin A), and also secretes a number of potential virulence factors, such as pneumolysin, neuraminidase and an IgA protease (Fig. P15). Pneumolysin is a pore-forming cytotoxin and is the major extracellular toxin of the pneumococcus.

Infected lungs take on an appearance similar to the liver (called 'hepatization'). The presence of fluid and pus cells in the alveoli is called consolidation and clinically gives rise to the physical signs of

Fig. P13 Macroscopic section of lung showing consolidation of lower lobe.

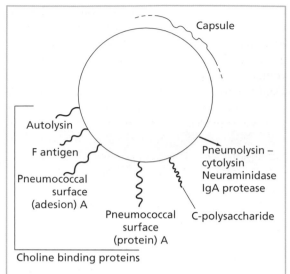

Fig. P15 Diagram showing virulence characteristics of the pneumococcus.

dullness to percussion and increased fremitus, the relatively solid organ acting as an efficient sounding board. The basis of recovery is a specific IgG antibody response, which allows the neutrophils to phagocytose the pneumococci. In an untreated first attack this takes about 7 days. Diagnosis is by isolation of the organism from blood, sputum or bronchoalveolar lavage; detection by PCR; or detection of antigen by immunoassays.

Management

Management includes antibiotics, e.g. penicillin or cefuroxime, and may require respiratory support on a ventilator. Serologically the capsule can be divided into at least 90 different capsular types. These can be used to type the organism and the capsular material is the basis of the pneumococcal vaccine, which, however, has to contain at least 35 serotypes to cover the common strains. Newer vaccines are likely to be based on cell wall proteins such as PspA.

PNEUMOCONIOSIS: Lung disease which develops secondary to long-term exposure to mineral dusts.

Aetiology and risk factors

In most instances pneumoconiosis develops as a result of industrial exposure to mineral dusts such as coal, silica, asbestos or beryllium. The clinical syndromes are named after the aetiological agent: anthracosis, silicosis, asbestosis or berylliosis. The development of pneumoconiosis depends on various factors including the amount of dust accumulated in the lungs, the physicochemical properties of the mineral and presence or absence of other irritants such as cigarette smoking.

Pathology

The most significant pathological feature of pneumoconioses is the fibrosis of lung parenchyma. It is thought that the inhaled mineral dusts activate alveolar and interstitial macrophages, which secrete a number of pro-inflammatory cytokines, inducing fibroblast proliferation and collagen deposition.

The pathological findings in coal worker's pneumoconiosis vary according to the amount and duration of exposure. Simple anthracosis is the mildest form of the disease. The inhaled carbon pigment accumulates in the macrophages and the local lymph nodes draining the lungs. Usually there is no inflammation or change in lung capacity. In simple coal worker's pneumoconiosis, the macrophages containing the carbon pigment form macules or nodules. These usually contain a delicate network of collagen fibres and dilatation of adjacent alveoli is observed. Around 10% of simple coal worker's pneumoconiosis cases go on to develop progressive massive fibrosis, numerous large scars measuring several centimetres in diameter being the main feature. This is associated with respiratory symptoms and reduction in lung capacity. There is no treatment for coal worker's pneumoconiosis other than prevention. Some cases of progressive massive fibrosis continue to progress even when exposure to coal dust is eliminated.

The pathology of asbestosis and silicosis is discussed under separate entries.

Management

Management is symptomatic, once the cause is established.

 Asbestosis; Inflammation; Silicosis

PNEUMOCYSTIS PNEUMONIA: Pneumonia caused by the fungus *Pneumocystis carinii*, which occurs predominantly in AIDS patients. It is believed that the infection can be acquired *de novo*, in an adult, by inhalation of the spores, rather than as a reactivation of previous colonization in the lungs as a child. The organism multiplies in the alveoli, damaging the surfactant layer, probably by means of degradative enzymes. *Pneumocystis* stimulates the induction of IL-8 and other pro-inflammatory mediators, which recruit neutrophils into the alveoli. Degranulation of neutrophils causes further alveolar cell damage. This leads to increase in capillary permeability, fluid accumulation in the alveoli, damage to the alveolar cells and a consequent reduction in oxygen transfer with a decrease in oxygen saturation, which can be exacerbated by exercise. Histologically, the alveoli appear to be filled with a foamy material composed of fluid

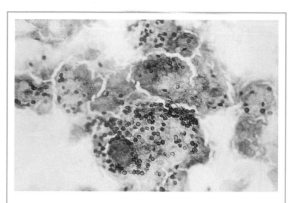

Fig. P16 Methenamine silver stain showing *Pneumocystis carinii* cysts in the lung.

and *Pneumocystis* organisms. Clinically the patient presents with shortness of breath, a non-productive cough, and fever. Radiological changes are usually evident but there is no characteristic appearance. The Po_2 and oxygen saturation are usually decreased. Diagnosis is by histology and demonstration of the cysts in the sputum or bronchoalveolar lavage fluid by silver staining (Fig. P16).

Treatment is with co-trimoxazole, clindamycin and primaquine or pentamidine.

POLIOMYELITIS: An infection with polio virus (an enterovirus) which is spread by faecally contaminated water or by the direct faeco-oral route. The virus multiplies in the lymphoid tissue of the oropharynx or small intestine and disseminates via the bloodstream. The patient may be asymptomatic or have a minor flu-like illness. The virus may localize in the neurons of the brain or spinal chord and the patient may present as an aseptic meningitis or progress to paralytic polio. The virus is a lytic virus and if the anterior horn cells of the spinal chord are destroyed, loss of reflexes and flaccid paralysis of the limbs occur, preceded by pain and fasciculation of the affected muscle groups. A more severe form of poliomyelitis is bulbar polio, when the neurons of the medulla are killed, leading to cranial nerve palsies, respiratory paralysis or autonomic disturbances, such as hypertension. Laboratory diagnosis is by isolation of the virus or serology. There is no specific treatment, but poliomyelitis is now a vanishing disease, thanks to the existence since the 1950s of two effective vaccines (Salk, Sabin).

POLYARTERITIS NODOSA: A systemic vasculitis involving medium-sized muscular arteries of visceral organs including kidneys, heart, gastrointestinal tract, CNS, and skin, but usually not the lungs.

The patients can present with fever of unknown origin with raised ESR and CRP and a variety of symptoms and signs which depend on the organs involved. Pathologically there is a necrotizing vasculitis involving medium-sized arteries. In acute lesions, fibrinoid necrosis of the arterial wall with accumulation of acute inflammatory infiltrate is seen. Later the lesions heal by fibrosis of the vessel wall. Weakening of the arterial wall can lead to formation of small aneurysms, which in the skin may be clinically palpable. Without treatment the disease is fatal.

The cause of polyarteritis nodosa is not known, but many cases follow infection with hepatitis B*, tuberculosis*, or streptococci, and an immune complex pathogenesis (type III hypersensitivity) is suspected. Immunosuppression is the only effective treatment, prednisone and cyclophosphamide being the drugs of choice.

 Vasculitis

POLYCYSTIC KIDNEY: Inherited disease of the kidneys characterized by development of numerous large cysts in the renal parenchyma often leading to renal failure.

The polycystic kidney diseases are divided into two types: adult and childhood. The adult type is relatively common and is inherited as an autosomal dominant trait. The childhood type is rare and has an autosomal recessive type of inheritance.

Adult polycystic kidney disease often presents late in life with slowly progressive chronic renal failure. Grossly, both kidneys are always involved. They show massive enlargement with numerous large cysts measuring several centimetres in diameter. The cysts contain clear sometimes haemorrhagic fluid and are lined by low columnar tubular-type epithelium. Cysts in other organs such as the liver, pancreas or spleen may also be present. Small berry aneurysms in the circle of Willis occur in around 20% of the patients. In childhood polycystic kidney disease, the kidneys are mildly enlarged and contain numerous small cysts, giving a sponge-like appearance. The prognosis is usually poor.

POLYCYSTIC OVARY: A disease characterized by enlargement of both ovaries by numerous follicle cysts. The patients usually have oligomenorrhoea and no ovulation and sometimes obesity and hirsutism (so-called Stein–Leventhal syndrome) The pathogenesis is unclear; however, abnormalities in enzymes regulating secretion of gonadotropic hormones are implicated. In 50–60% of patients,

P

serum luteinizing hormone, testosterone and androsterone are raised.

POLYCYTHAEMIA: Increase in red cell count, haemoglobin and haematocrit. This may be true polycythaemia, associated with an increased circulating red cell mass, or relative (sometimes known as pseudo-polycythaemia) due to a decreased plasma volume.

Relative polycythaemia is most commonly due to dehydration, which may be caused by fever (sweating), diarrhoea, vomiting or diuretic therapy. Rehydration restores the plasma volume, and hence the haemoglobin level, to normal. Some male patients with relative polycythaemia run a low plasma volume for no obvious cause. This is termed Gaisböck polycythaemia or stress polycythaemia as it tends to be found in busy overworked male executives.

True polycythaemia is associated with an increased red cell mass. The red cell mass and plasma volume can be measured by radio-dilutional methods. A sample of the patient's red cells is tagged with an isotope such as chromium-51 and re-injected into the circulation. After allowing time for mixing, a further sample is taken and its radioactivity measured and compared to the injected cells. The weaker this sample's radioactivity, the greater the patient's mass of red cells in which the labelled red cells have been diluted. A similar procedure can be applied to measure plasma volume by labelling a sample of the patient's plasma with iodine-131.

True polycythaemia may be primary or secondary. Primary polycythaemia, known as polycythaemia rubra vera, is one of the myeloproliferative disorders* and is associated with autonomous red cell overproduction by the bone marrow. Erythropoietin (EPO) levels are low and there is often an increase in neutrophils and platelets in the blood as well as red cells. The spleen may be enlarged and the disorder may burn out as myelofibrosis, or, less commonly, transform to acute myeloid leukaemia*.

Secondary true polycythaemia is due to increased EPO production from the kidneys (Fig. P17), which stimulates red cell production from the bone marrow. The stimulus to EPO production is hypoxia. Examples are chronic hypoxic chest disease such as emphysema and congenital cyanotic heart disease. Inhaled carbon monoxide in cigarette smoke combines irreversibly with haemoglobin to form carboxyhaemoglobin. This cannot release oxygen to the tissues and in response to this relative hypoxia, the kidneys release more EPO to stimulate the production of functional red cells. Smokers

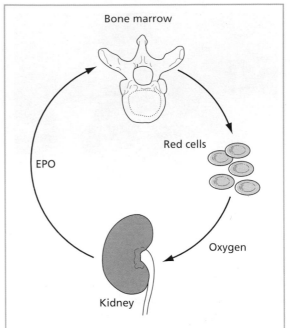

Fig. P17 Control of haemoglobin level is effected by renal secretion of erythropoietin (EPO). If the kidneys detect a relative oxygen deficiency, they secrete more erythropoietin to stimulate production of more red cells from the bone marrow to carry more oxygen.

therefore have higher haemoglobin levels than non-smokers.

If the circulation of blood through the kidney is impaired, renal EPO production increases. Increased pressure within the renal capsule from cysts or tumours may thus cause secondary polycythaemia.

Some tumours have the ability to secrete ectopic hormones and, rarely, such a secretion of EPO may cause polycythaemia. Tumours capable of secreting EPO include carcinoma of kidney, hepatoma and (surprisingly) giant uterine fibroids. Other causes of true polycythaemia are:

- primary: polycythaemia rubra vera
- secondary: smoking; hypoxic lung disease; congenital cyanotic heart disease; living at altitude; physiological in neonates; ectopic production of EPO by tumours; haemoglobinopathy with a high oxygen affinity haemoglobin.

Management

Increased haematocrit causes increased blood viscosity with stagnant flow. This may lead to thrombosis*, including coronary and cerebral thrombosis. The heart struggles to pump viscous blood around the circulation, leading to hypertension.

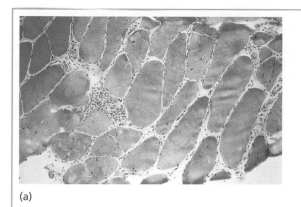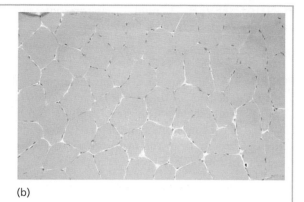

(a)   (b)

Fig. P18 Histology of muscle biopsy from a patient with polymyositis. (a) Note the reduction in fibres and perivascular interstitial mononuclear infiltrate compared with the normal tightly packed fibres (b).

If investigations show a cause for the polycythaemia, this should be removed – for example, surgical removal of a renal tumour or stopping smoking. The simplest method of reducing haemoglobin levels is by venesection. If this needs to be performed frequently, mild cytotoxic agents such as hydroxyurea may be given to cut down red cell production by the bone marrow.

POLYMYOSITIS: An inflammatory disease of muscles. Involvement of skin occurs in 50–60% of cases (see Dermatomyositis).

Aetiology and risk factors

Polymyositis is characterized by muscle pain, weakness and tenderness, proximal muscles being mainly affected. Biopsy shows degeneration of the muscle fibres with infiltrating mononuclear cells (Fig. P18).

Polymyositis is frequently associated with non-erosive peripheral arthritis (40% of cases). Other features include respiratory muscle weakness, myocarditis and diffuse interstitial pulmonary fibrosis. About 50% of the patients have a raised ESR and most have raised levels of serum muscle enzymes. Polymyositis can either be primary or secondary to other rheumatic diseases (Table P3).

Table P3 Classification of polymyositis

Primary polymyositis
Secondary polymyositis
  Polyarteritis nodosa
  Rheumatoid arthritis
  Sjögren syndrome
  Systemic lupus erythematosus
  Systemic sclerosis
Dermatomyositis
  Adults: can be associated with malignancy
  Children: rare, rapidly progressing

Although the aetiology is unknown, several viruses, including influenza, rubella and Coxsackie, have been implicated and cytotoxic T-cells from patients have been shown to kill muscle cells. Autoantibodies, which react with histidyl-tRNA have been found in 25% of the patients, especially those with diffuse interstitial pulmonary fibrosis. Their role in pathogenesis is not known. There is a weak association with HLA-B8 and DR3.

 Dermatomyositis; Polyarteritis nodosa; Rheumatoid arthritis; Sjögren syndrome; Systemic lupus erythematosus; Systemic sclerosis

POLYP; POLYPOSIS: The macroscopic description of a protruding tumour arising from an epithelial surface (Fig. P19).

Polyps can be neoplastic, hyperplastic, inflammatory or hamartomatous in nature. If numerous polyps are present in a given organ, this is called polyposis.

 Adenomatous polyposis coli

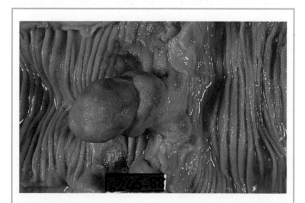

Fig. P19 A large intestinal polyp protruding into the small intestinal lumina.

PONTIAC FEVER: A mild respiratory infection caused by *Legionella pneumophila*.

 Legionnaires disease

PORPHYRIA: A group of disorders resulting from a partial deficiency of one of the enzymes involved in the biosynthesis of porphyrins. Porphyria can be classified according to its clinical presentation into acute or chronic, or to the major site of abnormal metabolism into hepatic or erythropoietic (Table P4).

Table P4 Classification of the porphyrias

Porphyria	Presentation	Site
Acute intermittent	Acute	Hepatic
Hereditary coproporphyria	Acute	Hepatic
Variegate	Acute	Hepatic
Cutaneous hepatic	Chronic	Hepatic
Congenital erythropoietic	Chronic	Erythropoietic
Erythropoietic protoporphyria	Chronic	Erythropoietic

Case

A 20-year-old female presented at the emergency unit with abdominal pain and vomiting. She thought that her abdominal pains were related to her periods and also complained of having occasional episodes of constipation. Her systemic review revealed that she had noticed her urine was red in colour on a number of occasions; this seemed to occur when she had abdominal pain. In addition, she had noticed that she had 'pins and needle sensation in both hands'. She was not on the contraceptive pill as it 'did not agree with her system'. On clinical examination, she had tachycardia and a moderately raised systolic blood pressure. All other system examina-tions were essentially normal. The doctor immedi-ately asked her if she had passed any urine since this episode of abdominal pain to which she replied no. He asked her to pass some urine and requested a screening test for urinary porphobilinogen.

> The urinary porphobilinogen screen was strongly positive. A quantitative analysis followed, which showed high levels of porphobilinogen, δ-aminolaevulinic acid, uroporphyrin and coproporphyrin.

This confirmed that the patient had acute inter-mittent porphyria.

Aetiology and risk factors

Acute intermittent porphyria is the most common type in the UK. Women are more commonly affected, and in over 90% of the individuals the disease remains clinically latent. There are a number of precipitating factors such as drugs (sulphonamides, oral contraceptives, barbiturates, alcohol), hormonal changes (pregnancy, menstrua-tion, puberty), stress, starvation and infection.

Table P5 Clinical manifestations of porphyria

Porphyria	Photosensitivity	Neurological
Acute intermittent	—	+
Hereditary coproporphyria	+	+
Variegate	+	+
Cutaneous hepatic	+	—
Congenital erythropoietic	+	—
Erythropoietic protoporphyria	+	—

+, positive; —, negative.

Table P6 Diagnosis of porphyria

Porphyria	Blood	Urine	Faeces
Acute intermittent	—	ALA, PBG	—
Hereditary coproporphyria	—	ALA, PBG, coproporphyria	Coproporphyria
Variegate	—	ALA, PBG, coproporphyria	Coproporphyria, protoporphyrinogen
Cutaneous hepatic	—	Uroporphyrinogen	—
Congenital erythropoietic	Uroporphyrinogen, protoporphyrinogen	Uroporphyrinogen, coproporphyria	Coproporphyria
Erythropoietic protoporphyria	Protoporphyrinogen	—	Protoporphyrinogen

—, negative.

Pathology

The porphyrias are a group of conditions, which arise as a consequence of the deficiency of one of the enzymes of porphyrin synthesis. This results in the accumulation of porphyrin precursors (ALA and PBG) and porphyrins. When precursors are in excess, the clinical manifestations are mainly neurological (seizures, depression, hysteria and psychosis) because they are neurotoxic. This patient did not have any neurological symptoms. However, she had abdominal pain, vomiting, constipation, paraesthesiae, tachycardia and hypertension, which are the typical gastrointestinal, cardiovascular and peripheral neuropathy symptoms. These symptoms and dark urine (precursors present) were precipitated in her case by her menstrual periods. In porphyria, when the porphyrins accumulate, the main clinical manifestation is photosensitivity (Table P5). She did not experience any photosensitivity because in acute intermittent porphyria there is accumulation of precursors but not porphyrins.

The porphyrias are diagnosed on the clinical features and the presence of the precursors and porphyrins in the blood, urine and faeces (see Table P6).

Management

The mainstay of treatment is the identification and avoidance of the precipitating factors, in the photosensitive porphyrias to avoid direct exposure to sunlight. In acute porphyrias, relatives of the affected patients should be screened.

POTT DISEASE: Tuberculosis of the spine causing bone destruction with vertebral collapse.

PRE-ECLAMPSIA: A disease of late pregnancy characterized by hypertension, proteinuria and oedema, also known as toxaemia of pregnancy.

The disease affects around 5% of all pregnancies and is usually discovered as a result of routine pregnancy follow-up. The symptoms, if present, are those of hypertension*. Some patients may progress to develop serious central nervous system symptoms such as convulsions and coma. This severe form of the disease is called eclampsia. The cause of pre-eclampsia is not known, but placental ischaemia is thought to play a role. Pathological features are usually subtle and are most commonly seen in the vessels, microthrombi and fibrinoid necrosis of the arterial wall being seen in the liver, brain and kidney. Pre-eclampsia can be controlled by rest, diet and antihypertensive drugs; the disease usually resolves a few weeks after delivery.

PRIMARY BILIARY CIRRHOSIS: A chronic progressive disease of the liver, characterized by destruction of intrahepatic bile ducts eventually leading to cirrhosis*.

Case

A 42-year-old woman presented with the complaint of pruritus (itching). She had increasing lethargy within the last 6 months, otherwise her past medical history was unremarkable. On examination her vital signs were normal. She had mild jaundice and scratch marks were observed on her lower extremities. There was mild sensitivity in the upper right quadrant of the abdomen and her liver was palpable 2 cm below the ribs.

Her peripheral blood count was normal. Liver function tests showed a cholestatic liver disease picture:

Total bilirubin 30 μmol/l
Alkaline phosphatase 300 U/l
Alanine aminotransferase 110 U/l
Aspartate aminotransferase 145 U/l
γ-glutamyltransferase 110 U/l
Cholesterol 7.2 mmol/l
Total protein 51 g/l
ANA negative
AMA positive
Anti-HAV negative
Anti-HBs negative
Anti-HBc negative
Anti-HCV negative.

Ultrasound scan showed diffuse parenchyma changes but no dilated bile ducts.
Endoscopic retrograde cholangiopancreatography was normal.
Liver biopsy showed prominent portal inflammatory infiltrate composed of lymphocytes, histiocytes and macrophages. The infiltrate surrounded the bile ducts, which showed vacuolation. In one portal tract a granuloma containing epithelioid histiocytes and giant cells was seen. In several portal tracts the inflammatory infiltrate was seen extending into the parenchyma, forming piecemeal necrosis. Moderate cholestasis was present in the liver acini. Although the overall architecture of the liver was preserved, there was periportal fibrosis. The features were strongly suggestive of primary biliary cirrhosis (Fig. P20).

In the presence of characteristic liver function tests, AMA positivity, normal ERCP findings and histopathology, the diagnosis of primary biliary cirrhosis (PBC) was established. The patient was treated to relieve the symptoms.

P

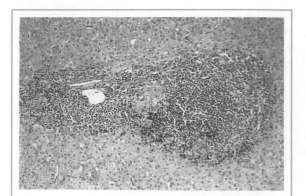

Fig. P20 Histological section of liver showing florid portal inflammation with a granuloma next to a bile duct.

Aetiology and risk factors

The aetiology of PBC is not known. However, autoimmunity* is thought to play a role, the anti-mitochondrial autoantibodies (AMA) probably being originally directed at bacterial enzymes. PBC is a rare disease with an incidence of 20 cases per million per year. It primarily affects middle-aged women, the female-to-male ratio being more than 6:1. A weak association with family history and certain HLA alleles, in particular HLA-DR8, has been reported.

Pathology

The critical pathology in PBC is loss of functional bile ducts, which leads to decreased excretion of bile, resulting in cholestasis*. As a result, blood levels of substances secreted into the bile, such as bile salts, bilirubin and cholesterol, are increased. The accumulation of bile salts is thought to cause the pruritus, the major presenting symptom in this case. Increased levels of bilirubin in the body manifests itself as yellow discoloration of the skin (jaundice). The blood chemistry reflects a cholestatic liver disease. Characteristically, serum alkaline phosphatase and γ-glutamyltransferase are increased several-fold. The cause of the debilitating lethargy observed in 85% of PBC patients is not known. The levels of amino-transferases are mildly increased secondary to hepatocyte injury. In any cholestatic liver disease, an obstructive extrahepatic lesion must be ruled out by appropriate imaging techniques such as ultrasonography or ERCP. In the absence of extrahepatic obstruction, a liver biopsy is indicated to identify the cause of cholestasis.

In PBC the diagnostic histological feature is the presence of a non-destructive granulomatous cholangitis. Some of the histological changes seen in the liver are described in the biopsy report above.

Classically the morphological changes are divided into four stages. In stage I, florid duct lesions with damage to bile duct epithelium and surrounding granulomatous inflammation are observed. In stage II the inflammation spreads from the portal tracts with biliary piecemeal necrosis into periportal hepatocytes. Stage III is characterized by progression of fibrosis and formation of porto-portal bridging. Stage IV shows established cirrhosis*. In many cases the progression of the disease does not follow the stages summarized above and the different stages can be observed in different segments of the liver. Nevertheless, most cases show progressive fibrosis and develop full-blown cirrhosis.

The pathogenesis of PBC remains uncertain. Histology suggests immunological destruction of the bile ducts, suggesting an autoimmune mechanism. A role of autoimmunity is supported by the fact that these patients have increased levels of serum immunoglobulins, particularly IgG and IgM, and the presence of many circulating autoantibodies. The most important autoantibodies in primary biliary cirrhosis are AMA found in 96% of all cases. AMA react with enzyme components of the inner mitochondrial membrane and are found in several other conditions. However, antibodies against the E2 component of mitochondrial pyruvate dehydrogenase are thought to be specific for PBC. Demonstration of AMA in cholestatic liver disease is considered to be virtually diagnostic of PBC (see Autoimmunity). Other autoantibodies occasionally detected include antinuclear and anti-smooth muscle antibodies.

A close association between primary biliary cirrhosis and certain other autoimmune diseases has been reported. Around 80% of the patients also suffer from Sjögren syndrome* and autoimmune thyroid disease is seen in a quarter. They also have increased risk of development of hepatocellular carcinoma*.

Management

There is no effective treatment for primary biliary cirrhosis. Most measures are directed towards relieving the symptoms. If end-stage liver disease develops, liver transplantation is indicated.

PRION DISEASE: Also known as transmissible spongiform encephalopathy. A neurodegenerative infection caused by a proteinaceous agent called a prion (see also Creutzfeldt–Jakob disease).

PROGRESSIVE MULTIFOCAL LEUCOEN-CEPHALOPATHY (PML): Central nervous system infection with the JC virus occurring in patients with AIDS or lymphoproliferative disease. There is demyelination and the production of abnormal giant oligodendrocytes. The patient presents with dementia, personality changes, seizures or weakness.

PROSTATIC CARCINOMA: A malignant tumour arising form the ducts or acini of the prostate gland.

Case

A 67-year-old man presented with difficulty in starting urination, frequency, urgency and nocturia. He was otherwise healthy. On physical examination his vital signs were normal. Rectal examination revealed an enlarged prostate and a hard solid nodule in the right lobe. Transrectal ultrasonography showed an area consistent with carcinoma in the right lobe. The tumour was limited to the prostate. The serum prostate specific antigen (PSA) level was elevated to 15 ng/ml (normal <4 ng/ml). Multiple transrectal trucut biopsies were performed to confirm the diagnosis.

> Histology: the trucut biopsies of the prostate showed an adenocarcinoma, Gleason grade 3 + 3 = 6. Some of the prostatic glands next to the invasive tumour contained foci of prostatic intraepithelial neoplasia (PIN).

CT scan of the pelvis and radionuclide bone scans did not show evidence of disease beyond the prostate. The patient was treated by radical prostatectomy and pelvic lymph node dissection.

> Histology: the radical prostatectomy specimen showed a prostatic adenocarcinoma identical to that observed in the needle biopsy. Adjacent glands showed PIN. The tumour was limited to the prostate and excision was complete. No tumour was found in the pelvic lymph nodes.

Postoperatively the patient recovered without complications. Serum PSA levels fell to normal limits and the patient remains free of disease.

Aetiology and risk factors

Prostatic carcinoma is the commonest type of cancer in man. It is estimated that in the sixth decade 25% and by the eighth decade 75% of men carry a focus of carcinoma in their prostate though the majority of these remain clinically silent. The cause of prostate cancer is not known; however,

hormones, ageing, genetic background and environment are thought to be contributing factors. Various chromosomal regions have been shown to be altered in prostate cancer, suggesting loss of several tumour suppressor genes.

Pathology

This patient presented with symptoms of prostate gland enlargement – 'prostatism' The enlarged prostate compresses the urethra, causing difficulty in emptying the bladder and reduces the capacity of the urinary bladder, leading to symptoms such as frequency, urgency and nocturia. Currently most prostate cancers are diagnosed incidentally as a result of routine testing of PSA serum levels. PSA is a protein secreted in the semen and is specific for the prostate tissue. An increased PSA level raises the strong possibility of prostate cancer but is not specific for this, since other benign diseases of prostate could also be responsible. In patients with raised PSA, histological confirmation of cancer is mandatory before treatment can be started. Once the cancer is histologically identified, PSA levels are very useful in following the effects of treatment, as demonstrated in this case.

Histologically, prostate cancers are almost always adenocarcinomas. The tumour cells usually form well-defined glands, which are arranged in a back-to-back fashion. Grading of glandular architecture according to the Gleason method has been helpful in predicting the behaviour of the tumour and is routinely performed. Most prostatic adenocarcinomas contain foci of *in situ* cancer – PIN adjacent to the invasive component. These lesions are characterized by glands with relatively normal architecture but cytological atypia, such as prominent nucleoli and hyperchromasia. They are considered to be precursor lesions for the development of invasive carcinoma. If PIN is the only histological finding in a prostatic trucut biopsy, close follow-up and repeated biopsies are warranted.

Management

The extent of tumour spread – the stage – is also critical in predicting prognosis and determining therapy. The majority of tumours are limited to the prostate at the time of diagnosis and respond very well to locally directed therapies such as surgery or radiotherapy. However, around a third of the cases have extensive local spread or distant metastasis, particularly to the bones. In these the prognosis is poor and endocrine therapy to suppress the androgens is the only treatment alternative available.

PROSTATIC HYPERPLASIA: Increase in the size of prostate gland secondary to hyperplasia of prostatic glands and stroma (Figs P21, P22). It is seen in

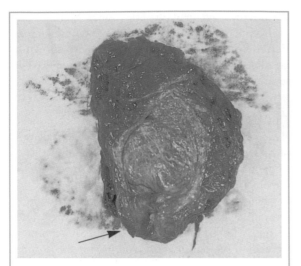

Fig. P21 Macroscopic specimen with prostatic hyperplasia (arrow) and bladder showing numerous trabeculi secondary to urinary obstruction. (Reproduced with permission from Lakhani SR, Dilly SA, Finlayson CJ. *Basic Pathology*, 2nd edn. London: Arnold, 1998)

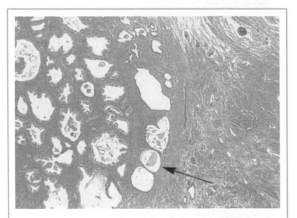

Fig. P22 Histological appearances of nodular hyperplasia of the prostate (arrow). (Reproduced with permission from Lakhani SR, Dilly SA, Finlayson CJ. *Basic Pathology*, 2nd edn. London: Arnold, 1998)

virtually every man over 50 years of age. The cause of the disease is not known, but hormonal influences have been implicated. In some individuals the enlargement can impede urinary outflow and medical or surgical treatment may be required.

Prostatic carcinoma

PROSTATITIS: An infection of the prostate which can be caused by a variety of different bacteria.

PSEUDOMEMBRANOUS COLITIS: An infection caused by the Gram-positive anaerobic organism, *Clostridium difficile.*

Aetiology and risk factors
Carriage of the organism in the normal healthy adult population is 1–3% but in healthy neonates it may be up to 20–70% and in hospitalized adult patients as high as 40%. It is a nosocomial pathogen, causing outbreaks as well as sporadic disease in hospitals. A significant factor in development of disease is a course of antibiotics. Although any antibiotic may induce PMC, cephalosporin and clindamycin are frequently to blame.

Pathology
The organism produces a number of toxins which are cytotoxic and increase vascular permeability. Some of the host damage may be linked to the bystander effect of misdirected cidal activity of neutrophil degranulation. Histologically, the colon and rectum are affected in a patchy distribution. Areas of ulceration in the lower intestine are covered by a fibrinous exudate consisting of fibrin, polymorphs and necrotic cells, which form the 'pseudomembranes' (Fig. P23).

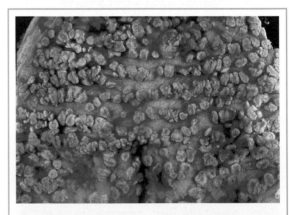

Fig. P23 Photograph of colon covered by pseudomembranes.

Clinically, the patient may present with mild, watery diarrhoea with abdominal pain, or severe diarrhoea with blood and mucus. Sigmoidoscopy is important to verify the presence of PMC. Complications are toxic megacolon and perforation. Laboratory diagnosis is by detection of the toxin in the faeces or culture of the organism, although this is used principally in epidemiological investigations. Treatment includes oral vancomycin or metronidazole.

P

PSITTACOSIS: An atypical pneumonia caused by *Chlamydia psittaci.*

Atypical pneumonia; Chlamydial disease

PSORIASIS: A common chronic inflammatory disease of skin most frequently involving knees, elbows and scalp (Fig. P24).

The cause of psoriasis is not known; however, genetic factors and immunological factors are thought to be critical, and there is an increased incidence of HLA-DR4, A26 and B27. Clinically, the involved areas show erythematous plaques and silver-coloured scales. In 5–7% of cases, the disease is associated with arthritis (psoriatic arthritis) clinically and pathologically mimicking rheumatoid arthritis*, but without nodules or rheumatoid factor. Biopsy of the skin lesions show characteristic histology with hyperplasia of the epidermis, marked parakeratosis, collections of neutrophils in the epidermis overlying the dermal papillae (Munro abscesses) and chronic inflammatory infiltrate in the dermis. Characteristic pitting of the nails may also occur.

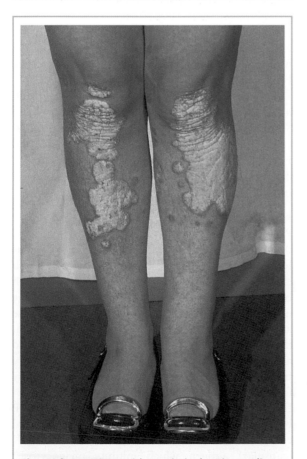

Fig. P24 A patient with psoriasis showing scaling lesions at and around the knees.

PSORIATIC ARTHRITIS: See Psoriasis.

PULMONARY HYPERTENSION: Increased blood pressure in the pulmonary vasculature.

In most instances pulmonary hypertension develops secondary to lung or heart diseases. The most important of these are:
- chronic obstructive or interstitial lung diseases which increase arterial resistance;
- recurrent pulmonary embolism which reduces the functional vascular bed;
- heart diseases such as mitral valve stenosis which increases the left atrial blood pressure and therefore also the pressure in the pulmonary vasculature.

Occasionally no cause can be identified – so-called idiopathic pulmonary hypertension.

Pathologically, in addition to changes related to the underlying disease, a number of specific changes in the pulmonary arteries and its branches are seen. Larger branches may show atheromatous plaques similar to those observed in systemic arteries. However, the most striking changes are usually present in small arteries and arterioles, where there is narrowing of the lumen, fibrosis of the intima and thickening of the media. In severe cases, capillary proliferation into the arterial lumen can occur, so-called plexogenic pulmonary arteriopathy. Clinically, the patients present with respiratory symptoms, with the eventual development of right ventricular failure and cor pulmonale.

Chronic obstructive airways disease; Embolism

PURPURA: Multiple small bruises, usually little larger than a pinhead, most frequently found in cases of thrombocytopenia* (Fig. P25). In contrast to telangiectases, they are not raised and do not blanch on pressure with a glass microscope slide.

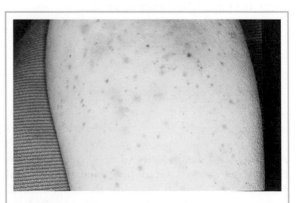

Fig. P25 Example of purpura in a case of thrombocytopenia.

In ambulant patients, purpura is most frequently seen on the lower limbs where hydrostatic pressure is highest. Occasionally purpura in a case of thrombocytopenia may be induced by congestion of capillaries induced by a sphygmomanometer.

Rarely, purpura may occur in the presence of a normal platelet count in congenital disorders of platelet function. In Henoch–Schönlein purpura*, the platelets and coagulation system are normal but red cells leak from capillaries damaged by an immunological vasculitis. Scorbutic purpura, found in scurvy*, is often confined to the hair follicles.

PYELONEPHRITIS: Bacterial infection of the kidney.

Case

A 26-year-old woman visited her GP complaining of frequency and burning on micturition (dysuria). She also complained of shaking chills (rigors) and a dull ache in her loin. On examination the GP found that she had a temperature and was tender in the right loin. Examination of the urine revealed blood and protein. The GP made the diagnosis of pyelonephritis, took a specimen of urine and started her empirically on antibiotics.

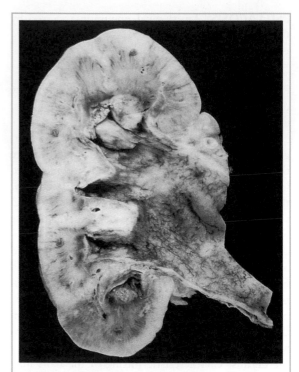

Fig. P27 Macroscopic view of a kidney showing pyelonephritis with papillary necrosis.

Microbiology: numerous pus cells and bacteria seen (Fig. P26).

Urine culture yielded > 10^5/ml of a pure growth of *Escherichia coli*.

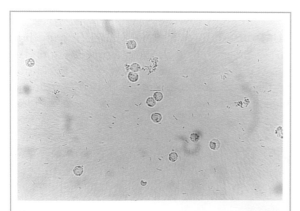

Fig. P26 Microscopy of urine showing presence of pus cells and bacteria.

Aetiology and risk factors

Escherichia coli is a Gram-negative bacillus and is part of the normal flora of the large bowel. Different strains of *E. coli* possess varying virulence characteristics, which are frequently coded for on plasmids. Some strains of *E. coli* produce toxins and are the cause of food poisoning or the haemolytic uraemic syndrome (see Gastroenteritis; Haemolytic uraemic syndrome).

The commonest cause of pyelonephritis is *E. coli*, although other numerically significant causes are *Staphylococcus saprophyticus* (in females), *Proteus* sp. (often associated with renal stones) and *Enterococcus* sp. Obstruction of the urinary tract, diabetes and pregnancy all increase the likelihood of infection.

Pathology

Pyelonephritis (Fig. P27) presents with frequency, dysuria, loin pain and haematuria. The patient is febrile and there is a peripheral neutrophilia with elevated serum levels of acute phase proteins. When bacteria gain entry to the bladder they attach to the uroepithelium, often by means of fimbriae. These adhesins bind to receptors on the uroepithelium, the amount of which may be genetically determined and thus predispose certain individuals to urinary tract infections. Some adhesins are commonly found on uropathogenic *E. coli*, such as the P-fimbria which has binding specificity for the P blood group antigen expressed on uroepithelial cells. Other virulence factors of *E. coli* are the K (capsular) antigen which inhibits phagocytosis, production of siderophores (iron-chelating compounds) and haemolysin production. P-fimbriate *E. coli* are particularly common in cases of pyelonephritis, in contrast to strains found in the faeces but not causing disease. The presence of the bacteria adhering to the bladder epithelium starts an acute inflammatory response and leads to the symptoms of cystitis. The bacteria do not invade the bladder wall, but they may pass up into the kidney, particularly if vesicoureteric reflux or some congenital abnormality is present, causing pyelonephritis. In cystitis there is poor or absent host immunological response with lack of IgG and IgA to the infecting organism. This may reflect the superficial nature of the infection and is in contrast to pyelonephritis. In some patients bacteria may colonize the bladder but the patient may be asymptomatic. This is important in children and pregnant women because asymptomatic bacteriuria may predispose to pyelonephritis.

Laboratory diagnosis of pyelonephritis is by semiquantitative culture of a midstream specimen of urine (MSU); $>10^5$ organisms per millilitre of urine is considered a significant bacteriuria. The infecting organism may also be found in blood cultures.

Management
Management may include hydration, alteration of urinary pH and/or appropriate antibiotics. In complicated or recurrent infections, radiological investigation is warranted.

PYOMYOSITIS: Acute suppuration of the muscles commonly occurring in the tropics and frequently caused by *Staphylococcus aureus*.

PYREXIA OF UNKNOWN ORIGIN (PUO): A condition in which a patient presents with a fever of 3 weeks' duration but where there is no obvious cause after preliminary investigation. The commonest cause of PUO are infections, the commonest of these being tuberculosis*. Other significant causes of PUO are neoplasm, collagen disease and drugs.

 Brucellosis

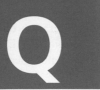

Q FEVER: An atypical pneumonia caused by *Coxiella burnetii*.

 Atypical pneumonia; Rickettsial disease

QUINSY: A peritonsillar abscess which can be caused by a number of different bacteria, e.g. *Staphylococcus*, *Streptococcus*, oral anaerobes.

RABIES: An encephalitis caused by the rabies virus.

Aetiology and risk factors

Rabies is acquired by contact with infected animals, usually via dog bites, but the virus is present in many wild animals, e.g. foxes, bats, wolves. The disease is endemic in most parts of the world excluding the UK, Iceland and parts of northern Scandinavia.

Pathology

The virus is neurotropic and, following a bite, multiplies locally and gains access to the peripheral nervous system. Travelling along the axon to the central nervous system, it replicates within neurons and from here spreads out to all body organs, e.g. heart, cornea, kidneys and salivary glands. Consequently, the virus can be found in urine and saliva and corneal grafts may be a source of human infection. The brain and spinal cord may show mild neuron degeneration with a perivascular mononuclear infiltrate. Characteristic intracytoplasmic eosinophilic bodies (Negri bodies) consisting of viral nucleic acid and cellular organelles can be seen most prominently in the hippocampus and cerebellar Purkinje cells. Cellular degeneration of some peripheral glands may be found, e.g. in the salivary and adrenal glands, and there may be a myocarditis in some patients. Because of this localization in the nervous tissue, there is no initial immune response against the virus.

Clinically, the incubation period can be from a few days to a year, depending in part where the virus was inoculated by the bite. Bites on the head have very short incubation periods. Initial symptoms are pruritus and paraesthesia at the site of the bite with non-specific systemic symptoms of malaise and myalgia. Clinically, there are two general presentations as follows:

- In **furious** rabies, the patient has hydrophobia and respiratory spasms, induced by the slightest external stimulus. The patient may hallucinate and become aggressive and may have evidence of autonomic nerve dysfunction. Cardiac or respiratory arrest may occur.
- In **paralytic** (dumb) rabies, the patient develops a flaccid paralysis extending to the respiratory muscles.

Laboratory diagnosis includes examination of the brain of the suspected animal vector and skin biopsy from the patient using immunofluorescent staining. The peripheral white count may be normal and the cerebrospinal fluid may show an increased number of mainly mononuclear cells.

Management

Management includes immune serum plus post-exposure immunization and intensive supportive care in an ITU, despite which the majority of patients will not survive. Note that rabies is the only disease in which, because of the long incubation period, post-exposure immunization is a possibility. Control is by pre-exposure vaccination in those at risk (e.g. vets) or by vaccination of domestic pets.

RADIATION INJURY: Changes observed in tissues secondary to ionizing radiation such as x-rays, gamma rays, or cosmic rays.

Normally, radiation changes are a result of radiotherapy, usually for malignant tumours. The clinical findings and pathology vary according to the type, intensity, duration of radiation and the organ affected. Common histological changes include endothelial necrosis, thrombosis and intimal thickening in arteries, so-called radiation fibrosis with bizarre fibroblasts and exfoliation of epithelium in various organs leading to ulceration, bone marrow suppression and sterility.

Note that, though not generally thought of as radiation injury, ultraviolet light can seriously damage skin.

RAMSAY–HUNT SYNDROME: Herpes zoster infection of the geniculate ganglion leading to formation of vesicles in the auricle and the palate, usually associated with ipsilateral facial nerve paralysis.

 Chickenpox

RAT-BITE FEVER: A rare infection caused by either *Streptobacillus moniliformis* or *Spirillum minus*, following the bite of a rat or occasionally with *Str. moniliformis* from contaminated milk. After an infection with *Str. moniliformis*, the patient has a fever with a macular or petechial rash involving the extremities, including the palms and soles. There is frequently a polyarthritis involving the large joints and a peripheral leucocytosis. In rat-bite fever caused by *Spirillum* there is a macular rash and commonly a lymphadenopathy local to the bite, but arthritis is uncommon. Complications include endocarditis. Laboratory diagnosis is by isolation of the organism (*Str. moniliformis*), microscopy or animal inoculation (*Spirillum*) and management is with penicillin.

RAYNAUD DISEASE:
Cyanosis of the fingers and toes secondary to spasm of small arteries and arterioles. The disease usually affects young women. No organic pathology can be found. The disease is thought to be an exaggerated physiological response to such events as cold or emotion. Similar signs seen secondary to organic pathology, leading to arterial narrowing, are called Raynaud phenomenon. The painful red mottling seen on re-warming distinguishes it from acrocyanosis.

REACTIVE ARTHRITIS:
A name given to sterile arthritides associated with infection, commonly venereal or intestinal (see Table R1) and probably immunologically mediated.

Table R1 Infections commonly associated with arthritis

Campylobacter
Yersinia
Salmonella
Shigella
Chlamydia

 Hypersensitivity; Seronegative arthritides; Urethritis

REITER DISEASE:
Also known as Reiter syndrome, is defined as the triad of seronegative arthritis, urethritis and conjunctivitis.

Presentation is usually with multiple painful joint swellings but there is often a recent history of urethral discharge and ocular symptoms. It is considered a 'reactive' arthritis since it often follows infection, but the joints themselves are sterile. Up to 80% of patients are HLA-B27 positive. Associated infections are commonly venereal (e.g. *Chlamydia*) or intestinal (e.g. *Shigella, Yersinia, Campylobacter*). Balanitis and mouth ulcers are also frequently present. It has been suggested that the pathogenesis is related to a type III hypersensitivity.

Histology shows a synovial infiltrate in which T-lymphocytes and monocytes are prominent.

 Hypersensitivity; Reactive arthritis; Seronegative arthritides; Urethritis

RELAPSING FEVER:
A spirochaetal infection caused by *Borrelia* species, characterized by cyclic periods of fever and systemic symptoms.

Aetiology and risk factors
The infection occurs following the bite of a tick (*Borrelia hermsii, Borrelia turicatae*) or louse (*Borrelia recurrentis*). Louse-borne disease is spread from human to human, usually in areas of deprivation or times of social upheaval such as wars, whilst the reservoir for tick-borne disease is wild animals.

Pathology
After the bite of the vector, the *Borrelia* multiply in the blood with the onset of systemic symptoms. There is sudden onset of headache with fever and myalgia. Hepatosplenomegaly may occur with elevation of liver enzymes and serum bilirubin in about a third of patients. Damage occurs to the vascular endothelium, leading to thrombocytopenia with epistaxis, haematuria and the development of a petechial rash. Disseminated intravascular coagulation* may occur. There is a peripheral leucocytosis. The organisms are found in the solid organs, e.g. heart, brain, liver, spleen, but confined to the vasculature. After 3 days to a week, specific antibodies are produced, resulting in a reduction of the number of organisms in the blood or retreat to immunologically privileged sites such as the eye or brain, and the febrile episode ends in a crisis. There is leucopenia, rigors, tachycardia, a rise in temperature, which is followed by profuse sweating, hypotension and a gradual fall in temperature. After about a week, antigenic variants of the *Borrelia* appear and proliferate in the blood again, producing further symptoms. Laboratory diagnosis is by demonstration of the *Borrelia* in the blood by microscopy and management is with tetracycline or penicillin. Antibiotic treatment is often associated with a Jarisch–Herxheimer reaction.

RENAL CELL CARCINOMA:
Adenocarcinoma of the kidney arising from tubular epithelial cells.

Most renal cell carcinomas are sporadic tumours and are seen in the 50–70 age group. A small proportion are hereditary and these have been important in understanding the oncogenesis of sporadic cases. Classically, patients present with three clinical features. These are haematuria, costovertebral pain and a palpable mass. However, due to increased use of imaging techniques, many patients are now being diagnosed at an earlier stage, before the development of the characteristic clinical features. Histologically, the tumours are classified into three main groups. The commonest type of sporadic renal cell carcinoma is the clear cell carcinoma. This type is also associated with von Hippel–Lindau (VHL) syndrome*. Both the sporadic and hereditary forms show abnormalities of chromosome 3, involving the putative tumour suppressor *VHL* gene. The next commonest histological type is the papillary renal cell carcinoma. Characteristic cytogenetic abnormalities in these are trisomies, in particular trisomy 7. Chromosome 7 contains the *MET* proto-oncogene, which is thought to be critical in development of this variant. The third and least common variant is the chromophobe renal cell carcinoma. Cytogenetically this differs from the other two by showing multiple chromosome losses and hypoploidy. Renal cell carcinoma is treated with nephrectomy. The prognosis predominantly depends on the stage at diagnosis.

RENAL CYST: An abnormal cystic dilation in the renal parenchyma, often lined by tubular epithelium.

The commonest type of renal cyst is the simple cyst, which develops secondary to obstruction of the tubules and accumulation of urine proximal to the obstruction. Other important cystic renal diseases include developmental disorders such as cystic renal dysplasia, hereditary diseases such as polycystic kidney* disease, acquired renal cystic disease secondary to long-term dialysis, and neoplasms.

 Polycystic kidney; Renal cell carcinoma

RENAL FAILURE: A condition occurring when there is a significant reduction in renal excretory or regulatory function with a resultant elevation in serum urea, creatinine, hydrogen ions and other metabolic products. Acute renal failure is characterized by a rapid loss of function over days or a few weeks with a marked diminution of urine output (< 400 ml/24 h). It is potentially reversible. Chronic renal failure appears when the number of functioning nephrons is reduced to about 25% and develops over a period of months or years and is irreversible.

Aetiology and risk factors
Renal failure, whether acute or chronic, may be due to pre-renal, renal or post-renal causes and in some cases to a combination of these:
- Pre-renal failure results from shock from hypovolaemia, renal vasoconstriction, a reduction in renal blood flow, burns, severe haemorrhage, hepatorenal syndrome, postoperative oliguria and dehydration.
- Renal failure can result from all types of glomerulonephritis, acute tubular necrosis, transplant rejection, acute cortical necrosis, snake bite, acute pyelonephritis and nephrotoxins.
- Post-renal failure can result from obstruction, renal tumours, prostatic hyperplasia, and calculus.

In addition, chronic renal failure may be seen in diabetes, hypertension, chronic glomerulonephritis, polycystic disease, amyloidosis, multiple myeloma, analgesic abuse and hypercalcaemia.

Pathology
In **acute renal failure**, the loss of excretory function results in retention of waste products (urea, creatinine and phosphate), giving rise to anorexia, vomiting and nausea. The loss of regulatory function results in retention of sodium chloride, water, and potassium and hydrogen ions, resulting in oedema, hypertension, cardiac arrhythmias and metabolic acidosis.

In **chronic renal failure**, the failure of renal function results in a significant increase in serum urea, creatinine and decrease in creatinine clearance. There is an inability to concentrate urine, resulting in polyuria, and an inability to excrete hydrogen ions, resulting in retention of these ions and giving rise to a metabolic acidosis. Due to a loss in renal ability to activate vitamin D, very little calcium is absorbed from the gut, resulting in hypocalcaemia. This in turn causes a compensatory parathyroid hyperplasia (secondary hyperparathyroidism). The abnormal calcium and phosphate metabolism produces a renal osteodystrophy (osteomalacia and osteitis fibrosa cystica) and metastatic calcification. Erythropoietin production is reduced in renal failure, giving rise to a normochromic normocytic anaemia; platelet function is also affected. The sodium and water retention results in hypertension; high levels of potassium are also seen later in development. The accumulation of nitrogenous waste products produces disturbances in conscious levels (uraemic encephalopathy).

Management
Management involves a general correction of fluid and electrolyte imbalance, acid–base balance, nutritional state and antibiotic cover. Other approaches include haemodialysis, continuous arteriovenous haemofiltration, continuous arteriovenous haemodialfiltration, peritoneal dialysis and, in renal cases, renal transplantation.

RENAL TRANSPLANTATION: A now common treatment for end-stage renal disease by grafting a foreign kidney.

Table R2 Clinical types of rejection

Type of rejection	Time after transplantation	Pathogenetic mechanism(s)
Hyperacute	Minutes–hours	Microhaemorrhages and thrombi result in cytotoxic antigens and obstruct small blood vessels; irreversible and the graft has to be removed; due to cytotoxic antibodies to HLA class I antigens of the donor kidney or ABO blood group antigens. Antibodies activate complement leading to type II/III hypersensitivity reaction; rare these days with cross-matching used
Acute rejection	Weeks–months	Rising serum and urine creatinine results from renal damage due to infiltrating cytotoxic CD8+ T cells recognizing the HLA class I antigens on the donor kidney; rejection may also be mediated through cyclosporin toxicity but this is distinguishable by carrying out a needle biopsy
Chronic rejection	Months–years	Progressive hypertension beginning after a long spell of good renal function. Histological picture is one of basement membrane thickening, hyalinization of glomeruli, interstitial fibrosis and proliferation of endothelial cells; the mechanism is unknown but probably both antibody (complexes) and cell-mediated mechanisms are responsible. May be due to minor MHC incompatibility.

Case

A 42-year-old man had suffered for two and a half years from renal failure due to chronic glomerulonephritis and had been carrying out his haemodialysis at home. He was put on the list for a kidney transplant when one became available. Blood was taken for ABO and HLA typing and he was examined for any contraindications for transplantation. He was found to be blood group A and was HLA-A10, A25, B6, B27, Cw3, Cw5 and DR3, DR4. Three months later he was admitted for his transplant operation. He was given a cocktail of immunosuppressive drugs which included azathioprine, prednisone and cyclosporin A. The renal transplant was from a donor who had died from a fatal road accident and was typed as HLA-A5, A11, B6, B11, Cw3, Cw6 and DR2, DR3 with the same blood group. A cross-matching test was done which was satisfactory. The surgery was successful and over the next few days his serum and urea levels of creatinine fell, indicating that the new kidney was functioning well. He returned home after a week and felt much better than he had for 3 years. Five weeks after the operation he developed a fever, his urine output dropped to 23 ml/h and his blood pressure increased to 140/115 mmHg. He had mild interstitial oedema. He was admitted into hospital for a renal biopsy, which showed a mononuclear infiltrate in the renal cortex. The patient was diagnosed as having acute rejection and was given parenteral prednisone. He began to improve on steroid treatment and was discharged. He was given cyclosporin A as a long-term treatment to prevent further rejection episodes.

Aetiology and risk factors

Rejection of transplants is mainly mediated through an immune response against transplantation antigens (see transplant rejection). It is particularly important in renal transplants that the donor's and recipient's ABO blood group antigens are matched. This is because the blood group antigens are also expressed by renal blood vessel endothelial cells. Cross-matching is also important and is carried out by mixing the recipient's serum with blood leucocytes from the donor. Binding of antibodies to the donor leucocytes (such as preformed HLA antibodies produced against a previously rejected transplant or if the recipient is female, by sensitization during pregnancy and delivery) would exclude the kidney for transplanting to that particular patient.

Pathology

There are three main clinical forms of rejection that can occur following a renal transplant. These are summarized together with the mechanisms of rejection in Table R2. The patient described had the features of an acute rejection episode.

Management

There is no treatment for hyperacute rejection and the donor kidney has to be removed. Acute rejection can be controlled in many cases by prednisone treatment and cyclosporin A. If there is chronic rejection, eventually the kidney will have to be replaced since no response would be expected to anti-rejection therapy.

 Glomerulonephritis; Hypersensitivity; Renal failure; Transplant rejection

RETICULAR DYSGENESIS: A severe form of immunodeficiency* due to a haemopoeitic stem cell defect. The function of T-cells, B-cells and granulocytes is grossly impaired.

RETINOBLASTOMA: A malignant tumour originating from neuroepithelial cells of the retina.

Retinoblastoma is a rare tumour of childhood. The vast majority of cases are diagnosed before the age of 8. The critical event in the pathogenesis of retinoblastoma is a defect in a tumour suppressor gene, the retinoblastoma (Rb) gene located on chromosome 13. In familial cases of retinoblastoma, the children are born with one defective allele and the second allele is lost later in life, when the tumour develops. In sporadic cases both alleles are lost by somatic mutation after birth. Macroscopically, the tumour arises from the retina and protrudes into the eye (Fig. R1). Microscopically, it is composed of small round undifferentiated cells, which form small

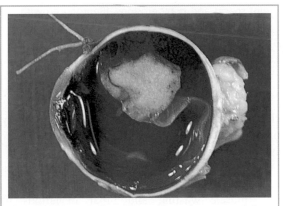

Fig. R1 Macroscopic appearances of eye containing tumour detaching the retina. (Reproduced with permission from Lakhani SR, Dilly SA, Finlayson CJ. *Basic Pathology*, 2nd edn. London: Arnold, 1998)

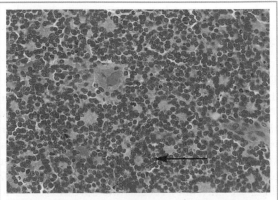

Fig. R2 Histological appearances with characteristic rosettes (arrow) of retinoblastoma. (Reproduced with permission from Lakhani SR, Dilly SA, Finlayson CJ. *Basic Pathology*, 2nd edn. London: Arnold, 1998)

rosettes mimicking neuroepithelial differentiation in the embryo (Fig. R2). The prognosis is very poor if the tumour spreads beyond the eye. Small tumours can be treated by radiation, but enucleation of the eye may be necessary for larger ones.

RETINOPATHY: Non-neoplastic, predominantly inflammatory disease of the retina, usually affecting vision.

Retinopathies can develop as a result of various clinical conditions. These include retinopathy of prematurity (retrolental fibroplasia), retinopathy of diabetes mellitus*, hypertension* and arteriolosclerosis*.

RETROPERITONEAL FIBROSIS: A progressive chronic inflammatory process of unknown aetiology, affecting the retroperitoneum and characterized by irregular fibrosis which encircles the lower abdominal aorta and ureters.

RHESUS DISEASE: A variety of haemolytic disease of the newborn* due to anti-D antibodies that cross the placenta from a mother previously sensitized against the D antigen. These antibodies may destroy the baby's red cells and cause haemolytic anaemia*, death *in utero*, or severe neonatal jaundice, resulting in damage to the basal ganglia of the brain – kernicterus.

The mother may be sensitized by an inadvertent Rhesus-positive blood transfusion or more commonly by leakage of Rhesus-positive red cells across the placenta, particularly at the time of a previous delivery.

Rhesus disease is becoming less common in Western countries due the programme of Rhesus prophylaxis, every Rhesus-negative mother receiving an injection of anti-D after the delivery of a Rhesus-positive baby. This destroys any circulating Rhesus-positive red cells that have crossed the placenta at the time of delivery, so preventing the mother being immunized against them. Haemolytic disease due to placenta-crossing IgG anti-A or anti-B is commoner, though usually milder, than Rhesus disease. Other Rhesus antibodies such as anti-c or anti-e may also be responsible.

Haemolytic disease of the newborn

RHEUMATIC FEVER: An uncommon (in the UK) late cardiac complication of an acute infection with the Gram-positive coccus, *Streptococcus pyogenes*.

Aetiology and risk factors
Certain M serotypes of *Strep. pyogenes* appear to be more closely linked to the development of

R

rheumatic fever. The most likely mechanism of pathogenesis is the production of cross-reacting antibodies by the host against either the carbohydrate Lancefield antigen, the protein M antigens or the hyaluronic acid of the *Streptococcus* and myocardial sarcolemma, myosin or a heart valve glycoprotein.

Pathology

The characteristic histological feature is the perivascular Aschoff nodules which are widespread in connective and myocardial tissue and consist of a necrotic core surrounded by giant multinucleate cells (Anichkov cells – histocytes) and lymphocytes.

The nodule eventually becomes fibrosed. This leads to distortion of the (principally) mitral valve, with regurgitation and stenosis. Clinically, the onset can be insidious or acute, with flitting polyarthritis and carditis. The arthritis affects mainly the large joints and there may be acute pain and erythema. The carditis may present as a pericarditis, myocarditis or valvular disease, as evidenced by a murmur and heart failure. In addition to the myocardial and connective tissue involvement, there may also be the neurological manifestation of Sydenham chorea, characterized by purposeless uncoordinated movements and dermatological manifestations of erythema marginatum or the appearance of rheumatic nodules over bony prominences. Diagnosis is clinical (Jones criteria), requiring two major criteria (polyarthritis/carditis/chorea/erythema marginatum/nodules) or one major and two minor (fever/ previous rheumatic or scarlet fever/prolonged PR interval/elevated acute phase proteins), plus laboratory evidence of a recent streptococcal infection based upon isolation or serology. Management is supportive with anti-inflammatory drugs and penicillin given as treatment and subsequent prophylaxis.

RHEUMATOID ARTHRITIS: A common chronic symmetrical polyarthritis with extra-articular features.

Case

A 38-year-old woman complained of pain and stiffness in her hands and wrists for the past 3–4 months, worst in the morning. On examination, her wrists and metacarpophalangeal joints were tender and slightly swollen and other joints apparently normal. Her blood count was normal apart from slight anaemia (Hb 9.8 g/dl), but her ESR was significantly raised (35 mm/h), as was her serum C-reactive protein (33 mg/l). Serological investigation showed a positive rheumatoid factor but no antinu-

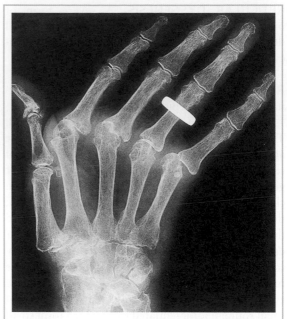

Fig. R3 Radiograph of hand showing narrowing of joint spaces and bony erosions. (Reproduced with permission from Curtis J, Whitehouse G. *Radiology for the MRCP.* London: Arnold, 1998)

clear or other autoantibodies. She was initially prescribed aspirin, but this did not control her symptoms and she was switched to indomethacin.

A year later she had developed pain and stiffness in her knees and her hands showed slight deformities (muscle wasting and ulnar deviations of fingers). A painless subcutaneous nodule was found on one forearm. Radiographs of hands, wrists and knees showed extensive erosion of bone (Fig. R3). She now fulfilled many of the ARA criteria for rheumatoid arthritis and a firm diagnosis was made. At this visit her treatment was changed to ibuprofen, which has maintained her in reasonable health.

Aetiology and risk factors

The cause of rheumatoid arthritis is not known, though claims have been made at various times for micro-organisms, including mycoplasma and virus, as causative agents. The incidence is 1–3% of the population, with a female:male ratio varying from 13:1 (Japan) to 2:1 (UK). The disease is rare in black Africans. Onset is usually between 25 and 60 (but see juvenile rheumatoid arthritis*). The possession of HLA-DR4 increases the risk sevenfold. There is a 30% concordance in identical twins, suggesting involvement of both genetic and environmental factors.

Pathology

The pathological appearance of the joints is of an inflammatory synovitis. The synovial membrane is thickened, vascular and oedematous, with an infiltrate mainly of T-lymphocytes and macrophages but also plasma cells, some of which can be shown to be making rheumatoid factor (anti-IgG autoantibody). Note that rheumatoid factor is only found in about 75% of cases, and is not itself diagnostic. The hypertrophied synovia ('pannus') may contain typical lymphoid follicles, and may grow over the articular cartilage, which, together with the adjacent bone, may be severely eroded (see Fig. R3). The synovial fluid contains predominantly neutrophils, their released enzymes and pro-inflammatory cytokines such as TNF and IL-1. Rheumatoid nodules, most commonly seen at pressure sites such as elbow and forearm, are highly characteristic and are not found in other forms of arthritis. There is a central necrotic area surrounded by chronic inflammatory tissue containing numerous macrophages. Similar areas of necrosis are found in advanced cases in blood vessels, and there may be nodules and/or fibrosis in the lung and, particularly in males, pleural effusion. As in other chronic inflammatory conditions, secondary amyloidosis (AA type) may develop. About 5% of patients develop splenomegaly and leucopenia; this is known as Felty syndrome*.

Management

Rest, physiotherapy, splinting where needed and anti-inflammatory drugs are the mainstay of treatment, but there is no cure. Drugs commonly used are aspirin, indomethacin and ibuprofen and if these fail, steroids, gold and penicillamine. In severe cases, immunosuppressives such as azathioprine or cyclophosphamide may be used.

 Amyloidosis; Felty syndrome; Juvenile rheumatoid arthritis

RHINITIS: Inflammation of the nasal mucosa, the main cause of which is one of the common cold viruses, e.g. rhinovirus. This is an RNA virus that has over 100 serogroups and attaches to either the ICAM-1 or low-density lipoprotein receptor (LDL) of the host cell. The virus inhibits host cell protein synthesis by inactivation of an initiation factor and replicates in the respiratory epithelium of the upper respiratory tract. The viruses are transmitted principally by hand contact, rather than droplet infection. Similar 'colds' are produced by adenovirus, Coxsackievirus and ECHO virus. Infection of the nasal mucosa is also produced by *Klebsiella rhinoscleromatis*, which causes rhinoscleroma, a chronic granulomatous infection which sometimes involves the underlying bone or cartilage. Chronic atrophic rhinitis (ozaena) is caused by *Klebsiella ozaenae*. Other organisms that affect the nasal mucosa are *Mycobacterium leprae* and *Treponema pallidum*.

RICKETS: A bone mineralization defect in children with abnormal bone growth.

Failure of mineralization occurs when there is a long-standing low blood level of calcium (dietary deficiency of calcium or vitamin D, fat malabsorption syndromes, failure of 25α-hydroxylation in liver, failure of 1α-hydroxylation in kidney, drugs) or phosphate (dietary phosphate deficiency, renal tubular phosphate loss). The main causes are nutritional deficiency, vitamin D-resistant rickets, end-organ insensitivity to vitamin D and vitamin D-sensitive rickets. In children, the failure of mineralization affects new bone growth and subsequently leads to softening and growth retardation of the affected bones. Clinically, the children present with bowing of the tibias and abnormal curvatures in vertebra and pelvis. The biochemical abnormalities are similar to those seen in osteomalacia.

 Osteomalacia; Vitamin deficiencies

Table R3 Organisms causing rickettsial disease

Disease	Organism	Vector/Route	Reservoir	Distribution
Rocky Mountain spotted fever	*R. rickettsii*	Tick	Rodents, dogs	North America
Boutonneuse fever	*R. conorii*	Tick	Rodent, dogs	Africa, S. France
Rickettsialpox	*R. akari*	Mite	Rodent	USA, Africa, former Soviet Union
Epidemic typhus	*R. prowazekii*	Louse	Human	World wide
Murine typhus	*R. typhi*	Flea	Rodents	World wide
Scrub typhus	*R. tsutsugamushi*	Mite	Rodents	Asia, Australia
Q fever	*Coxiella burnetii*	Aerosol, milk	Cattle, sheep	World wide

RICKETTSIAL DISEASE: Infection with one of the species of *Rickettsia*.

Aetiology and risk factors

Rickettsiae are obligate intracellular parasites and are transmitted by insect vectors, with the exception of Q fever*, which can also be acquired by the aerial route. The organisms causing disease are shown in Table R3.

Pathology

Rickettsiae enter the bloodstream after inoculation and bind to receptors on endothelial cells of the blood vessels. They are taken up by a phagocytic process and escape from the phagosome, replicating in the cytoplasm. Damage to the endothelial cells is probably due in part to proteases and phospholipases that are released from the organism and it leads to a widespread vasculitis and activation of the kallikrein system. There is increased vascular permeability leading to hypovolaemia and hypotension. Vascular lesions can be found in all viscera and in the skin, leading to the development of a characteristic rash. In severe cases of vasculitis, gangrene of the fingers and toes can develop. There is frequently a thrombocytopenia, although the white count may be normal. Clinically, the patient presents with an acute onset of fever, myalgia, headache and a rash. There may be clinical evidence of pulmonary, liver, cardiac or central nervous system involvement. Laboratory diagnosis is mainly by serology and management includes tetracycline or chloramphenicol.

RINGWORM: A superficial fungal infection of the stratum corneum of the skin.

Aetiology and risk factors

Ringworm is caused by a group of fungi called dermatophytes (see Table R4) which may also infect the nails and hair. These infections occur world wide but some of the fungi have a regional distribution. Predisposing factors for ringworm infection are humidity and maceration of the skin.

There are three sources of infection:
- another person (anthropophilic fungus);
- an animal (zoophilic fungus);
- the environment (geophilic fungus).

Transmission is by contact.

Pathology

The arthrospores of the dermatophytes adhere to keratinized cells and germinate, invading the stratum corneum (ringworm or tinea), nail (onychomycosis) or hair. Virulence factors of the dermatophytes are keratinases and proteases. Ringworm presents as slowly spreading, scaling,

Table R4 Fungi causing ringworm

Dermatophyte	Disease
Trichophyton rubrum	Tinea corporis. tinea cruris, tinea pedis (athlete's foot), onychomycosis
Trichophyton interdigitale	Tinea pedis
Trichophyton violaceum	Tinea capitis
Trichophyton schoenleinii	Favus
Trichophyton verrucosum	Tinea capitis
Microsporium audouinii	Tinea capitis
Microsporium canis	Tinea capitis
Epidermophyton floccosum	Tinea cruris

annular, raised plaques with an erythematous border and clearing in the middle. Infection with zoophilic dermatophytes can lead to a severe inflammatory reaction with oedema, pustule formation and scarring (kerion). In some instances an immune reaction occurs, producing a vesicular eruption (severe inflammatory reaction) which correlates with a strong DTH response. Histologically, the appearance is of eczema. Erythema nodosum* may also occur. In athlete's foot there is scaling and maceration between the toes, and in tinea capitis infection scaling of the scalp with hair loss. A severe form of scalp ringworm is favus where there is a strong inflammatory reaction and scab formation, leading to hair loss. If the fungus infects the nails, they become hypertrophic and discoloured (see onychomycosis). Laboratory diagnosis is by microscopic examination of specimens and isolation of the fungus (Fig. R4).

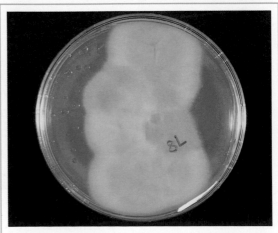

Fig. R4 *Microsporium canis* growing on agar.

Management

Treatment is with topical keratolytics, azoles (clotrimazole, ketoconazole) or terbinafine. Occasionally oral therapy with terbinafine, griseofulvin or azoles is required.

RUBELLA: German measles, an exanthematous disease of childhood caused by the rubella virus.

Aetiology and risk factors

Rubella is spread by the aerial route. It has an incubation period of 10–21 days. If acquired by a pregnant female. it is spread transplacentally to the fetus and can cause multiple congenital abnormalities.

Pathology

Infection acquired postnatally may be clinically inapparent or present with fever, coryza, sore throat and a rash, which begins on the head and neck and spreads to the trunk. Cervical lymphadenopathy occurs. Complications include arthralgia, thrombocytopenia, encephalitis and the Guillain–Barre syndrome*. Congenitally acquired infections typically lead to cataracts*, deafness and cardiac abnormalities, although other congenital abnormalities may occur (e.g. microcephaly, mental retardation). The mechanisms of fetal damage are unknown, although the rubella virus, by replicating in fetal cells or those of the placenta, may lead to chromosomal damage, mitotic arrest, cell death or vasculitis. The risk of congenital abnormalities depends upon the stage of pregnancy at which the infection occurs. In the first trimester the risk is about 60–90%, in the second trimester about 17% and in the final trimester about 3%. Maternal reinfection may occur, although it is rare and the risk of congenital abnormalities unlikely. Laboratory diagnosis is mainly by serology; virus isolation or *in situ* hybridization may be used but are not routine.

Management

Pregnant women who have been in contact with a case of rubella may be given immunoglobulin, although this does not stop the viraemia and therefore the possibility of congenital abnormalities. Rubella vaccination is part of the MMR (attenuated measles, mumps and rubella) triple vaccine. Adult women who are given the vaccine should not become pregnant during the following 3 months.

R

S

SALPINGITIS: Infection of the Fallopian tubes.

 Pelvic inflammatory disease

SARCOIDOSIS: A disease characterized by a chronic granulomatous inflammation of unknown aetiology involving multiple organs.

Case

A 35-year-old female patient was seen in the local surgery complaining of cough and 5 kg weight loss within the last 3 months. There was no sputum production. She was not a smoker. Her past medical history and social history were unremarkable. There was no history of exposure to industrial pollutants.

On examination, her temperature was 37.6°C, and her respiration rate was increased (25/min); other vital signs were normal. Her respiratory sounds were within the normal range. She had bilateral cervical microlymphadenopathy and her liver was just palpable. Other systems were unremarkable.

Her blood count was normal but the ESR was mildly elevated (30 mm/h). Liver function tests showed slightly raised transaminases. Blood gases were within normal limits.

Due to the long history of respiratory complaints a chest radiograph was performed.

> The chest x-ray showed bilateral prominent hilar lymphadenopathy and patchy interstitial shadowing in both lungs.

FNA of the cervical lymph node contained lymphocytes and occasional clusters of epithelioid histiocytes consistent with granulomatous lymphadenitis.

Cervical lymph node biopsy showed numerous non-caseating granulomas formed predominantly by epithelioid histiocytes and Langhans giant cells. Staining for acid-fast bacilli was negative (Fig. S1).

Bronchoscopic and liver needle biopsies showed similar granulomatous inflammation.

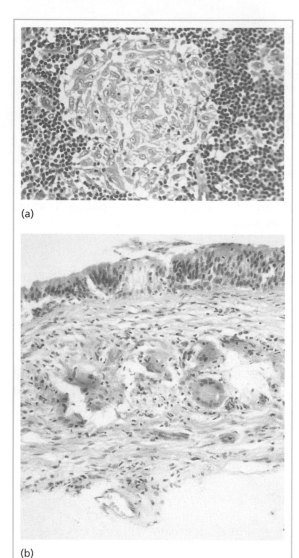

(a)

(b)

Fig. S1 (a) Section of lymph node showing a well-defined epithelioid granuloma; (b) granuloma in bronchial sarcoid.

Microbiological cultures obtained from blood, urine, cervical lymph node and liver biopsies did not yield any organisms.

> Skin testing: tuberculin test negative, Kveim test positive.

The patient was diagnosed as having sarcoidosis and was put on steroids.

Aetiology and risk factors

The aetiology of sarcoidosis is not known. It is thought to be a consequence of a cell-mediated immune response, but despite many efforts no responsible antigen has so far been identified. The disease is relatively common in northern Europe but very rare in the Far East. Generally females are more likely to be affected than males.

Pathology

In many cases sarcoidosis is discovered accidentally in an asymptomatic individual during a routine chest x-ray which shows characteristic bilateral hilar lymphadenopathy. However, around 30% of the patients present with respiratory symptoms as seen in this case. The respiratory symptoms usually result from obstruction of major airways by the enlarged mediastinal lymph nodes or direct involvement of the lung parenchyma. The disease characteristically involves multiple organs and tissues. Lymph nodes and liver are often involved. Other commonly involved organs include skin, eyes, spleen and salivary glands. The fever and raised ESR is a consequence of immunological activation and the release of acute phase reactants into the circulation. Histologically, numerous non-caseating granulomas formed by epithelioid histiocytes and occasional Langerhans giant cells are seen in the involved organs. As similar granulomatous inflammation can develop in a number of conditions including tuberculosis*, fungal infections and berylliosis, the diagnosis of sarcoidosis can only be established by exclusion. In this case the absence of caseation necrosis, the absence of acid-fast bacilli in biopsy specimens and negative microbiological cultures, and the lack of history of exposure to beryllium helped to establish the diagnosis of sarcoidosis. Furthermore, the patient did not show tuberculin reactivity and responded to Kveim test. The Kveim test is performed by intradermal injection of an antigen extract obtained from human sarcoid tissues. If the test is positive, the skin at the injection area shows sarcoid granulomas at the end of 4 weeks. It is considered to be a reliable way of distinguishing sarcoidosis from other granulomatous inflammatory disorders. Sarcoidosis has a chronic but benign clinical course. Around 75% of all patients will recover spontaneously or after administration of short-term steroid therapy. The remainder may develop permanent respiratory or visual impairment as a result of chronic fibrosis. Progressive pulmonary disease may result in respiratory failure and death in a small number of patients.

Management

Many cases do not require treatment. If symptoms are severe, oral corticosteroid treatment can be administered with good results.

SARCOMA: A malignant tumour arising from tissues which develop from the fetal mesenchyme. Specific types, named according to the major line of differentiation, include leiomyosarcoma (smooth muscle), rhabdomyosarcoma (striated muscle), osteosarcoma (bone), liposarcoma (fat) and fibrosarcoma (fibrous tissue).

SCABIES: Infestation with the mite *Sarcoptes scabiei*. Person-to-person transmission is facilitated by close proximity and family outbreaks are common. The mite burrows into the skin, particularly between the fingers or toes or in the axilla, wrists or ankles, and lays its eggs. The eggs hatch and adults mature within 10–14 days and, after fertilizing the females, the males die off. The gravid females lay further eggs and the cycle is repeated. Within the skin there is a perivascular lymphocytic infiltrate with the presence of eosinophils and IgE may be detected in the blood vessel walls. After about 3–6 weeks, sensitization to the mite faeces or saliva occurs and the patient complains of itching, particularly at night. This may be severe enough to lead to excoriation, which may become secondarily infected. Macroscopically, the lesions are papulovesicular, which may become crusted. Severe scabies can present in institutionalized or immunocompromised patients, e.g. AIDS patients, in which there are widespread hyperkeratotic crusted nodules, intraepidermal pustules and the presence of tens of thousands of mites on and in the skin. This severe variety is called Norwegian scabies. It is highly contagious and hospital outbreaks have been seen. Laboratory diagnosis is by microscopy of skin scrapings. Treatment is with topical permethrin or for Norwegian scabies, ivermectin.

SCALDED SKIN SYNDROME: Infection by some strains of *Staphylococcus aureus* which secrete exfoliative toxins. These are serine proteases and act on the stratum granulosum layer of the skin. The stratum granulosum is disrupted by splitting of the desmosomes between the cells, leading to the formation of intraepidermal blisters. The superficial layers of the skin slough off if touched (Nikolsky sign). The exfoliating toxins are also superantigens and may lead to pathology by stimulating the massive release of cytokines, causing fluid to leak into the stratum granulosum. The patient presents with the formation of bullae, an erythematous rash and a generalized exfoliation exacerbated by touching the skin. Complications can include hypovolaemia. Laboratory diagnosis depends upon isolation of *Staph. aureus* and demonstration of toxin production. Treatment is with antistaphylococcal antibiotics. The denuded areas normally heal within a week.

S

SCARLET FEVER: A skin rash associated with a *Streptococcus pyogenes* sore throat and caused by erythrogenic toxins secreted by the streptococcus. It is currently uncommon in the UK. The patient presents with fever and a fine punctate rash that spreads over the whole body and is either bright or dusky red in colour. Characteristically, the rash is absent around the mouth and the tongue takes on the typical 'strawberry' appearance – red with elevated papillae. Eventually exfoliation of the skin occurs. There is a peripheral neutrophilia and laboratory diagnosis depends upon serology or isolation of a toxin-producing strain of *Strep. pyogenes*. Management is with penicillin.

SCHISTOSOMIASIS: Infection with one of the schistosome blood flukes.

Aetiology and risk factors

Schistosomiasis is caused by *Schistosoma haematobium*, *Schistosoma mansoni* and *Schistosoma japonicum* and is acquired by contact with water contaminated by the cercarial stage of the parasite. Eggs are passed in the faeces and if discharged into fresh water, hatch and infect snails, undergoing a developmental stage before being released into the water again as the infective stage for the final host. *Schist. mansoni* has a global distribution, being endemic in the Far and Middle East, Africa and South America; *Schist. japonicum* is found in the Far East and *Schist. haematobium* in Africa.

Pathology

The cercariae penetrate the skin, mucous membranes or conjunctiva of the host, developing into schistosomula. Once in the host, these migrate to the lungs and then to the liver, where the flukes mature and mate, migrating once more as a copulating pair of adults to their final destination, the venules of the large intestine (*Schist. mansoni*, *Schist. japonicum*) or bladder and ureters (*Schist. haematobium*). Disease is caused principally by the host reaction to the presence of the ova in the tissues. An adult female can lay up to 3000 ova a day and the adults live about 7 years. The host response to the presence of the highly antigenic ova in the tissues of the hepatoportal system or bladder is the development of T-cell-mediated granuloma and fibrosis, leading to the signs and symptoms of disease. There is some evidence for the slow development of protective immunity, as judged by diminishing faecal egg counts in repeatedly infected patients.

- The patient may complain of a dermatitis associated with penetration of the cercaria through the skin (swimmers' itch).
- Symptoms may also develop as the schistosomes migrate through the lungs, giving rise to pulmonary eosinophilia. Similarly, an allergic reaction can occur during the maturation stage of the adult with fever, cough, rash, myalgia and a peripheral eosinophilia.
- The early symptoms of infection in the bladder are haematuria accompanied by a sterile pyuria. Eventually an obstructive uropathy develops due to the fibrosis. A complication of chronic infection is squamous carcinoma of the bladder.
- Infection of the intestine and liver produces presinusoidal periportal fibrosis, portal hypertension, hepatosplenomegaly and oesophageal varices, with eventual haematemesis.

Ova may sometimes be distributed to other organs, e.g. lung, spinal cord, leading to pulmonary fibrosis and hypertension or myelitis and paraplegia, respectively. The laboratory diagnosis is by histology, demonstration of the ova in the faeces or urine and serology.

Management

Treatment is with praziquantel. An experimental vaccine has proved effective in farm animals.

SCHWANNOMA: A benign neural tumour arising from Schwann cells of the peripheral nerves.

Neurofibromatosis

SCLERODERMA: Often used synonymously with progressive systemic sclerosis, but strictly referring only to the skin changes – thickening, hardening, and depigmentation.

Systemic sclerosis

SCURVY: Deficiency of vitamin C causes scurvy, which is characterized by perifollicular haemorrhages, bleeding gums, poor wound healing, failure of hair follicle eruption and anaemia.

SEMINOMA: A malignant germ cell tumour of the testis.

Aetiology and risk factors

Seminomas account for 50% of germ cell tumours of the testis. They are most commonly seen in the third and fourth decades. The cause is not known. However, abnormalities of germ cell development are thought to be important, as cryptorchism and syndromes resulting in testicular dysgenesis, such as Klinefelter* or testicular feminization, are critical risk factors.

Pathology

The commonest clinical presentation is painless swelling of the testis. Occasionally the first

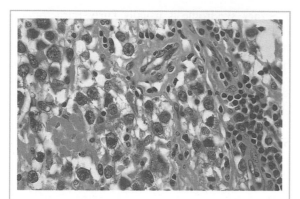

Fig. S2 Histological appearances of seminoma, large tumour cells with clear cytoplasm and a lymphocytic infiltrate in the stroma.

symptoms may relate to secondary spread of the tumour. Macroscopically, the testis contains a solid, relatively well circumscribed tumour nodule. Histologically, the nodule is composed of large polyhedral seminoma cells with clear cytoplasm and large central nuclei. These are arranged in nests separated by a fibrovascular stroma containing numerous lymphocytes (Fig. S2). Serum β-hCG is raised in about one-third of patients, but AFP is normal unless there is a teratomatous component. Seminomas tend to remain localized to the testis for long periods and when they spread this tends to be via the lymphatics. They are usually very sensitive to chemotherapy and radiotherapy and most patients can be cured.

Management
Treatment consists of surgery and radiotherapy.

 Ovarian cyst; Teratoma

SEPTIC ARTHRITIS: Pyogenic infection of the joints which can be caused by many different bacteria but principally *Staphylococcus aureus*. Other important pathogens are *Streptococcus pneumoniae* and *Neisseria gonorrhoeae*. The organism spreads to the joint by the bloodstream, following trauma or from a contiguous area of osteomyelitis. Bacteria that gain entry to the joint space induce an acute inflammation of the synovium, with proliferation of the synovial lining cells and an influx of neutrophils. Pro-inflammatory cytokines are induced, enhancing the inflammatory response and the accumulation of pus in the joint space. The presence of both bacterial and neutrophil proteases leads to destruction of the cartilage. The knee and hip joint are the two most commonly affected joints. The patient presents with acute onset of pain, swelling and erythema of the affected joint

with loss or diminished function. Patients also show a systemic response with elevated acute phase proteins and a peripheral neutrophilia. Laboratory diagnosis is by isolation of the organism from the joint space or blood and management is by joint drainage and appropriate antibiotics.

SEPTIC SHOCK: See Meningococcal meningitis.

SERONEGATIVE ARTHRITIDES: A heterogeneous group of arthritides in which autoantibodies, including rheumatoid factor, are absent (Table S1).

Table S1 Seronegative arthritis

Condition	Associated with
Reiter disease, Crohn disease	Ankylosing spondylitis, ulcerative colitis, psoriasis, Behçet disease

 Behçet disease; Psoriasis; Reiter disease; Ulcerative colitis

SERUM SICKNESS: An acute systemic self-limiting (7–10 days) immune-complex-mediated reaction to an extrinsic antigen; also known as serum disease since it was common following the injection of heterologous antiserum used to provide immediate passive immunity against toxins (e.g. tetanus) or for immunosuppression before transplants (antilymphocyte globulin). A mild form can also occur following treatment with drugs such as penicillins or cephalosporins, which can modify plasma proteins. It is a type III hypersensitivity reaction resulting in fever, dermatitis, lymphadenopathy and joint symptoms. For treatment, aspirin and antihistamines are usually effective but short-course, high-dose corticosteroids may be required for more severe reactions.

SEVERE COMBINED IMMUNODEFICIENCY DISEASE (SCID): An inherited immunodeficiency disease affecting both T-cell- and antibody (B-cell)-mediated immunity.

Affected children have prolonged diarrhoea due to rotavirus or bacterial infection of the gastrointestinal tract, and usually die of overwhelming infections within the first 2 years of life. Infants also show retarded growth. The thymus contains stromal cells but few lymphocytes. SCID is commoner in males than females. There are two main causes of the disease:
• In >50% of the cases, the disease is caused by a defective gene on the X chromosome. This is

the chain of the IL-2 receptor which is also used by other cytokine receptors, e.g. IL-4, 7, 11 and 15. Lymphoid stem cells fail to proliferate and differentiate since they cannot receive all the necessary signals.

- In at least 25% of the cases the disease is due to defects in the recessive genes coding for the DNA salvage pathway enzymes adenosine deaminase (ADA) or purine nucleoside phosphorylase (PNP). These enzymes are important in the degradation of purines adenosine and guanosine and deficiency results in accumulation of dATP and dGTP, respectively, which are toxic for lymphoid stem cells, and through inhibition of the enzyme ribonucleotide reductase, inhibit DNA synthesis and therefore cell proliferation.

This disease mainly affects T-cells but since antibody production is mainly dependent on T-cell help, antibodies are also deficient. The treatment of choice is a bone marrow transplant. ADA deficiency has been successfully treated using gene therapy.

 Adenosine deaminase deficiency; Immunodeficiency

SÉZARY SYNDROME: A chronic T-cell lymphoma involving blood and skin. The skin involvement frequently manifests as an itchy erythroderma, sometimes with exfoliation. In the blood, Sézary cells are seen. These lymphocytes have cleaved nuclei (Fig. S3) and show the immunophenotype of T-cells (CD2, 3, 5 and 7 positive), usually T-helper cells (CD4). Lymph nodes may be involved, as in other types of T-cell lymphoma. This disorder forms a spectrum with mycosis fungoides* in which cutaneous plaques and tumours of T-cells are usually present.

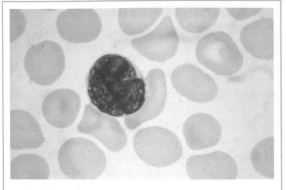

Fig. S3 Sézary cell showing cleaved cerebriform nucleus, resembling the brain as seen on a CT scan.

Sézary syndrome is usually fairly refractory to chemotherapy. The cutaneous manifestations may respond to ultraviolet light, particularly if the lymphocytes have been sensitized by psoralen exposure (PUVA). UVA may also be used to irradiate the blood directly: extracorporeal photochemotherapy.

SHINGLES: Reactivation of latent varicella-zoster virus.

Chickenpox

SHOCK: This refers to a state of circulatory collapse. The patient with 'shock' tends to be severely ill and the condition needs intensive treatment to correct the cause of the circulatory failure and its complications due to hypoperfusion. In cardiogenic shock, there is poor perfusion due to cardiac failure. Hypovolaemic shock results from a drop in blood volume as may occur following trauma and severe loss of blood. Septic shock results from overwhelming infection, usually due to Gram-negative bacteraemia. Finally, anaphylactic shock results from an acute hypersensitivity reaction with resultant vasodilatation and vascular permeability.

SICKLE CELL DISEASE: A common haemoglobinopathy associated with precipitation of abnormal haemoglobin S within red cells, which causes the cells to change to a sickle shape and obstruct small blood vessels.

Case

An 18-year-old Jamaican man was visiting his relatives in the UK with his bride-to-be. His brother took him to a local night club where he overindulged in alcohol. Approximately an hour after returning home he developed abdominal and back pains. An ambulance was called and he was brought to the hospital A&E department at 5 a.m. There was no significant medical or family history and he was taking no medication. On examination he was found to be sweating and anxious. In his abdomen a generalized tenderness with guarding was found. Bowel sounds were normal. The duty surgical registrar reviewed him at 6 a.m. and ordered some investigations and preparations were made for an exploratory laparotomy.

The blood count revealed:

WBC 8.6×10^9/l
RBC 2.81×10^{12}/l; Hb 8.5 g/dl; Hct (ratio) 0.253

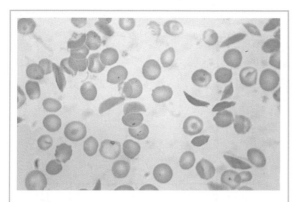

Fig. S4 Blood film in sickle cell disease showing sickle cells, target cells and Howell–Jolly bodies.

MCV 89.9 fl; MCH 30.4 pg
MCHC 33.7 g/dl; RDW 15.4 %
Plt 417 × 10⁹/l.

The white cell differential count was normal but examination of the blood film showed sickle cells, target cells, and Howell–Jolly bodies (Fig. S4). A sickle solubility screening test was positive.

He was given an injection of pethidine for his abdominal pain and a dextrose–saline infusion was set up. Further investigations included haemoglobinopathy screening by HPLC, which showed haemoglobin S predominant, with HbA_2 3.2%, HbF 6.5%. The reticulocyte count was 6.2% (normal <2%).

A diagnosis of sickle pain crisis in homozygous sickle cell anaemia was made and he was treated with intravenous fluids and opiate analgesia. The proposed laparotomy was cancelled and his pains became more generalized but settled over the next week. Haemoglobinopathy screening of his fiancée was normal.

Aetiology and risk factors

The sickle cell diseases consist of homozygous sickle cell anaemia, haemoglobin SC disease and haemoglobin S thalassaemia. Haemoglobin S is inherited from one parent and an interacting haemoglobin, in this case also haemoglobin S, from the other parent.

Inheritance of a single gene for haemoglobin S (heterozygosity), with the gene for normal haemoglobin A on the other chromosome results in sickle cell trait, in which 30–40% of the circulating haemoglobin will usually be haemoglobin S. This protects against falciparum malaria* as parasitized red cells sickle and are rapidly removed from the circulation by the reticuloendothelial system. The gene for sickle haemoglobin, and hence sickle cell

disease, is most common in areas of the world where falciparum malaria is endemic, particularly central and western sub-Saharan Africa. Persons with sickle trait are asymptomatic and have normal blood counts unless they are exposed to low oxygen tensions. Such a situation may arise in unpressurized aircraft or during anaesthesia. Black patients having an anaesthetic should be tested for sickle haemoglobin preoperatively so appropriate precautions can be taken to avoid hypoxia or dehydration during anaesthetic. If the partner of a patient with sickle trait also has sickle trait or an equivalent interacting haemoglobinopathy such as HbC trait or thalassaemia trait, then one in four of the couple's offspring will have homozygous sickle cell disease. For this reason haemoglobinopathy screening of antenatal patients is usual in areas with a high proportion of black mothers. If a pregnant patient has sickle trait then her partner should be tested. If he is a carrier then placental villus sampling can be performed to establish if the fetus will suffer from sickle cell disease. If so, therapeutic termination of pregnancy can be offered.

Pathology

The clinical manifestations of sickle cell disease are due to vascular occlusion by logjams of sickled red blood cells. This process may be triggered by dehydration (increasing the haematocrit and blood viscosity, leading to stagnant flow), infection, or hypoxia. Often no precipitating cause is found. Obstruction of blood vessels by sickled red cells leads to local tissue hypoxia and acidosis. This causes more sickling of red cells and more vascular obstruction so that a vicious cycle is set up, resulting in local tissue infarction*.

The most common site for tissue infarction is red bone marrow. This results in the clinical picture of deep-seated bone pain. This may be difficult to localize and may present as an acute abdomen, chest pain or pain in the limbs. Sickling in lung tissue may result in hypoxaemia, particularly when associated with infection.

Infarction of brain, causing stroke, although rare, is one of the most lethal manifestations of sickle cell disease. Infarction of kidneys results in haematuria and papillary necrosis with renal colic as the dead tubular tissue is passed down the ureter. Repeated minor infarction of the kidney damages the renal tubular urine concentrating apparatus so that patients with sickle cell disease become dehydrated easily, increasing the risk of sickle crisis. In women, infarction of the placenta results in increased risk of miscarriage, premature delivery and small-for-date babies. In males, sickling in the corpora cavernosa

S

of the penis may result in priapism (sustained painful erection) and eventual impotence.

The molecular abnormality of sickle haemoglobin
Haemoglobin is made up of an iron-containing portion, haem, and a protein portion, globin. The globin part of the molecule consists of two pairs of polypeptide chains. The three major haemoglobins of man, fetal haemoglobin (HbF), adult haemoglobin (HbA) and the second adult haemoglobin HbA$_2$ all contain a pair of α chains. They differ in the nature of their other pair of polypeptide chains. HbF contains a pair of γ chains, HbA a pair of β chains, and HbA$_2$ δ chains. At birth most of the circulating haemoglobin is HbF and during the first year of life this changes to haemoglobin A.

Congenital abnormalities of haem are termed the porphyrias*. Congenital abnormalities of haemoglobin are called haemoglobinopathies. There are dozens of haemoglobinopathies but sickle haemoglobin is the most important. In sickle haemoglobin there is a single amino acid substitution (valine for glutamic acid) in the β chain of globin. This structural abnormality results in crystallization of the haemoglobin S molecule, which forms long, thin, needle-like structures termed tactoids. These tactoids distort the red cell membrane, resulting in the characteristic sickle shape and make the red cell rigid so that it will not pass easily through small blood vessels, and logjams tend to form. Children with sickle cell disease are normal at birth, as most of their circulating haemoglobin is HbF, which does not contain the abnormal β (sickle) chains. However, very small amounts of sickle haemoglobin present in cord blood at delivery may be detected by sensitive techniques such as HPLC, prompting follow up in the paediatric clinic.

The anaemia of sickle cell disease is well tolerated because haemoglobin S has a relatively low oxygen affinity compared to HbA (Fig. S5). This means that oxygen is easily given up to cells that require it and transfusion for correction of anaemia is rarely required. Repeated severe pain crises or life-threatening sickling events can be treated by exchange transfusion using non-sickling (haemoglobin A containing) red cells. An increased concentration of haemoglobin F in the red cells protects against sickling. Some patients have a hereditary persistence of haemoglobin F and this makes their sickle cell disease milder. The cytotoxic agent hydroxyurea causes increased amounts of haemoglobin F to be manufactured and is being used therapeutically for this purpose.

The spleen in sickle cell disease In childhood the spleen may be enlarged. Occasionally,

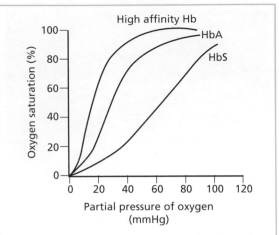

Fig. S5 Oxygen dissociation curves of sickle and adult haemoglobin. HbS has a relatively low affinity.

sequestration crises may occur when the spleen and liver swell rapidly and very severe anaemia with a higher reticulocyte count than usual are found. Mothers may be taught to look out for this problem, as transfusion may be lifesaving.

Repeated minor episodes of infarction eventually results in atrophy of the spleen and hyposplenism with increased risk of septicaemia with capsulate organisms such as *Pneumococcus* or *Haemophilus*.

Management

Factors known to precipitate sickle crisis such as dehydration should be avoided. The treatment of pain crisis involves bed rest, vigorous hydration, treatment of any precipitating infection, effective pain relief and correction of hypoxaemia. Prophylactic penicillin tablets with pneumococcal and haemophilus immunization are required to counter infective risk resulting from hyposplenism.

SIDEROBLASTIC ANAEMIA: A biochemical block in haem synthesis resulting in failure to incorporate iron into the haemoglobin molecule so that it accumulates within mitochondria. The iron-poisoned mitochondria come to lie in a ring around the nucleus of the normoblast. The diagnostic feature of the condition is therefore the ring sideroblast (Fig. S6). In the peripheral blood, iron granules may be found in the red cells, where they are known as Pappenheimer bodies.

Sideroblastic anaemia may be congenital (rare) or acquired. Primary acquired sideroblastic anaemia is one of the myelodysplastic disorders. Secondary sideroblastic anaemia may be seen in lead poisoning, malignant disease, collagen diseases and as a side-effect of drugs such as antituberculous treat-

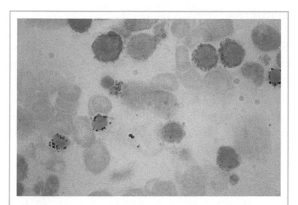

Fig. S6 Ring sideroblasts in a bone marrow aspirate stained by the Perls stain for iron. Iron granules lie around the nucleus of the normoblast, like satellites around the earth.

ment. Management depends on removing the cause, if possible. Some cases of primary acquired sideroblastic anaemia respond to high doses of the vitamin pyridoxine, which acts as a co-enzyme in the incorporation of iron into haemoglobin.

SILICOSIS: A chronic occupational lung disease caused by inhalation of silica.

Silicosis develops after exposure to silica dust for many years, usually in mine workers. World-wide it is the commonest type of pneumoconiosis. Pathologically it is characterized by development of fibrous nodules in the lung parenchyma. Eventually progressive massive fibrosis can develop, leading to severe respiratory impairment.

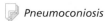 *Pneumoconiosis*

SINUSITIS: Infection of the paranasal sinuses (maxillary, frontal, ethmoid and sphenoid) usually following a viral upper respiratory tract infection. Hyperaemia of the mucosa may cause blockage of mucus drainage and proliferation of bacterial pathogens, particularly *Streptococcus pneumoniae*, *Haemophilus influenzae* or *Moraxella catarrhalis*. In cases of chronic sinusitis, anaerobic organisms are frequently present and in AIDS patients, *Pseudomonas* is a frequent pathogen. In chronic sinusitis the usual ciliated respiratory epithelium becomes stratified squamous epithelium. The patient presents with fever, a purulent nasal discharge and facial pain. The patient may also complain of frequent sore throats and a postnasal discharge. Complications include osteomyelitis, brain abscess and cavernous sinus thrombosis. Laboratory diagnosis is by isolation of the organism from an antral puncture although, as with otitis

media, the pathogens are so consistent that empirical antibiotics covering the recognized pathogens can be used.

SJÖGREN SYNDROME: An autoimmune chronic inflammatory condition involving the salivary and lacrimal glands. Patients characteristically have a dry mouth (xerostomia) and/or eyes (keratoconjunctivitis sicca), classically called sicca complex or syndrome. This can occur in isolation (primary Sjögren syndrome) or together with non-organ-specific autoimmune diseases, notably rheumatoid arthritis or other connective tissue diseases (secondary Sjögren syndrome).

Aetiology and risk factors

The aetiology of Sjögren syndrome (SS) is unknown but viral particles have been seen in biopsies and EBV may be associated with the disease. It occurs mainly in middle-aged women (F:M = 9:1) but the disease can occur in children. Commonly, dryness is also seen in the vagina, nose, trachea, bronchus and skin. There is an increased risk of developing lymphomas, which are normally outside the exocrine glands of the gastrointestinal, respiratory and genital tracts. An increased frequency of HLA-DR3 and HLA-B8 is associated with primary SS and secondary SS with SLE.

Pathology

The main immunological findings are:
- hypergammaglobulinaemia
- antibodies to the nuclear antigens Ro and La
- cryoglobulins (more rarely)

The exocrine glands become infiltrated with lymphocytes and Fig. S7 shows the histological picture of the labial salivary gland seen in about 75% of SS patients. Note the infiltrating T-cells (CD4+) between the salivary ducts as shown with immunohistochemical staining.

S

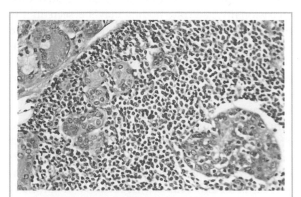

Fig. S7 Histological picture of a labial salivary gland.

Management

For the sicca syndrome the treatment is symptomatic, using artificial tears and stimulating salivation.

SPARGINOSIS: Infection with the tapeworm *Spirometra* (see Tapeworm infections). It is acquired by drinking water contaminated with infected copepods (zooplankton) or eating uncooked frogs or snails and is common in the Far East. If the larval stage is eaten by humans, it penetrates the intestine, migrates through the peritoneal cavity and localizes in subcutaneous tissue, the eye, or the central nervous system. A granulomatous reaction occurs and the patient may present with erythema and pruritus at a nodule that disappears only to reappear at another location. If in the central nervous system, epilepsy may occur. Laboratory diagnosis is by histology and treatment is surgical.

SPINA BIFIDA: See meningocele.

SPONGIFORM ENCAPHALOPATHY: A disease of the brain characterized by progressive dementia and spongiform change in neurons, without signs of inflammation. The human disease is known as Creutzfeldt–Jakob disease*, but similar diseases occur in animals.

SPOROTRICHOSIS: An infection with the dimorphic fungus *Sporothrix schenckii*, which is found in soil and on vegetation (e.g. flowers, trees), an occupational hazard of gardeners. The fungus is introduced following abrasions and produces a subcutaneous infection. The disease is endemic in North and South America and Africa. The yeast form of the fungus proliferates in the tissues and histologically there is granuloma formation and an acute inflammatory infiltrate with neutrophils. Occasionally asteroid bodies may be seen in the tissue, where the yeast is surrounded by a stellate arrangement of eosinophilic PAS-positive material. The patient may present with a painless subcutaneous nodule, which may ulcerate. The infection can remain localized or spread along the lymphatics to produce a line of ulcerating nodules on the skin. Rarely, *Sporothrix* may produce systemic disease involving the central nervous system, joint or lungs. The pulmonary form presents with a low-grade fever, weight loss and pulmonary cavities, suggestive of tuberculosis. Laboratory diagnosis is by isolation of the fungus and treatment is with potassium iodide, itraconazole or amphotericin for systemic disease.

SPRUE: See Tropical sprue.

SQUAMOUS CELL CARCINOMA: The most common tumour arising from squamous epithelium in sun-exposed skin.

Aetiology and risk factors

Apart from sunlight, other risk factors include arsenic poisoning, industrial chemicals such as tar and radiation. In the mouth, tobacco and betel nut chewing are implicated.

Pathology

The tumours may be *in situ* or invasive. *In situ* carcinomas appear as red plaques whereas invasive cancers tend to be nodular and/or ulcerated. In the mouth, they may appear as white plaques (leucoplakia). The differentiation of the tumours is variable ranging from very well differentiated lesions that may be difficult to separate from benign lesions to overtly cancerous. Without complete excision, the tumour tends to recur locally. It is very unusual for the tumour to metastasize.

Management

The management of squamous cell carcinomas is surgical. Most can be resected as they tend to present early while still small.

Basal cell carcinoma; Malignant melanoma

STEM CELL TRANSPLANTATION: The restoration of haemopoiesis and immunological function to a patient with a hypoplastic bone marrow by intravenous transfusion of haemopoietic stem cells.

Case

A 42-year-old woman was diagnosed with Philadelphia-positive chronic myeloid leukaemia*. Whilst in chronic phase her blood count and splenomegaly were brought under control by treatment with hydroxyurea tablets. Tissue typing of herself and her siblings was performed (Fig. S8). She had two grown-up twins and did not desire further children. An HLA matched T-cell-depleted bone marrow transplant was performed 6 months after diagnosis using total-body irradiation and high dose cyclophosphamide conditioning. Both patient and donor were CMV antibody positive. Neutrophil engraftment was apparent on day 16 post-transplant and she had no evidence of graft-versus-host disease*. One month after discharge from hospital, she required readmission for treatment with ganciclovir for persistent CMV positivity, as measured by PCR on blood. No clinical evidence of CMV infection was present at any time.

Two years after her transplant, she relapsed back into chronic phase chronic myeloid leukaemia. She

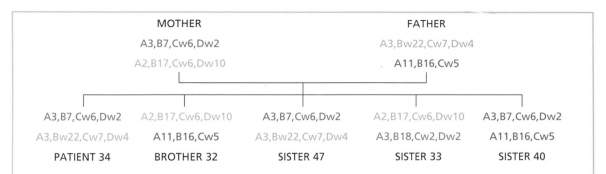

Fig. S8 Inheritance of HLA antigens. Each child receives one of two alternative packages of HLA antigens from its parents. In this family's case the 47-year-old sister of the patient requiring an allogeneic stem cell graft is an HLA match. His 33-year-old sister has inherited an HLA haplotype from a different father.

received an infusion of her brother's peripheral blood lymphocytes, following which she developed mild skin graft-versus-host disease, controlled by topical steroid creams. Her peripheral blood counts gradually normalized and regular monitoring of her bone marrow for *BCR-ABL* transcripts and Philadelphia chromosome was restarted, with a view to further infusions of her brother's peripheral blood lymphocytes if there was further evidence of relapse.

Types of stem cell transplant

Autologous stem cells These are the patient's own. Autologous transplantation is commonly used to allow the patient to have otherwise lethal doses of chemotherapy or radiotherapy that would result in permanent bone marrow aplasia (see Aplastic anaemia). Stem cells may be frozen before the procedure, high-dose chemotherapy given to cure the malignancy under treatment, then the stem cells thawed and transfused to repopulate the bone marrow. Because the stem cells are the patient's own, there are no problems of mismatch in tissue type such as graft-versus-host disease or graft rejection. Care needs to be taken that the harvested stem cells are not contaminated by the malignant cells of the disease under treatment.

Allogeneic stem cells These are obtained from a human leucocyte antigen (HLA) matched stem cell donor. Commonly this may be a brother or sister, but because of the way in which the HLA antigens are inherited there is only a one in four chance of any individual sibling being a match (Fig. S8).

One or even two HLA antigen mismatch transplants can be performed with effective post-transplant immunosuppression when the clinical circumstances demand it, albeit with increased risk of graft-versus-host disease* (GVHD).

With the trend to smaller families, many patients requiring a stem cell transplant do not have a suitable HLA-matched sibling donor. To accommodate these patients national and international computerized panels of volunteer unrelated donors (VUD) have been set up. These donors have had their blood tested to determine tissue type and are available to donate stem cells for suitable recipients. Even with the most modern tissue typing, there is increased risk of GVHD and graft rejection from a matched VUD donor compared to a matched sibling donor.

Syngeneic stem cells These are obtained from an identical twin. As the HLA type will be identical, there will be no problems of GVHD or graft rejection.

Source of stem cells

Stem cells may be obtained from the donor's bone marrow or peripheral blood. Bone marrow for transplantation is obtained under a general anaesthetic by repeated aspiration from the iliac crests and sometimes the sternum. For adult transplantation, approximately a litre of bone marrow is required. Much of the aspirated bone marrow is blood, so a red cell transfusion is usually given during or after the procedure, usually of the donor's own autologous blood collected in the weeks prior to the procedure. For allografting (see below) a nucleated cell dose of approximately 2×10^8 nucleated cells per kilogram of recipient is required. Ideally the bone marrow is then transfused to the recipient without further manipulation, but sometimes graft processing may be required to remove T-cells to prevent graft-versus-host disease* or to remove red cells/plasma if the donor and recipient are of different blood groups.

Stem cells are increasingly being obtained from the donor's peripheral blood, avoiding the requirement for a general anaesthetic. Under normal conditions, less than 1% of the peripheral blood mononuclear cells are stem cells. Under certain

S

Table S2 Uses of stem cell transplantation

Leukaemias
  Acute myeloid leukaemia*
  Acute lymphoblastic leukaemia*
  Chronic myeloid leukaemia*
  Chronic lymphocytic leukaemia* (rare in those
    young enough to benefit from transplant)
  Myelodysplastic syndromes*
Congenital anaemias (otherwise require life-long
    transfusion, die of iron overload)
  Thalassaemia* major
  Sickle cell disease*
  Fanconi anaemia*
Severe aplastic anaemia*
Congenital enzyme deficiencies and storage diseases
Congenital immune deficiency

conditions this proportion can be increased, making it possible to harvest sufficient stem cells for transplantation from the peripheral blood using a cell separator. Peripheral blood stem cells are increased in the blood recovery phase after cytotoxic treatment. However, cytotoxic drugs cannot be given to healthy donors, so an alternative is to give an injection of the cytokine granulocyte colony-stimulating factor to stimulate bone marrow production of stem cells.

Indications for stem cell transplantation

As there is a 5–10% mortality rate associated with stem cell transplantation, it is only performed when the underlying disorder is not amenable to cure using less drastic therapy. For example, more than 60% of cases of childhood leukaemia can be cured by conventional chemotherapy; bone marrow transplantation would only be performed if the disease relapsed, making cure by conventional chemotherapy unlikely. It is necessary to carefully weigh up the potential risks and benefits of the procedure in each individual case. Table S2 shows the diseases potentially curable by marrow transplantation.

Conditioning regimens

In order to 'make space' in the recipient's bone marrow for the donor stem cells to engraft and immunosuppress the recipient so that the donor cells will not be rejected, a regimen of total-body irradiation (TBI) and/or powerful chemotherapy is administered to the recipient. Following this, the donor stem cells are administered by intravenous infusion. The conditioning regimen also helps to eradicate residual cells of disease if the transplant is being performed for haematological malignancy. Conditioning regimens including total-body irradiation will usually result in permanent infertility in the recipient. In most cases the delay between trans-

fusing stem cells and blood count recovery is of the order of 2–3 weeks. During this period there is a severe pancytopenia with dependence on support and antibiotic and antifungal treatment for intercurrent infection.

STEVENS–JOHNSON SYNDROME: Inflammation of mucosal surfaces caused by some drugs and some infections.

 Erythema multiforme

STILL DISEASE: A non-specific systemic seronegative chronic arthritis in children with an early onset (usually before 5 years of age) and without a gender bias; it represents about 15% of cases of children with juvenile chronic arthritis (see Juvenile chronic arthritis for classification of childhood chronic arthritides). There is also an adult form of the disease.

STRONGYLOIDIASIS: Infection with the intestinal nematode *Strongyloides stercoralis* acquired by contact with contaminated soil containing the larval stage, which penetrates the skin. The nematode then migrates to the lungs via the bloodstream, moves up the bronchi and trachea and is eventually swallowed, maturing in the small intestine (Fig. S9). The females produce ova that are passed in the faeces and develop into infective larvae in the soil. Autoinoculation can also occur when the larval stage develops on soiled skin of the perianal region or even within the intestine; this is commonest in immunocompromised individuals. The presence of the worm in the intestine leads to inflammation and blunting of the villi, malabsorption and a protein-losing enteropathy. In severe cases there may be a haemorrhagic colitis. The nematode may migrate to other organs, e.g. lungs, giving rise to a haemorrhagic pneumonitis.

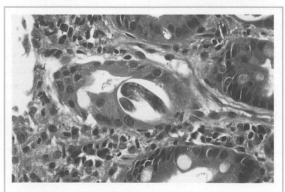

Fig. S9 Histological section of nematode in the intestine.

Clinically the patient may present with minimal gastrointestinal symptoms or those of malabsorption. There is a peripheral eosinophilia. Laboratory diagnosis is by detection of the ova/larvae in the faeces and serology, and treatment is with thiabendazole.

STURGE–WEBER SYNDROME: A rare congenital disorder characterized by venous angiomatous masses in the leptomeninges, port wine naevi on the face, and mental retardation.

SUBACUTE SCLEROSING PANENCEPHALO-MYELITIS (SSPE): A neurological complication occurring in children following infection with the measles virus. There is a deficient cell-mediated immune response allowing continuous viral replication. Histologically, there is encephalitis with perivascular cuffing, demyelination and neuronal cell death. The patient presents with dementia, seizures or pyramidal signs.

SUDDEN INFANT DEATH SYNDROME (SIDS): Sudden death of an infant under the age of 1 year, which remains unexplained after a thorough case examination including an autopsy.

Case

The mother of a 5-month-old baby boy had noticed that the baby was not breathing when she got up to check him at 5 a.m. She had immediately called the ambulance service. When the paramedics arrived, no heart sounds were present and the baby was not breathing. No response was obtained despite attempts to resuscitate. The baby was pronounced dead. The baby was born weighing 2300 g after 38 weeks of normal gestation (small for gestational age). No perinatal or postnatal problems were reported and the development since had been normal. He had been sneezing the day before he died but was otherwise healthy. He had been sleeping in a prone position after feeding at midnight that night. The mother was a 19-year-old healthy, unemployed, single woman. She had been smoking 30 cigarettes/day for the last 4 years, including during the pregnancy and postpartum period. She had had one abortion but no other live births.

> At the postmortem the physical development of the baby was at the lower end of expected normal for the age. No macroscopic external or internal abnormalities were seen. Histologically, the only abnormality observed was mild gliosis in the brain stem. No significant abnormalities were present to explain the cause of death.

An examination of the death scene and an interview performed with the mother revealed no suspicious circumstances.

A postmortem examination was performed.

Aetiology and risk factors

By definition, the aetiology of sudden infant death syndrome is not known. It has been suggested that inborn errors of metabolism play a role in some cases. The maternal risk factors for SIDS are teenage pregnancy, low socioeconomic status, short interval following a previous pregnancy, smoking and drug abuse. Other risk factors include premature or low birth weight delivery, male sex, twin pregnancy, and history of SIDS in previous child.

Pathology

The diagnosis of SIDS is made by exclusion of all other possible causes. Therefore a thorough examination of the death scene and exclusion of unnatural causes of death are required. A full autopsy usually discloses a number of minor non-specific findings. There may be evidence of inflammation in the upper respiratory tract or lungs, suggesting a recent infection. In the brain stem increased number of glial cells can be seen. Various subtle abnormalities such as increase in thickness of pulmonary arteries, right ventricular hypertrophy, histological changes in the cardiac conduction system have been reported. However, these findings fall short of explaining the cause of death and are likely to be secondary events. It has been suggested that abnormal or immature temperature control may play a role in some cases. These observations indicate that SIDS is a heterogenous disorder. In recent years, public health measures directed at the risk factors mentioned above have had a dramatic effect on the incidence of SIDS, the number of victims having fallen by nearly 70% between 1988 and1992. It is thought that campaigns to promote supine instead of prone sleeping and changes in cigarette smoking habits have been critical in this fall of the incidence of SIDS.

SYMPATHETIC OPHTHALMIA: A progressive autoimmune-mediated inflammation in the second eye following trauma to the first; also known as sympathetic ophthalmitis, sympathetic uveitis.

Following penetrating injury to one eye (usually 1–2 months later), the 'sympathizing' eye develops minor symptoms of anterior uveitis which progresses to a granulomatous panuveitis. The retina remains uninvolved except for perivascular cuffing of retinal blood vessels with inflammatory cells. There may be accompanying vitiligo and/or poliosis. The sympathetic uveitis is prevented if the

S

injured eye is removed within 10–20 days of injury. The histological picture shows that the uvea contains T-lymphocytes (CD4+), macrophages, epithelioid cells and giant cells, characteristic of a giant cell granuloma. The autoimmune-induced granuloma formation (type IV hypersensitivity) is induced by the release of soluble lens antigen (S) following the initial trauma to one eye. This results in sensitization of CD4+ T-lymphocytes, probably due to the fact that tolerance has not been induced to these antigens in the thymus (see Autoimmunity). Vogt–Koyanagi–Harada syndrome shares clinical and immunological features, the autoimmune reaction being against retinal antigen, but does not involve direct trauma.

Treatment is with corticosteroids, locally applied or, in more severe cases, systemically. Cyclosporin has been promising in treating corticosteroid-resistant uveitis.

SYPHILIS: A chronic multisystem infection caused by the spirochaete *Treponema pallidum*.

Aetiology and risk factors
Syphilis is usually transmitted by sexual contact but can also be transmitted congenitally.

Pathology
The treponemes penetrate through the skin or mucous membranes and disseminate via the bloodstream to all organs. The disease presents in three stages:
- Primary syphilis presents with a painless ulcer (chancre) on the genitals. Histologically there is periarteritis and endarteritis obliterans (concentric proliferation of endothelial cells and fibroblasts) with enlarged regional lymph nodes showing follicular hyperplasia.
- Secondary syphilis occurs when there is a high treponemal antigen load in the tissues and presents with a macular skin rash covering the body, including the palms and soles, with widespread lymphadenopathy. Mucosal ulcers may also be present (snail track ulcers). Other organs may be affected such as the liver and kidneys, leading to hepatitis or glomerulonephritis.
- Tertiary syphilis has a variety of clinical presentations depending upon the organ system most affected. The characteristic histological lesion is the gumma, which shows a necrotic centre, periarteritis and endarteritis obliterans and an intense peripheral cellular infiltrate consisting mainly of mononuclear cells and giant cells. This may present on the skin as a chronic granulomatous punched-out ulcer; on the

mucosa causing destruction of the palate and nasal septum; in the bones producing an osteomyelitis; in the viscera, e.g. liver, producing a granulomatous hepatitis. Endarteritis obliterans can lead to aneurysm formation in the vascular system (e.g. aorta) and meningovascular neurosyphilis in the CNS with cerebellar signs (tabes dorsalis) or personality changes (general paresis).

Laboratory diagnosis is by microscopy, histology and serology and treatment is with penicillin.

SYSTEMIC LUPUS ERYTHEMATOSUS: A multisystem autoimmune disease mainly affecting young women.

Case
A 28-year-old woman presented to her GP with a mild fever, muscle and joint pains and swollen finger joints. She was given a course of ibuprofen. She returned a month later saying that she had only got mild relief from the drug. She now mentioned occasional bouts of fatigue and arthralgia lasting 2–3 days over the last year which had not been relieved by aspirin. A blood test was carried out and ESR but not CRP levels were higher than normal and she was mildly anaemic. Her haemoglobin and white blood cell count (WBC) were also low, even though her neutrophil count was slightly elevated.

ESR 40 mm/h; CRP 4.0 mg/l; haemoglobin 11.0 g/dl; WBC 3100/l

Her urine was normal and she had no increase in serum creatinine. Results of autoantibody tests were negative. She returned for her test results and was put on a low dose corticosteroid treatment. One month later she returned and a further blood test was carried out. This showed a high ANA (1:640) and anti ds-DNA (1:40) with a positive test for anticardiolipin and rheumatoid factor. On returning for her test results she was asked if she had had any spontaneous abortions or major thrombotic episodes, which she reported as negative. She now complained of a rash on her face (Fig. S10) and chest and no major improvement of her symptoms.

Further tests were done which showed an increased ESR, a weakly positive VDRL and decreased levels of both C3 and C4.

ESR 65 mm/h; C3 58 mg/dl; C4 11 mg/dl

Her serum creatinine level was now increased and a urine sample showed red blood cells. An EDTA

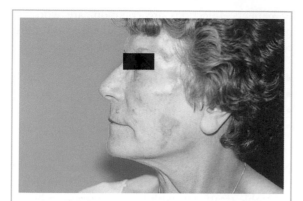

Fig. S10 Classical malar rash (seen in 3–40% of SLE patients).

creatinine clearance test was carried out which showed a decrease in renal function. She was admitted for a renal biopsy, which showed diffuse proliferative lupus nephritis (Fig. S11) and a diagnosis of systemic lupus erythematosus (SLE) was made.

Aetiology and risk factors

The cause of SLE is at present unknown but there is some evidence of a viral aetiology. The disease affects predominantly young women of child-bearing age and the prevalence varies from country to country. In the UK this is about 1/10 000 of the population with a female: male ratio of 6–9:1. Blacks and Chinese are particularly susceptible, one in 250 female blacks of child-bearing age being affected in the USA.

There is an increased risk if a family member has had SLE and there is 25% concordance in monozygotic twins (3% in dizygotic twins). A genetic deficiency in C2 may predispose to SLE since an increased incidence has been reported in this group of individuals. Associations with particular HLA haplotypes, HLA-B8, DR2 and DR3, have been described for SLE but the relative risk for either DR2 or DR3 is low (3) in Caucasian patients.

Pathology

The patient presented with a mild fever which is either due to an infection or more likely to overproduction of particular cytokines, e.g. IL-1 resulting from an ongoing inflammatory response. The muscle and joint pain is due to tendonitis and the swollen fingers are also due to tendon inflammation rather than true synovitis. Acute inflammation also accounts for the increased erythrocyte sedimentation rate (ESR) which is probably due to the large increase in acute phase proteins in the bloodstream. These coat the erythrocytes, making them heavier, and thus they sediment more rapidly. The reported bouts of fatigue were probably the result of anaemia but also could have

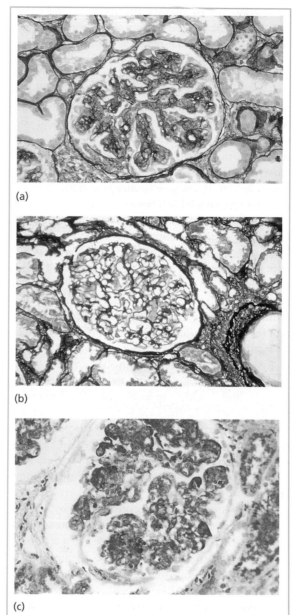

(a)

(b)

(c)

Fig. S11 Lupus glomerulonephritis with increased mesangial cellularity and thickened basement membranes (a), compared with the normal glomerular tuft (b). In the lupus patient, there are characteristic deposits of immunoglobulins as complexes (brown stain), seen in the capillary walls and mesangium using immunohistochemical enzyme-based techniques (c).

been due to accompanying hypothyroidism, the disease activity itself or even the treatment with NSAIDs. The mild anaemia and reduced haematocrit might have been caused by reduced uptake in dietary iron or due to inflammatory cytokines, e.g. TNFα, which can suppress erythropoiesis. The mild leucopenia might also be due to cytokine effects on haematopoiesis or due to anti-leucocyte antibodies. The patient was asked about spontaneous abortions and thrombotic events since she had anti-cardiolipin antibodies. Anti-cardiolipin (a phospholipid) is detected in the serum of some patients with SLE and since it interferes with blood clotting can lead to recurrent venous and arterial thromboses and abortions. Anti-phospholipid syndromes can also be primary but are most often secondary, occurring in association with SLE (in about 10% of cases) or other autoimmune rheumatic diseases. Anti-phospholipid autoantibodies bind to lipids on treponemes and thus give rise to a false-positive VDRL test.

Measurement of antinuclear antibodies is made by immunofluorescence on tissue sections and high levels are not unique to SLE. However, a particular pattern of staining with the patient's serum is highly suggestive of SLE. Anti-dsDNA is virtually confined to patients with SLE. The presence of serum rheumatoid factors (antibodies to IgG, RF) is common in a number of autoimmune diseases, including rheumatoid arthritis, SLE and Sjögren syndrome. The facial rash was erythematous and probably due to small immune complexes attaching to the vessel endothelial wall and resulting in local vasculitis. The reason for the location in the face is related to the photosensitive nature of the lupus rash. It has been shown experimentally that UV irradiation increases apoptosis in cultured human keratinocytes, the products of which could form immune complexes with autoantibodies and deposit in the facial blood vessels. Low C3 and C4 levels are due to consumption by immune complexes in the kidney. Erythrocyte ghosts in the urine are indicative of renal damage and a creatinine clearance confirmed renal damage. The histological picture of diffuse proliferative lupus nephritis is pathognomonic for SLE.

Body systems affected in SLE SLE is a multisystem disease and although the commonest presentation of SLE is a musculoskeletal complaint, patients may also present with other symptoms such as the facial rash which occurred later in the patient described. Skin lesions appear most often in sun-exposed areas. Pericarditis frequently occurs during acute exacerbations and myocardial disease is common. Renal involvement, which occurs in about 60% of cases, if severe, can be followed by hypertension. Vasculitis can lead to scleritis, infarction and Raynaud phenomenon. The respiratory system may be compromised. Pleurisy is common and bacterial pneumonia often seen. Disorders of mental function and seizures are not uncommon and there is CNS involvement of some sort in about 50% of the patients with renal involvement. Autoimmune haemolytic anaemia is seen in a small proportion of patients. Infections are common, are worse in patients on therapy, and are the second most common cause of death after renal failure.

Syndromes related to SLE are:
- discoid lupus erythematosus
- overlap syndromes
- antiphospholipid syndrome
- drug-induced lupus.

Management

Non-steroidal anti-inflammatory drugs are used for symptomatic relief. Low doses of corticosteroids are the stable treatment, with higher doses (in a bolus) used for treating flares. Antimalarials are of use for rashes and arthritis. Immunosuppressive drugs such as azathioprine are also effective. Patients should avoid sunlight and all non-essential drugs.

 Autoimmunity/autoimmune disease/autoantibodies; Glomerulonephritis; Rheumatoid arthritis

SYSTEMIC SCLEROSIS: A chronic disease characterized by progressive fibrosis, affecting primarily the skin but also visceral organs. The skin changes are also known as scleroderma.

Aetiology and risk factors

The aetiology of systemic sclerosis is not known. T-cell-mediated fibroblast activation and microvascular injury are thought to contribute. Most patients have circulating anti-DNA antibodies, suggesting a role for antibody-mediated immunity. Women are three times more likely to be affected than men.

Pathology

In systemic sclerosis any organ system can be involved and presenting symptoms vary accordingly. Skin changes in the form of fibrous atrophy of the dermis are present in the majority of cases. In advanced cases, extensive sclerosis may cause limitation in movement of fingers or extremities. Sclerosis can involve any level of the gastrointestinal tract. The oesophagus is particularly susceptible. Sclerosis of the muscle layer results in severe dysphagia. Fibrosis of the synovial tissue and inflammation of the skeletal muscle may cause difficulty in movement. The majority of patients show renal involvement with thickening and degeneration of medium-sized arteries. Some develop malignant hypertension and eventual renal failure. Interstitial fibrosis is seen in the lung of around half of the cases and myocardial fibrosis may be a feature. It is a chronic, progressive disease, with a 5-year survival rate of about 40%.

Management.

Steroids and penicillamine are of benefit to the skin manifestations.

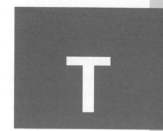

TAPEWORM INFECTION: Infection with cestode helminths involving the gastrointestinal tract or tissues (cysticercosis).

Aetiology and risk factors

The tapeworms include *Echinococcus* (see Hydatid disease); *Taenia*, *Hymenolepis*, *Diphyllobothrium* and *Spirometra*. The worm consists of a scolex (head) with which it attaches to the gastrointestinal wall, and body segments (proglottids) which are self-sustaining hermaphrodite units that produce the infective stage (ova). The definitive host is infected with the adult tapeworm and the intermediate host with the cyst stage. Humans can be both definitive and intermediate hosts (see Table T1).

Taenia is acquired by eating undercooked meat. With *Taenia solium* the human can act as both definitive and intermediate host and may develop cysticerci in any organ (see cysticercosis). This is due to autoinfection in the intestine when ova hatch and develop into oncospheres. *Hymenolepis* is acquired by direct faeco-oral transmission or contact with rodent faeces. *Diphyllobothrium* is acquired from eating undercooked fish and is common in Japan and Scandinavia. In the UK, sushi bars are a potential source of infection. *Spirometra* is acquired by drinking water contaminated with infected copepods (zooplankton) or eating uncooked frogs or snails (see Sparginosis).

Pathology

The oncospheres penetrate the intestinal wall to enter the portal circulation. The cyst may locate anywhere but particularly in striated muscle, brain or eye. When the cyst dies, an acute inflammatory reaction occurs and the cyst may calcify. With *Diphyllobothrium* infection, vitamin B12 deficiency may develop and the patient may present with megaloblastic anaemia*, the blood film showing macrocytosis. The patient may be asymptomatic with the adult worm or present with gastrointestinal symptoms of abdominal pain, malabsorption, diarrhoea and pruritus ani. The proglottids may be seen in the faeces. There is little evidence of effective immunity. Laboratory diagnosis is by demonstration of the worms or ova in the faeces. Treatment is with niclosamide or praziquantel.

TEMPORAL ARTERITIS: See Vasculitis.

TERATOMA: A tumour arising from pluripotential germ cells present in the gonads but also occasionally outside the gonads.

Teratomas mimic the development of normal embryo and can show differentiation towards endodermal (e.g. gut), mesodermal (e.g. connective tissue) or ectodermal (e.g. skin) structures. They are separated into three categories according to their maturity:

- 'teratoma, differentiated' containing only mature elements;
- 'malignant teratoma, intermediate' containing a mixture of mature and immature elements;
- 'malignant teratoma, undifferentiated' containing malignant undifferentiated cells.

Serum hCG and AFP levels are usually raised, and both markers are useful in monitoring treatment. Surgical excision is usually sufficient for the treatment of mature teratomas, but malignant teratomas require additional aggressive chemotherapy.

 Ovarian cyst

Table T1 Hosts and treatment of tapeworms

Tapeworm	Intermediate host	Intermediate host	Definitive host	Treatment
Echinococcus granulosus		Human and sheep	Carnivores	Albendazole and surgery
Echinococcus multilocularis		Human and sheep	Carnivores	Albendazole and surgery
Taenia saginata		Cattle	Humans	Niclosamide or praziquantel
Taenia solium		Pigs, humans	Humans	Niclosamide or praziquantel
Hymenolepis nana		Human	Human	Praziquantel
Diphyllobothrium latum	Crustaceans	Fish	Human	Praziquantel
Spirometra mansonoides	Crustaceans	Fish, frogs, humans	Dog	Praziquantel

TESTICULAR TUMOURS: Benign and malignant neoplasms of the testis.

Testicular tumours usually present as painless enlargement of the testicles and most commonly affect young adults. They can be divided into two groups according to histogenesis. The majority are germ cell tumours (95%) and the rest are so-called sex-cord stromal tumours. The germ cell tumours include seminomas* and teratomas* which are discussed as seperate entries.

TETANUS: A disease caused by the toxin produced by *Clostridium tetani*.

Aetiology and risk factors

Tetanus is acquired, usually following trauma, when the wound becomes contaminated with the organism. In certain parts of the world, neonates may get tetanus in association with the cultural practice of pasting the umbilical stump with dung. *Clostridium tetani* is a Gram-positive, anaerobic sporulating organism (Fig. T1) naturally found in the soil and faeces.

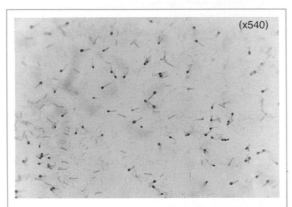

(x540)

Fig. T1 *Clostridium tetani* stained to show the spores.

Under anaerobic conditions, e.g. devitalized tissue in a wound, the spore germinates to produce the vegetative bacillus and during germination also produces the toxin.

Pathology

The toxin is very similar to botulinum toxin (see Botulism). The tetanus toxin binds specifically to receptor(s) on the motor end plate. The mechanism of action of tetanus toxin is identical to that of botulinum toxin but acts on different VAMPs. The net result of the toxin action is to prevent neurotransmitter (γ-aminobutyric acid) release at inhibitory synapses in the spinal cord. This in turn means that contraction of one muscle group (e.g.

the biceps) is not accompanied by the physiological normal relaxation of the opposing muscle group (e.g. the triceps). Clinically, the patient will develop spasmodic contractions of all muscles under the slightest stimulus. The patient may initially complain of trismus and difficulty in mastication ('lockjaw'). Prolonged contraction of the facial muscle elicits the characteristic 'risus sardonicus' appearance. As the disease progresses, other muscle groups may be involved and generalized convulsions may occur. In addition, the muscles of respiration may be involved. If the lateral horn cells of the spinal cord are involved, cardiac dysrhythmias may occur. Laboratory diagnosis is by isolation of the organism from the wound, although tetanus can follow inapparent injuries, e.g. thorn pricks.

Management

Management consists of (1) supportive therapy, (2) human immune globulin combined with toxoid vaccination, and (3) antibiotics to eliminate the organism. Prevention is by toxoid vaccination (with diphtheria and pertussis in DPT), a booster being recommended every 5–10 years.

THALASSAEMIA: A group of inherited disorders common around the Mediterranean, usually characterized by anaemia and microcytosis, due to inability to make the globin chains of haemoglobin. Inheritance is usually autosomal recessive.

Normal haemoglobin

The haemoglobin molecule consists of haem, the iron-containing part, and globin, the protein component. Globin is made up of two pairs of polypeptide chains (Fig. T2), the type of chains differing between the different haemoglobins.

The three normal haemoglobins (Hb) of man are fetal Hb (HbF), adult haemoglobin (HbA) and the second adult haemoglobin HbA$_2$. All three types of

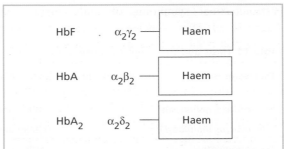

Fig. T2 The three major normal haemoglobins of man are fetal Hb (HbF), adult haemoglobin (HbA), and the second adult haemoglobin (HbA$_2$). They differ only in the second type of polypeptide chain making up the globin part of the molecule.

Hb contain a pair of α chains. They differ in their second pair of polypeptide chains. Fetal haemoglobin has a pair of γ chains, HbA β chains and HbA$_2$ δ chains. At birth, the majority of circulating haemoglobin is fetal haemoglobin. During the first year of life haemoglobin F is gradually replaced by haemoglobin A. Approximately 3% of circulating haemoglobin is the second adult haemoglobin A$_2$.

In the thalassaemias, structurally normal globin chains are produced, in contrast to the haemoglobinopathies where abnormal chains are manufactured. The problem is that not enough chains can be manufactured. In α-thalassaemia α chains cannot be manufactured, in β-thalassaemia β chains cannot be manufactured.

Case

A 1-year-old boy of Greek parents was noted to be pale and slightly jaundiced by his GP. Both spleen and liver were palpable. His developmental milestones had been normal and he had no siblings. Blood count was performed:

WBC 13.0 × 10⁹/l
RBC 3.09 × 10¹²/l; Hb 6.9 g/dl; Hct (ratio) 0.188
MCV 61.4 fl; MCH 22.5 pg
MCHC 36.7 g/dl; RDW 12.9 %

Blood film examination showed numerous target cells, occasional spherocytes, and the presence of nucleated red cells. Reticulocyte count was modestly elevated at 5% (<2%). White cells and platelets were normal. Serum iron, total iron-binding capacity and ferritin were normal. Blood counts performed on both parents showed a mild microcytic hypochromic anaemia.

Pathology

His microcytic hypochromic anaemia would fit a diagnosis of iron deficiency, except that the measurements of iron status were normal. Also, nucleated red cells are not usually a feature of iron-deficiency anaemia. Analysis of haemoglobin by high-pressure liquid chromatography (HPLC) showed HbF and normal levels of HbA$_2$ but no HbA. By a year of age only a small percentage of Hb should be HbF, indicating deficient manufacture of HbA in this case.

A diagnosis of β-thalassaemia major was made. A programme of life-long blood transfusions was embarked upon, with desferrioxamine iron chelation therapy to prevent secondary haemosiderosis*. His parents, both carriers of β-thalassaemia trait,

were offered antenatal diagnosis by amniotic villus sampling for future pregnancies, but decided to have no further children.

Haemoglobin defect in β-thalassaemia

The gene for control of β-chain manufacture is on chromosome 11. Loss of the function of one gene (heterozygous) causes β-thalassaemia trait. This results in a microcytic hypochromic anaemia difficult to distinguish from iron deficiency, except that the haemoglobin level is rarely below 9 g/dl and measurements of iron status such as serum ferritin are normal. Increased amounts of HbA$_2$, which does not require β chains for its manufacture, are found in the blood.

Loss of the function of both β-globin genes (homozygous) causes β-thalassaemia major, with severe impairment of haemoglobin A production.

Haemoglobin defect in α-thalassaemia

There are two α-globin chains on each chromosome 16, so that control of α-globin chain manufacture is under the control of a total of four genes. The clinical picture of α-thalassaemia is thus very heterogeneous, depending on how many genes, and on which chromosome, are affected. Deletion of all four genes results in inability to make any haemoglobin containing α chains (Fig. T2). Death *in utero* results. Deletion of only one gene causes a mild microcytic hypochromic blood picture that may not be clinically detectable. Deletion of intermediate numbers of genes may result in haemoglobin H disease, a microcytic hypochromic anaemia associated with splenomegaly. Haemoglobin H is a polymerization of surplus β chains which are unpaired by α chains and so combine together to form tetramers (β$_4$). These may be detected in the blood by haemoglobin electrophoresis or HPLC.

Management of the thalassaemias

β-Thalassaemia major usually presents in childhood with progressive anaemia and enlargement of liver and spleen in a patient of Mediterranean or Asian origin. Blood transfusion is required on a regular basis for life. The iron overload that this produces will result in cirrhosis*, cardiomyopathy and endocrine failure without iron chelation therapy with desferrioxamine. Bone marrow transplant, if performed before iron overload becomes a problem, cures some cases.

Patients with β-thalassaemia trait should be counselled about the risks of having children with thalassaemia major if their partner has thalassaemia trait or an interacting haemoglobinopathy. Iron treatment for their microcytic hypochromic anaemia should not be given without confirmation

T

that they are truly iron deficient, usually by finding a low serum ferritin.

 Sickle cell disease

THROMBOCYTOPENIA: A reduction in platelet count below normal.

The normal range extends from $140 \times 10^9/l$ to $500 \times 10^9/l$, but nature overprovides platelets as with many other systems in the body. Haemorrhage in response to trauma is not usually seen until the count drops below $70 \times 10^9/l$, and spontaneous bleeding is rare at counts above $20 \times 10^9/l$. False low platelet counts may be found when the blood sample has clotted, or EDTA-induced platelet clumping has occurred. Examination of the sample and blood film will allow these causes of artefactual thrombocytopenia to be excluded.

The causes of thrombocytopenia may be conveniently divided into marrow underproduction or increased peripheral destruction. Some of these are shown in Table T2. Bone marrow aspiration provides a simple way of distinguishing between these two types of thrombocytopenia. In peripheral platelet destruction, the number of megakaryocytes will be normal or increased, but in marrow underproduction they will be reduced and some marrow disease will usually be evident (Fig. T3).

In peripheral platelet destruction, the circulating platelets are relatively young and healthy but in marrow disease they are old and ineffective. This means that for a particular platelet count, bleeding manifestations will be fewer in peripheral platelet destruction than marrow underproduction. Young platelets, like young red cells, carry a residual RNA framework in their cytoplasm, which can be stained by fluorescent dyes and detected by flow cytometry. This reticulated platelet count is increased in peripheral platelet destruction.

Table T2 Some causes of thrombocytopenia

Marrow underproduction	Peripheral platelet destruction
Aplastic anaemia*	Immune thrombocytopenia*
Acute and chronic leukaemias*	Disseminated intravascular coagulation*
Marrow infiltration with secondary cancers	Thrombotic thrombo-cytopenic purpura* and haemolytic uraemic syndrome*
Marrow lymphomas* or myeloma*	Extracorporeal circulation, e.g. heart–lung bypass
Myelodysplasia*	Hypersplenism

THROMBOCYTOSIS: An increased platelet count. The normal range is $(140–500) \times 10^9/l$. Common causes are bleeding, trauma, inflammation and iron deficiency. A thrombocytosis may also be found in the myeloproliferative disorders*, particularly essential (primary) thrombocythaemia.

THROMBOEMBOLISM: Detachment of an arterial or venous thrombosis from the endothelium of a blood vessel. The clot is carried by the bloodstream through the arterial or venous systems and may cause symptoms by vascular obstruction where it is arrested in the arterial tree. Other substances that may cause harmful emboli are air, amniotic fluid or fat; these are dealt with elsewhere in this volume.

Pulmonary embolism usually arises from deep venous thrombosis in the legs or pelvis, the embolus lodging in and obstructing the pulmonary artery.

Cerebral embolus may originate from thrombus in the left atrium in patients with atrial fibrillation. The clot forms because the atria do not empty completely as they do not contract. The thrombus may pass to the brain, causing stroke or to the legs, causing obstruction of lower aorta, femoral or popliteal arteries.

Case

A 25-year-old woman fell from the balcony of her alpine hotel following an après-ski party, sustaining a compound fracture of the femur and a double fracture of the pubic ramus. There was no significant previous medical history and the combined oral contraceptive pill was her only medication. Immediate internal fixation of the femoral fracture was performed, but her postoperative course was

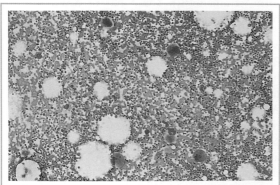

Fig. T3 Stained smear of normal bone marrow aspirate showing normal numbers of megakaryocytes. At this low magnification the only cells to be distinguished with certainty are the giant megakaryocytes. The cytoplasm of these cells fragments once the cell has reached maturity and each fragment becomes a blood platelet.

T

complicated by bleeding from a branch of the femoral artery and wound infection. She was evacuated to the UK by air-ambulance.

Twelve hours after arrival she experienced right-sided pleuritic chest pain. On auscultation a pleural rub was heard. Allowing for the previous orthopaedic operation, examination of her legs was normal. Chest radiograph and electrocardiogram were normal and there was no fever. Ventilation and perfusion scans (Fig. T4) showed multiple areas of hypoperfusion of lung parenchyma, without associated ventilatory defect.

A diagnosis of multiple small pulmonary emboli was made and she restarted anticoagulation with heparin, prophylactic heparin having previously been stopped after her episode of arterial haemorrhage. She made a slow but uneventful recovery except for one episode of haemoptysis. Oral anti-coagulation with warfarin was prescribed until 3 months later, when she was fully mobile. It was decided not to perform screening tests for thrombophilia*.

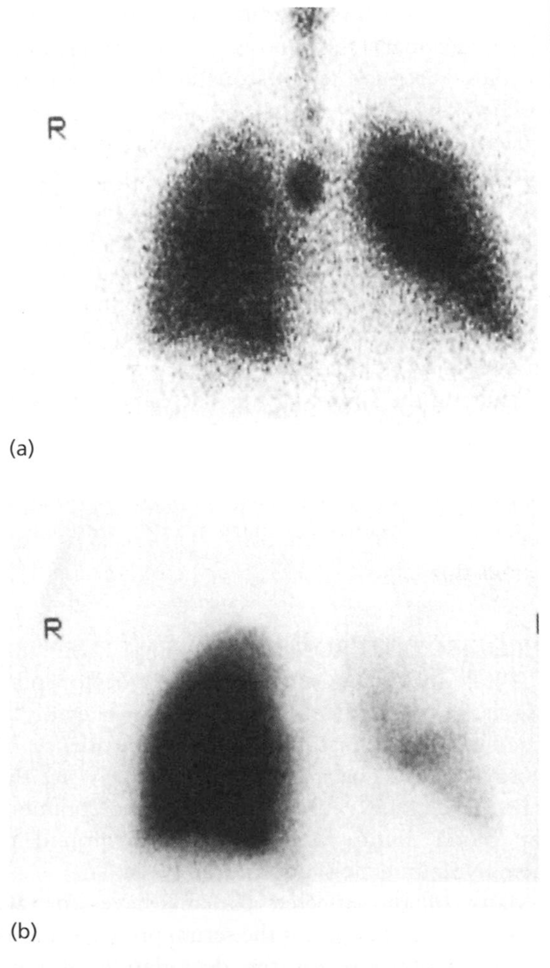

Aetiology and risk factors

This woman had several predisposing causes for venous thrombosis including trauma, operation, immobilization, and oestrogen therapy. Other risk factors for venous thromboembolism are previous thrombosis, malignancy, pregnancy, increasing age and congestive cardiac failure. Most patients in her situation would receive prophylactic heparin treatment to prevent venous thromboembolism.

Pathology

Venous thrombosis most commonly starts in the valve pockets of the veins of the lower limbs and gradually extends proximally to involve large veins. The affected leg is often, but not always, swollen and painful. Emboli from these areas of thrombosis may be single and massive, obstructing the main pulmonary artery, sometimes straddling the bifurcation ('saddle embolus') and causing sudden death (Fig. T5). Alternatively, they may coil up within a

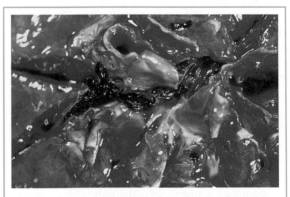

Fig. T5 Macroscopic appearance of lung showing a massive embolus blocking main pulmonary arteries.

single pulmonary artery, causing unilateral chest pain, hypoperfusion of one lung on the chest radiograph and a ventricular strain pattern on the electrocardiogram. Small emboli impact in the terminal arterioles of the pulmonary vasculature, causing infarction of a pyramidal segment of lung supplied by that arteriole (Fig. T6). Inflammation resulting from this infarction causes pleuritic pain and the infarcted area may liquefy and be coughed up. It then shrinks to form a scar manifested by an area of linear atelectasis on the chest radiograph.

Management

Avoidance of venous stasis prevents thrombosis. Early mobilization after operation and elastic

(a)

R

(b)

R

Fig. T4 Ventilation/perfusion lung scan showing homogeneous ventilation in both lungs (a) but decreased perfusion in left lung (b). (Reproduced with permission from Lisle DA. *Imaging for Students*. London: Arnold, 1996)

T

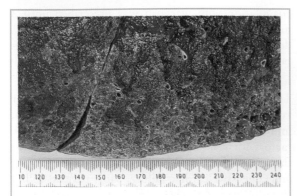

Fig. T6 V-shaped pale infarction in lung secondary to thromboembolism.

stockings to improve venous return from the legs are simple measures that can be taken. For high-risk situations such as hip surgery low doses of heparin anticoagulant can be given prophylactically.

Treatment of established thrombosis is with heparin and warfarin anticoagulation. Once thrombosis has been prevented, the body's own fibrinolytic system will gradually dissolve thrombus and embolus. In life-threatening situations such as coronary thrombosis or massive pulmonary embolus, fibrinolytic agents may be used, but they do carry a risk of inducing bleeding.

THROMBOPHILIA: A predisposition to venous and arterial thrombosis, which may be inherited or acquired. Young patients presenting with repeated thromboembolism without the usual clinical risk factors for thrombosis* should be investigated for thrombophilia, particularly if there is a family history of thrombosis.

Acquired causes of thrombophilia include polycythaemia*, thrombocytosis* and the lupus anticoagulant. The lupus anticoagulant is detected in the laboratory by prolongation of phospholipid-dependent coagulation tests such as the activated partial thromboplastin time. *In vivo*, however, the clinical picture is of repeated venous thromboembolism and recurrent miscarriage due to placental infarction. It is an autoimmune disease associated with the presence of antiphospholipid antibodies in the serum. As the name suggests, some patients with the lupus anticoagulant have systemic lupus erythematosus*, although most do not.

Inherited thrombophilia is due to deficiency of one of the natural anticoagulants of the blood: protein C, protein S and antithrombin; or to a structural abnormality of the coagulation factors that makes them relatively insensitive to degradation once they have been activated. One of the best

characterized of these abnormalities is factor V Leiden. An inherited abnormality of factor V makes it resistant to inactivation by protein C. Similar structural abnormalities of prothrombin have been described.

THROMBOSIS: The formation of an intravascular clot, usually qualified by its site, e.g. deep venous thrombosis, coronary thrombosis, etc. Besides causing symptoms due to vessel obstruction, the clot may detach from the vessel wall and migrate in the vascular system forming an embolus. Clots consist of a meshwork of fibrin, activated platelets and entrapped red blood cells.

Most cases of thrombosis can be explained by the classical Virchow triad of stasis, factors in the vessel wall, and factors in the blood itself. For example, stasis due to venous compression by tumour or pregnancy predisposes to venous thrombosis. Intimal plaques of atheroma* may ulcerate and trigger coronary thrombosis. In polycythaemia*, the blood is thick and viscous and flows slowly, predisposing to thrombosis.

Clots are dissolved by the fibrinolytic system. An inactive precursor, plasminogen, is converted to plasmin which splits fibrin into soluble fibrin degradation products. Stimuli to plasminogen conversion include urokinase, an enzyme present in normal urine designed to ensure the urinary system does not become obstructed by clot, and streptokinase, produced by streptococci to prevent the body obstructing the spread of this bacterium by laying down fibrin. Therapeutic plasminogen activators ('clot busters') such as tissue plasminogen activator are frequently used in the early stages of myocardial infarction to dissolve coronary artery thrombosis.

 Thromboembolism

THROMBOTIC THROMBOCYTOPENIC PURPURA (TTP): Peripheral consumption thrombocytopenia* associated with a microangiopathic haemolytic anaemia* blood picture and clinical evidence of microvascular obstruction, particularly in the brain. Fever and neurological signs are common. The blood picture is similar to that found in haemolytic uraemic syndrome*.

Many of the affected patients have an IgG antibody directed against the serum protease that is usually responsible for the degradation of high molecular weight von Willebrand factor (vWF). Normally, such large multimers are secreted by the endothelial cell beneath the intima of the blood vessel and promote platelet aggregation if the subendothelial layer is exposed by vascular damage. It is thought that these large multimers accumulating in the plasma in TTP cause the formation of platelet aggregates and platelet thrombi. These deplete the platelet count and cause the symptoms of microvascular obstruction.

In contrast to disseminated intravascular coagulation*, in which thrombocytopenia and microangiopathic red cell changes are also found, the coagulation tests are usually normal. Management is usually by large volume plasma exchange for fresh frozen plasma, which may replace the protease responsible for successful vWF degradation, and remove high MWt vWF.

THYROIDITIS: Acute or chronic inflammation of the thyroid gland.

Inflammation of the thyroid can have various causes, and the pathological features depend on the inciting agent. Common varieties are:

- infectious thyroiditis: various infectious agents can infect the thyroid, usually via the haematogenous route. These include bacteria, viruses, and fungi. Hashimoto thyroiditis, an autoimmune disease, is discussed as a separate entry.
- de Quervain thyroiditis*: a subacute thyroiditis which is thought to be caused by a granulomatous inflammatory response against a viral infection.

THYROTOXICOSIS: A metabolic disease due to increased levels of thyroid hormones.

Case

A 33-year-old woman presented with complaints of palpitations and reduced exercise capacity which had become worse during the last 6 months. She had lost 8 kg in weight during the last year and felt increasingly anxious. She had been well till 6 months ago though she remembered complaining of excessive sweating 3 years ago. She had no visual complaints apart from 'grittiness' of the eyes. Her social and past medical histories were unremarkable.

On examination her pulse was 120 beats/min, her blood pressure was 170/90 mmHg and respiration rate 12/minute. Her skin was moist. Her left eye showed mild exophthalmos and there was upper lid lag in both eyes. On palpation, both lobes of her thyroid gland were diffusely enlarged and a bruit was clearly audible. Her peripheral blood count was normal.

She was diagnosed as having thyrotoxicosis secondary to Graves disease and was treated with the antithyroid drug, carbimazole. After a year of treatment, the drug was stopped; however, the

Serum free thyroxine: 46.7 pmol/l (normal 9–24)
Serum free tri-iodothyronine: 26.0 pmol/l (normal 4.7–8.2)
Serum TSH: <0.2 mU/l
Antithyroid antibodies: thyroglobulin, positive; thyroid microsomes, positive; thyroid-stimulating antibody, positive

hyperthyroidism recurred. After the patient had been rendered euthyroid for a second time, a subtotal thyroidectomy was performed to control the excess hormone secretion.

Histopathology: Macroscopically the thyroid was diffusely enlarged and weighed 75 g. The cut surface was colloid-rich and no focal lesions were seen. Microscopically the overall architecture of the gland was preserved. The follicles were lined by tall columnar hyperplastic thyroid epithelium. The edge of the colloid in the follicles had a scalloped appearance. These features were consistent with Graves disease (Fig. T7).

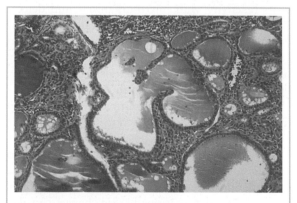

Fig. T7 Histological section of thyroid showing follicles lined by high columnar epithelium suggestive of hyperfunction.

Postoperatively the patient became euthyroid and remains well.

Aetiology and risk factors

There are three main causes of thyrotoxicosis. In around two-thirds of the cases the cause is Graves disease or autoimmune diffuse thyroid hyperplasia, which was the diagnosis in this case and is discussed in detail below. The other two are toxic nodular goitre and follicular adenoma of the thyroid. Graves disease affects the 30–50 years age group with a 5:1 female to male ratio. About half the patients have a family history of thyroid disease. Caucasians with Graves disease have an increased frequency of HLA-DR3.

Pathology

Thyroid hormones act on many systems, thus hyperthyroidism affects many organs and tissues. The major effect of excess thyroid hormone is an increase in the metabolic rate. This manifests itself as irritability, weight loss, increased heart rate, increase in pulse pressure, decrease in exercise capacity, excess sweating and heat intolerance, all of which were present in this patient. In Graves disease the increase in thyroid hormone secretion is immunologically mediated. These patients have circulating antibodies against the TSH-receptor and detection of the autoantibody serum is critical in establishment of the diagnosis. These antithyroid antibodies mimic the effects of TSH and induce diffuse enlargement of the gland and the hyperplastic changes described in the biopsy report above. The levels of antithyroid antibodies fluctuate and development of the classical picture of thyrotoxicosis may take a few years as observed in the above case. The reasons for the generation of antithyroid antibodies are not clear. Genetic factors, antigenic cross-reactivity with micro-organisms and defects in T-cell suppressor activity have all been implicated. The excess of thyroid hormones in the blood suppresses TSH secretion in the pituitary by negative feedback, and characteristically no or very little TSH can be detected in the circulation.

Around half the cases of Graves disease develop ophthalmopathy with characteristic exophthalmos and associated complications such as corneal ulceration. Retro-orbital inflammation, possibly also immunological, is considered to be the cause of the exophthalmos, though the precise pathogenesis is not understood. Occasionally skin changes can also be observed (so-called pretibial myxoedema). These are itchy, raised, pink-coloured plaques on the anterior part of the leg and the dorsum of the foot.

Management

The first line of treatment for Graves disease is suppression of hormone secretion by antithyroid drugs such as carbimazole. If this fails, ablation of the gland with radioactive iodine administration or surgery is the choice.

 Goitre

TONSILLITIS: An acute inflammation of the pharynx/tonsils (also called sore throat or pharyngitis) and caused most commonly by viruses (e.g.

adenoviruses, rhinoviruses, enteroviruses). Severe tonsillitis can be caused by EBV. The commonest bacterial cause of tonsillitis is *Streptococcus pyogenes*.

TOXAEMIA OF PREGNANCY: See Pre-eclampsia.

TOXIC SHOCK SYNDROME: Infection by some strains of *Staphylococcus aureus* (or *Streptococcus pyogenes*) which secrete toxic shock syndrome toxin (TSST-1). Like exfoliative toxin (see Scalded skin syndrome) and the enterotoxins of food-poisoning, strains of *Staph. aureus* (see Gastroenteritis), TSST-1 is a superantigen which stimulates large numbers of T-cells to release cytokines. The syndrome can occur in either gender and all ages, but is most common in menstruating females, probably related to a specific type of tampon. Presentation is acute, with diarrhoea, myalgia, vomiting, fever, hypotension and an erythematous rash. In a few days the skin begins to desquamate, particularly on the palms and soles. Complications can include renal failure. Clinical investigations demonstrate a peripheral neutrophilia with thrombocytopenia, elevated serum creatinine, blood urea and creatinine phosphokinase and elevated hepatic enzymes and bilirubin. Laboratory diagnosis is by isolation of the micro-organism and demonstration of toxin production. Management is supportive, including dialysis if required, together with antistaphylococcal antibiotics.

TOXOPLASMOSIS: Infection with the protozoon *Toxoplasma gondii*.

Case

An otherwise healthy 29-year-old woman presented to her GP complaining of a sore throat, fatigue, headache and myalgia of 1 week's duration. She had noticed a lump in her neck and on examination the GP found generalized cervical and axillary lymphadenopathy with discrete and non-tender lymph nodes. The patient had a low-grade fever. The GP arranged for a throat swab, full blood count, monospot test and lymph node biopsy.

Microbiology: throat swab, no Group A streptococcus isolated; monospot negative.
Haematology: Hb 13 g/dl; WBC 8000 × 10⁶/l; differential normal.
Film: no atypical cells seen.
Lymph node biopsy: showed reactive follicular hyperplasia with focal distension of sinuses and epithelioid macrophage infiltration of germinal centres (Fig. T8).

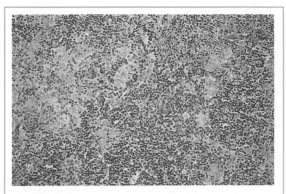

Fig. T8 Reactive follicular hyperplasia with focal distension of sinuses and epithelioid macrophage infiltration of germinal centres.

Aetiology and risk factors

Toxoplasma gondii is an ubiquitous coccidian parasite that is found naturally in cats and can be acquired directly from cat faeces or by eating undercooked meat or vegetables contaminated with the oocysts. The transmission cycles are shown in Fig. T9.

Most infections are acquired by ingesting the oocyst stage which excysts in the gastrointestinal tract, releasing the tachyzoite which is then distributed to all body organs via the bloodstream. Once in the tissues the parasite multiplies intracellularly within a vacuole in the cell and, if taken up by a macrophage, is not killed by the oxidative burst, avoiding phagolysosomal fusion. The infected cell lyses and the released tachyzoites can infect other adjacent cells. Eventually a tissue cyst is formed as the host begins to respond immunologically to the tachyzoite. TNF and IFN-γ are important mediators of toxoplasmacidal activity. The tissue cysts are found particularly in the brain and striated muscle, where they may remain for the lifetime of the individual, although any organ can be affected. If an individual becomes immunocompromised (e.g. in AIDS or following immunosuppressive drug therapy), the tissue cysts reactivate, giving rise to symptoms. In the brain there are focal areas of necrosis surrounded by tachyzoites and an intense inflammatory infiltrate with perivascular cuffing. In the lungs there is a necrotizing pneumonitis with both extracellular and intracellular tachyzoites. Infection in pregnant females can lead to congenital infection of the fetus as the tachyzoite spreads transplacentally. The different clinical presentations are shown in Table T3.

Laboratory diagnosis is by serology, demonstration of tachyzoites or tissue cysts by histology, isolation of tachyzoites from placenta, blood or CSF or by PCR. Treatment is with antimicrobials: pyrimethamine and sulphadiazine in the immunocompromised, spiramycin or sulphadiazine (± pyrimethamine and folinic acid) in pregnant

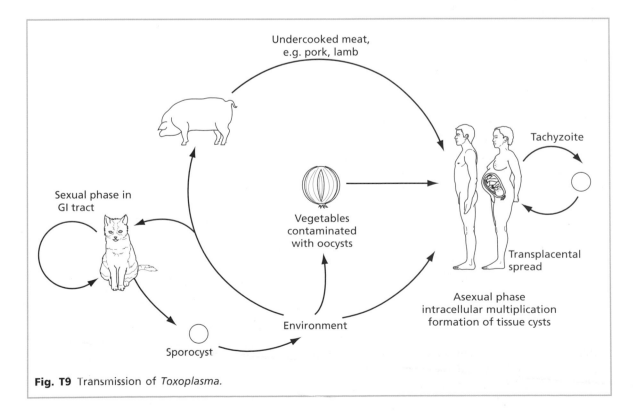

Fig. T9 Transmission of *Toxoplasma*.

Table T3 Presentation of toxoplasmosis

Presentation	Usual host	Symptoms
Asymptomatic	Immunocompetent	Most infections
Acute symptomatic	Immunocompetent	10–20% of infections present with lymphadenopathy and are frequently self-limiting
Ocular	Mostly fetus in congenital infections†	Necrotizing retinitis
Congenital	Fetus	Chorioretinitis, blindness, anaemia, jaundice, epilepsy, microcephaly, hydrocephalus intracerebral calcification
CNS	Mostly immunocompromised	Wide range of symptoms including: encephalitis, space-occupying lesion, fits, coma, altered personality
Lungs	Mostly immunocompromised	Necrotizing pneumonitis
Liver	Mostly immunocompromised	Necrotizing hepatitis
Heart	Mostly immunocompromised	Myocarditis

†About 15% of fetuses become infected if the mother acquires an infection in the first trimester compared to 90% if infected in the 3rd trimester; however, about 85% of fetuses will have severe congenital abnormalities if infected in the first trimester compared with 10% if infection occurs in the third trimester.

women, but this is not generally required for the acute symptomatic presentation in immunocompetent individuals unless symptoms are severe or ocular toxoplasmosis is present.

TRACHOMA: Infection of the eye with *Chlamydia trachomatis*.

 Chlamydial disease

TRANSPLANT REJECTION: The rejection of donor organ or tissue grafts mediated by the recipient's immune system.

Risk factors

Transplants may fail for surgical reasons or because of infection or the recurrence of diseases in the transplant, but rejection in most cases is due to the histoincompatibility between the donor and recipient of the graft. Transplantation antigens are recog-

Table T4 Organs and tissues used in transplantation

Organ/tissue	Main reason(s) for transplantation	Typing	Main rejection mechanism(s)
Kidney	End-stage renal failure	ABO, HLA	Antibodies and cell-mediated immunity, CD4 and CD8 T cells (depends on type of rejection – see Renal transplantation)
Heart (increasingly with lung)	Heart failure, infarction, cardiomyopathies, congenital diseases	Not required and usually impractical	Cell-mediated immunity
Liver (also with pancreas)	Liver failure	HLA not of major value	Uncertain
Pancreas†	IDDM	HLA	Cell-mediated
Bone marrow	Stem cell replacement used for immunodeficiencies, malignancies and metabolic diseases	ABO, HLA	Antibodies (note: risk of graft-versus-host disease*)
Blood transfusion	Severe blood loss, leukaemias, various anaemias, HDN	ABO	Antibodies
Cornea	Opacity due to trauma, infections	Usually not typed, (HLA)	Cell-mediated if graft becomes vascularized‡
Skin	Wounds, burns	Not usually needed as short-term	T-cells

HDN, haemolytic disease of the newborn; IDDM, insulin-dependent diabetes mellitus.
†Pancreatic islet cells now in clinical trials.
‡Usually accepted unless vascularized.

T

Table T5 Strategies for prevention of graft rejection

Blood group typing	Important for blood transfusions and some transplants, including bone marrow and kidney
Transplantation within families	Acceptance is complete between genetically identical twins of the same sex since there are no differences in their HLA genes; HLA is inherited in mendelian fashion and co-dominant, therefore a good match is more likely within a family, with a complete match between sibs in 1 of 4 cases
Tissue typing	This is necessary in most cases; serological and molecular techniques are used to check donor and recipient HLA
Immunosuppression	There is some degree of rejection in most cases; this is prevented and treated with drugs including azathioprine, cyclosporin A and prednisone

nized by the host's immune system and an immune response ensues, the severity of which is dependent on the extent of the mismatch of the donor and host's transplantation antigens. Transplantation antigens are the blood group antigens and major histocompatibility complex antigens – human leucocyte antigens (HLA). Although there are only a few blood group antigens, there are many HLA and the combinations within an individual result in the chance of a completely identical set of HLA (apart from family members) of greater than 1 in many millions. Typing of histocompatibility antigens is therefore essential to minimize rejection (see management).

A variety of organs and tissues are now transplanted from one individual to another, and this is often the only way of successfully treating the patient's disease. Table T4 summarizes the important features. Note that the exact mechanisms of rejection are complex and not yet fully established.

Management
Graft rejection is minimized by (1) typing blood groups and HLA in most cases and (2) preparation of the patient with immunosuppressive drugs (summarized in Table T5).

TRAVELLER'S DIARRHOEA: Diarrhoea associated with travel abroad (from the UK) and most frequently due to pathogenic strains of *Escherichia coli* or *Giardia*.

TRENCH FEVER: An infection, common in times of social upheaval such as wars. Currently its true prevalence is unknown but it is probably rare. The disease is caused by *Bartonella quintana* and the organism is transmitted by the louse. Little is known about the pathogenesis of the infection but it presents with fever, headache and severe pains in the legs. There is sometimes a macular rash. Splenomegaly may occur and there is a peripheral neutrophilia. Diagnosis is by culture of the organism and treatment is with chloramphenicol or tetracycline.

TREPONEMATOSIS: Endemic non-venereal infection with treponemes that are serologically and morphologically indistinguishable from *Treponema pallidum*.

TRICHINOSIS: Infection with *Trichinella spiralis* and other *Trichinella* species, associated with eating undercooked meat containing the larvae, which excyst in the stomach and develop into adult worms in the intestine. The worms mate and new larvae are distributed, mainly to skeletal muscle by the blood supply, where they encyst, thus completing the life cycle. When the worm is in the intestine there are an associated partial villous atrophy and a submucosal infiltrate with neutrophils, eosinophils, macrophages and mast cells. In the skeletal muscle the muscle fibres degenerate. Coiled larvae are enclosed in a cyst wall derived from the host cell and surrounded by an infiltrate of lymphocytes and eosinophils. With time, the cysts may calcify. Clinically, the infection may be asymptomatic or, if the inoculum is heavy, the patient may present with diarrhoea due to the adult worms in the intestine, or a systemic illness characterized by periorbital oedema, headache, fever, myalgia, rash and splinter haemorrhages, due to dissemination of the larvae causing a myositis. Complications include myocarditis and encephalitis. There is peripheral eosinophilia and elevated serum creatinine phosphokinase and lactic dehydrogenase. Laboratory diagnosis is by histology and serology. There is no effective management other than NSAIDs for the myositis, although thiabendazole and albendazole have been used.

TROPICAL SPRUE: Chronic malabsorption following an infection acquired in the tropics leading to mucosal damage, an altered microbial flora and giving rise to vitamin deficiency, megaloblastic anaemia* and hypoalbuminaemia.

Table T6 Trypanosomiasis – location of causative organisms and their hosts

Species	Vector	Reservoir	Geography
Try. brucei var rhodesiense	Glossina (tsetse fly)	Wild game and domestic animals	East and southern Africa
Try. brucei var gambiense	Glossina	Human	West and central Africa
Try. cruzi	Reduviid bug	Humans and domestic animals	S. America

TRYPANOSOMIASIS: Infection with species of the haemoflagellate protozoan *Trypanosoma*.

Aetiology and risk factors
There are three main species, one occurring in South America, which causes Chagas disease* (see separate entry for Pathology) and two in Africa, which cause 'sleeping sickness' (Table T6).

The flagellate trypanosomes are taken up into the intestine of the tsetse fly during feeding where they multiply and, after some weeks, migrate to the salivary gland of the fly and undergo further development to the infectious form. These are inoculated into the next human host.

Pathology
The trypanosomes multiply at the site of inoculation, producing a sore, characterized histologically by oedema and a perivascular mononuclear infiltrate in the skin with regional lymph node enlargement. They then enter the lymphatics and eventually the bloodstream, avoiding the host immune defences by periodically expressing variant surface glycoproteins and thereby giving rise to waves of parasitaemia. The trypanosomes are spread to all organs, producing inflammation, e.g. heart and kidneys. Immune complexes and hypocomplementaemia are evident and autoantibodies can be detected, e.g. anti-DNA. Erythrocytes coated with immune complexes are lysed and there is thrombocytopenia with leucocytosis. The parasite eventually enters the central nervous system, causing a meningoencephalitis, characterized by a perivascular mononuclear cell infiltrate including the typical foamy plasma cells containing IgM (morula cells of Mott). Oedema of the brain occurs, with signs of raised intracranial pressure. There is evidence of autoantibody production (e.g. anti-myelin basic protein), demyelination, altered levels of neurotransmitters and neuronal cell death.

Clinically, the patient may notice the ulcerating papule at the inoculation site. The two forms of African trypanosomes produce slightly different diseases, *Trypanosoma gambiense* giving mild symptoms and a protracted course whilst *Trypanosoma rhodesiense* produces a severe disease with rapid progression to CNS disease. Disease is characterized by episodes of fevers, chills, and general malaise with widespread lymphadenopathy and hepatosplenomegaly. There may be an erythematous rash and evidence of myocarditis with arrhythmias and heart failure. In CNS disease the patient develops neurological signs and symptoms with changes in consciousness, ataxia, apathy and eventually coma ('sleeping sickness'). Laboratory diagnosis relies on demonstration of the parasite in the appropriate specimen (by microscopy or histology) or serology. Treatment is with suramin, melarsoprol or eflornithine, depending upon the stage of disease.

TUBERCULOSIS: Infection with *Mycobacterium tuberculosis*.

Case
A nurse was admitted to hospital complaining of generalized malaise, fever, cough and weight loss over a period of 2 months. A chest radiograph was performed and sputum sent for culture. Tuberculosis being suspected, the patient was placed in source isolation and started on antituberculous therapy.

> Radiology: areas of consolidation with cavitation seen at the left apex (Fig. T10).
> Microbiology: acid-fast bacilli seen in the sputum (Fig. T11). Ligase chain reaction for *M. tuberculosis* positive.

After 3 weeks of incubation, *M. tuberculosis* grew from the sputum specimen.

Aetiology and risk factors
The genus *Mycobacterium* comprises about 30 different species, of which *M. tuberculosis* (causing tuberculosis) and *M. leprae* (causing leprosy) are the most important. Other species that are found in the environment also cause disease as indicated in Table T7. See also Mycobacteriosis (p. 170).

All mycobacteria have a thick waxy cell wall, rich in mycolic acids which retain the red colour of carbol fuchsin dye even after exposure to mineral acids (hence acid-fast bacilli) – the Ziehl–Neelsen (ZN) stain. Contact with mycobacteria leads either to a protective response associated with resolution

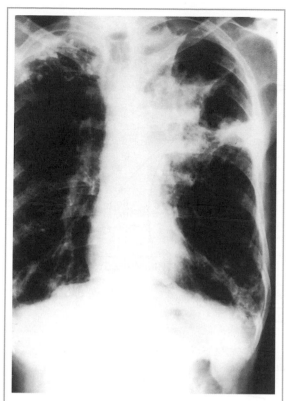

Fig. T10 Chest radiograph showing cavitation at left apex.

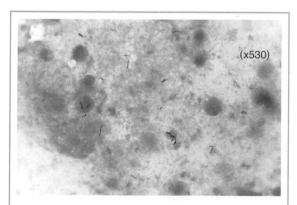

(×530)

Fig. T11 ZN stain showing presence of acid-fast (red) bacilli.

Table T7 Mycobacteria causing disease

Mycobacterial species	Disease
M. avium	Disseminated disease in AIDS patients
M. kansasii	Tuberculosis and disseminated disease in AIDS patients
M. xenopi	Tuberculosis and soft-tissue infections associated with endoscope disinfector contamination
M. ulcerans	Buruli ulcer
M. scrofulaceum	Lymphadenitis
M. marinum	'Fish-tank' granuloma
M. chelonei/fortuitum	Soft-tissue infections associated with endoscope disinfector contamination

of disease or a tissue-destructive response; these different responses may be activated by separate mycobacterial antigens. *M. tuberculosis* is spread mainly by droplet infection, rarely nowadays by ingestion, and initial contact with the tubercle bacillus in the lungs gives rise to primary tuberculosis.

Pathology

Bacilli are taken up into alveolar macrophages, stimulating a local inflammatory reaction with recruitment of further macrophages. The bacilli are transported to the regional lymph nodes in the macrophages, which are then activated by CD4 T-cells, IFNγ and vitamin D3. In some cases the activated macrophages are able to kill the mycobacteria but some bacteria remain viable. The focal pulmonary lesion is called the Ghon focus and this, with the regional lymphadenopathy, is the primary complex. At this stage the bacilli may be circulated to other organs of the body, e.g. brain, bone, kidneys, within the macrophages. In the majority of cases the protective response occurs with areas of focal infection contained by granuloma formation. A granuloma consists of a central area of necrotic tissue surrounded by epithelioid cells, giant cells (fused macrophages) and lymphocytes and encapsulated by fibrous tissue. Cytokines such as TNF are important for granuloma formation. The majority of the bacilli are killed, although some may survive within the granuloma to cause post-primary tuberculosis later in life. About 2 months after exposure to the bacillus, delayed hypersensitivity to mycobacterial antigens develops, which is the basis of the Mantoux test. Reactivation of disease may occur at any time and usually presents, as in this case, with the principal damage occurring in the well-oxygenated apices of the lungs, leading to extensive caseous necrosis. Tissue destruction is mediated in part by TNF released by activated macrophages and leads to cavity formation in the lungs. With the abundant supply of oxygen, the tubercle bacilli proliferate in the walls of the cavity and large numbers of organisms may be expectorated in sputum, thus potentially infecting another person (Fig. T12).

T

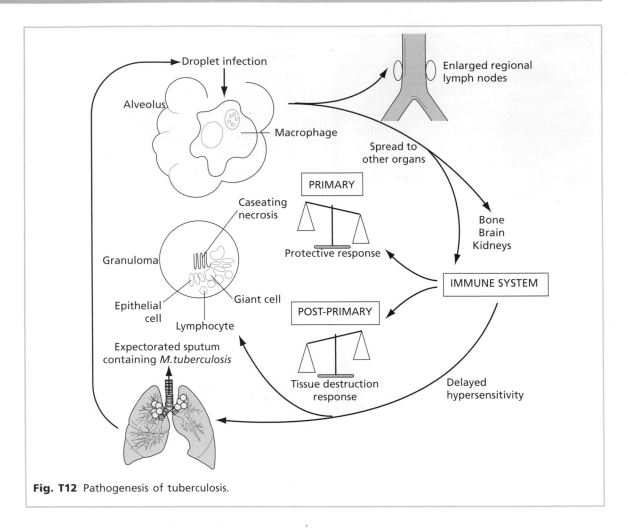

Fig. T12 Pathogenesis of tuberculosis.

Laboratory diagnosis is by ZN stain (or auramine, which is an equivalent stain) of sputum or other appropriate specimen, isolation on Lowenstein–Jensen (LJ) medium or detection by the ligase chain reaction (similar to PCR). It is worth noting that *M. tuberculosis* is very slow growing and can take 2–4 weeks to give visible colonies on LJ medium. More rapid detection is possible by growth in liquid medium and its detection by the evolution of labelled $^{14}CO_2$ from ^{14}C-palmitic acid.

Management
Management includes source isolation (when in hospital for the first 2 weeks of treatment), contact tracing (if appropriate), notification to the relevant authority (as it is a statutorily notifiable disease) and antibiotics. The usual regimen is a combination of rifampicin, isoniazid and pyrazinamide for 2 months followed by a combination of rifampicin and isoniazid for a further 4 months.

TUBEROUS SCLEROSIS: An autosomal dominant syndrome characterized by the development of cortical hamartomas in the brain, renal angio-myolipomas, retinal hamartomas, cardiac and pulmonary myomas, and skin lesions.

TULARAEMIA: Infection with *Francisella tularensis*.

Aetiology and risk factors
Tularaemia has a worldwide distribution. It is widespread in animals and is a zoonosis acquired by direct contact with an infected animal or following a tick bite.

Pathology
The organism multiplies at the site of inoculation, spreading to the regional lymph nodes and via the bloodstream to many organs. It is an intracellular parasite and can survive in macrophages (by preventing phagolysosome fusion) and also in other cell types, e.g. endothelial cells.

There are several clinical presentations:
- typhoidal: acute onset of systemic symptoms with high fever, headache, myalgia, cough and diarrhoea; absence of regional lymphadeno-pathy;

- ulceroglandular: ulceration at the site of inoculation and regional lymphadenopathy;
- glandular: regional lymphadenopathy only;
- oculoglandular: corneal ulcers and regional lymphadenopathy;
- pneumonic: systemic symptoms, cough, pleuritic chest pain, mediastinal lymphadenopathy;
- pharyngeal: sore throat, pharyngeal ulcers, enlarged cervical nodes.

Diagnosis is by serology although the organism can be cultured with difficulty. Treatment is with streptomycin.

TYPHOID FEVER: Infection with *Salmonella typhi*.

Case

Shortly after returning from his elective period in India, a 24-year-old medical student became unwell with a cough, temperature and constipation. Several days later his condition deteriorated and he developed diarrhoea. He was admitted to hospital where he was noted to have a rash and splenomegaly. A blood culture, faeces, chest radiograph and full blood count were ordered and he was placed in source isolation.

Haematology: Hb 10 g/dl; WBC 4000 × 10^6/l; differential normal.
Radiology: chest radiograph showed patchy consolidation in both bases.
Microbiology: blood cultures and faeces both yielded *Salmonella typhi* (Figs T13, T14).

Aetiology and risk factors

Salmonella is a Gram-negative rod and the genus consists of *Salmonella enteritidis*, which can be subdivided into about 200 named serovars and

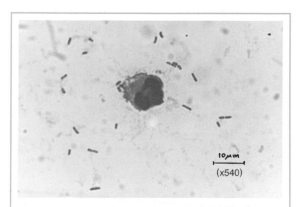

Fig. T13 Gram stain of blood culture showing Gram-negative bacilli.

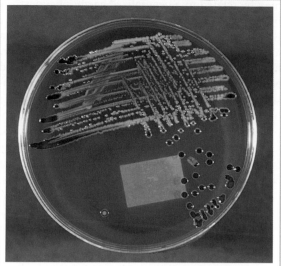

Fig. T14 Culture of faeces showing black colonies of *Salm. typhi* due to the production of H$_2$S.

which are the cause of gastroenteritis; *Salmonella typhi*, which is the cause of typhoid fever, and *Salmonella paratyphi* species, which cause paratyphoid fever. Typhoid and paratyphoid fever are clinically similar and are generally called enteric fever. *Salmonella typhi* carries a virulence plasmid similar to that carried by *Yersinia* species. Important virulence properties of *Salm. typhi* are the proteins involved in penetration of the macrophage, which acts as a sanctuary for the organism, the lipopolysaccharide and a surface antigen (Vi antigen), which masks the organism from the host immune defences. Infection is acquired by drinking contaminated water or eating contaminated food. The infection is endemic in many tropical countries and is associated with poor sanitary conditions and lack of clean potable water supplies.

Pathology

The bacteria penetrate to the lamina propria of the intestine by passage through the M cells overlying the gut-associated lymphoid tissue (Peyer patches) in the small intestine. They are ingested by macrophages, inducing pinocytosis and preventing acidification of the phagosome, where they are able to multiply intracellularly. They are then spread through the lymphatics to the bloodstream, where they seed the reticuloendothelial system and the bone marrow. Here they undergo further multiplication either within the cells of the reticuloendothelial system or possibly in the parenchymal cells of the liver, leading to a second bacteraemia. The ability to induce pinocytosis by macrophages

T

may be related to a generalized haemophagocytosis by macrophages occurring in the bone marrow, which in turn may be responsible for the anaemia and neutropenia often seen in typhoid fever. Furthermore, by penetrating macrophages and endothelial cells, the salmonellae avoid phagocytosis by PMNs, which rapidly kill the organism. The organisms are spread throughout the body to many other organs such as the bones, lungs and kidneys. Continued multiplication in the Peyer patches may eventually lead to necrosis and perforation. Other complications include cholecystitis, pyelonephritis, osteomyelitis, pneumonia and splenic rupture. A small number of patients become chronic carriers of *Salm. typhi* in their gastrointestinal tract. Laboratory diagnosis is by isolation from the appropriate specimen, usually blood culture or faeces.

Management

Management is with an antibiotic, usually ciprofloxacin, and it is a notifiable disease.

TYPHUS: Systemic infection with rickettsial sp.

 Rickettsial disease

T

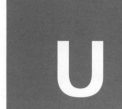

ULCERATIVE COLITIS: A chronic, ulcerating, inflammatory disease of the colon affecting the mucosa and submucosa of the rectum and often the rest of the proximal colon in a contiguous fashion.

Case

A 38-year-old woman presented with a complaint of diarrhoea for the last week. She had had a similar episode 6 months ago, which lasted for 3 weeks. This time she had noticed the presence of blood and mucus-like material in the stool and was concerned. The frequency of stools was also increased, reaching 15 on some days. She described lower abdominal discomfort and pain and felt generally weak and ill.

On examination she was dehydrated with increased skin turgor and dry mucous membranes. Her pulse was 110 beats/min, temperature 37.8°C, respiratory rate 18/min and blood pressure 110/60 mmHg. There was ill-defined lower abdominal sensitivity on palpation.

In the absence of any microbiological explanation for the diarrhoea, a rectosigmoidoscopy was performed. This showed hyperaemia in the rectal

Haematology: Hb 90 g/l; Hct 30%; WBC 1.3×10^9/l; 80% neutrophils; ESR 62 mm/h.
Microbiology: direct microscopic examination of the stool; no parasites or amoebae identified.
Stool cultures: no pathogenic organisms identified.

mucosa, loss of normal vascular pattern and numerous superficial ulcers and foci of bleeding.

Several colonic biopsies were obtained.

Histopathology: colonic biopsies showed ulceration and active chronic inflammation of the colonic mucosa characterized by distortion of glandular architecture, goblet cell depletion, a diffuse inflammatory infiltrate in the lamina propria, numerous crypt abscesses and foci of ulceration (Fig. U1).

The patient was treated with steroids in the acute phase. She responded well and the symptoms subsided. However, the disease relapsed after 6 months despite maintenance treatment with sulphasalazine. This episode was characterized by severe symptoms and severe inflammation involving the whole colon. No response was obtained by steroids and a total colectomy was performed to control the disease.

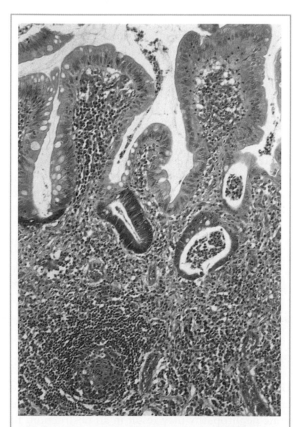

Fig. U1 Histological appearances of colonic mucosa in ulcerative colitis showing distortion of glandular architecture, goblet cell depletion, a diffuse inflammatory infiltrate in lamina propria and numerous crypt abscesses.

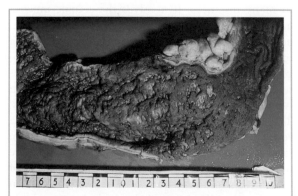

Fig. U2 Macroscopic appearances of ulcerative colitis resection specimen. Note the irregular mucosal surface.

Histopathology: colectomy specimen showed severe ulcerative colitis involving diffusely the whole of the colonic mucosa and submucosa (Fig. U2).

Aetiology and risk factors

The aetiology of ulcerative colitis is not known. No infectious agent has so far been identified. The florid inflammation is thought to be secondary to an antibody-mediated immune response to as yet unknown antigens. The strong association between ulcerative colitis and primary sclerosing cholangitis support a role for misdirected immune response. The disease predominantly affects young adults and is more common in females than males and in Caucasians than blacks.

Pathology

Ulcerative colitis and Crohn disease are both chronic inflammatory bowel diseases. In ulcerative colitis, although the disease is localized to the colon, it is always associated with systemic as well as local symptoms and signs. Acute phase reactants and inflammatory mediators released from the inflamed colon lead to the development of fever and increased ESR, and loss of blood through chronic colonic bleeding may cause anaemia, as observed in this patient. Locally the inflammatory process destroys the mucosal epithelium, leading to diarrhoea, secondary to decreased water absorption and bleeding, secondary to exposure of mucosal blood vessels. The reasons for epithelial damage are not clear, but proteases released by activated macrophages and cytotoxic cytokines such as TNFα released by the macrophages are thought to be critical.

The inflammation in ulcerative colitis, in contrast to Crohn disease*, always starts from the rectum and extends proximally, affecting the whole colon in many instances. It involves the colonic mucosa and submucosa but not the deeper layers. In the active phase, the inflammatory cells comprise a mixture of lymphocytes, plasma cells, macrophages, neutrophils and eosinophils. Characteristically, collections of neutrophils are seen within the crypt lumina, forming crypt abscesses. The goblet cells are depleted of their mucin as a result of excessive secretion due to inflammation. Granulomas, the hallmark of Crohn disease, are not observed in ulcerative colitis. The diagnosis of ulcerative colitis requires a close interaction between the clinician and the pathologist and can only be made in the presence of characteristic clinical features, histopathology and negative microbiological investigations.

Although in most instances the inflammation can be controlled with medical treatment, sometimes extensive inflammatory reaction associated with pan-colonic involvement may necessitate surgery as observed in this case. A rare but life-threatening complication of ulcerative colitis is development of toxic dilatation of the colon. This occurs as a result of toxic damage to the muscularis propria; the nerves and neuromuscular unit cannot operate and acute dilatation of the colonic wall results. Emergency total colectomy is the treatment of choice. Histology shows extensive necrosis of the mucosa and gangrene of the bowel wall.

The disease usually has a prolonged natural history with remissions and relapses. In remission, the histology of the colon shows a mild chronic inflammatory infiltrate in the lamina propria and atrophic changes in the mucosal glands. No acute neutrophils or crypt abscesses are seen. An important complication of long-standing ulcerative colitis is development of colorectal carcinoma. The risk seems to be highest in patients with pan-colitis for 10 or more years.

Management

The management depends on the severity of disease. Medical treatment includes administration of local and systemic steroids and sulphasalazine. Those patients who fail to respond to medical treatment may require colectomy.

 Crohn disease

URAEMIA: An elevation in serum urea levels (reference range 3.3–6.7 mmol/l). The term is often used synonymously with renal failure. The term azotaemia refers to the retention of nitrogenous waste products, including urea and creatinine.

A number of factors will cause an increase in blood urea levels, e.g.:

- increased production from a high protein diet; increased catabolism (surgery, infection, trauma); steroid therapy; tetracycline usage
- decreased excretion from glomerular disease; reduced renal blood flow (hypotension, dehydration); urinary obstruction; nephritis.

URATE NEPHROPATHY: The deposition of urate crystals in the kidney tubules. In gout, an acute urate nephropathy may result in an obstruction. In patients with chronic gout, this accumulation of urate crystals in the kidney produces a tubulointerstitial inflammation and subsequently fibrotic changes; the clinical presentations are usually mild and gradual.

URETHRITIS: Infection of the urethra, the two main causes being *Neisseria gonorrhoeae* and *Chlamydia trachomatis*.

 Chlamydial disease; Gonorrhoea; Pelvic inflammatory disease

URTICARIA: A common disorder characterized by recurring episodes of dermal oedema and clinically by itchy wheals. In general, any substance producing a sudden increase in local vascular permeability can cause urticaria. Oedema occurring in the deep dermis, subcutaneous tissues, or mucous membranes, is called angioedema and often coexists with urticaria. Acute urticaria is caused by mast-cell degranulation, which can be of immune or non-immune origin (Table U1). Urticaria lasting for more than 2 months (chronic) may have a physical cause (e.g. exposure to cold, heat, etc.) but in most cases the cause is unknown.

Table U1 Causes of acute urticaria

Immune mechanisms (40%)	Non-Immune mechanisms (60%)
Type I hypersensitivity (IgE)	Direct activation of mast cells by: physical stimuli, antibiotics, acetylcholine
Atopy Type III hypersensitivity (immune complexes; complement)	

Management
Treatment with antihistamines is generally more effective for acute than for chronic urticaria. Corticosteroids can suppress the chronic state.

UVEITIS: Inflammation of the iris, ciliary body or choroid.

Case
A 26-year-old, HIV-positive homosexual male attended the STD clinic complaining of blurred vision and the presence of 'floaters' in the eye. On examination it was noted that there was a loss of visual acuity and a diminution of the peripheral fields. Visualization of the retina showed localized diffuse opacities and a diagnosis of retinitis caused by cytomegalovirus was made.

Table U2 Causes of uveitis

Non-infectious	Infectious
Sarcoidosis	Cytomegalovirus
Reiter syndrome	Herpes simplex virus
Still disease	Toxoplasmosis
Ankylosing spondylitis	Toxocariasis
Behçet syndrome	Tuberculosis

Aetiology and risk factors
Inflammation of the eye can occur in the anterior uveal tract (iritis or iridocyclitis) or in the posterior chamber (retinitis). In some cases a pan-uveitis may develop. The causes can be infectious or non-infectious; some examples are shown in Table U2.

Cytomegalovirus is a herpesvirus and the commonest cause of retinitis in AIDS* patients. It is usually acquired in childhood by direct contact with secretions from an infected person.

Pathology
The primary cell target is the white blood cell and infection can be transmitted by blood transfusion. This is particularly important in transplant patients. CMV binds to the host cell protein $\beta2$-microglobulin, which acts as a receptor for the virus. As with other herpesviruses, it remains dormant in the target cell and becomes reactivated when the cell-mediated immune defences become compromised. Replication of the virus occurs in the retinal pigment epithelial cells with spread to adjacent cells through the lateral membrane. This leads to cell death and desquamation into the vitreous, giving rise to the symptoms of decreased visual acuity and the presence of 'floaters'. In addition to retinitis in AIDS patients, CMV can cause oesophagitis, colitis or pneumonitis. In addition, it can cause a mononucleosis-like picture (see Glandular fever) in adults and congenital malformations following intrauterine infection. Laboratory diagnosis is by isolation of the virus, immunofluorescent detection of early antigen expression on infected cells, detection by PCR or the presence of the characteristic 'owl-eye' intranuclear inclusion in histopathological sections. Serology can be used as a screening test. Treatment is with ganciclovir or foscarnet.

U

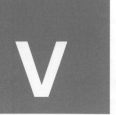

VACCINATION: Strictly, immunization against smallpox using vaccinia, but generally used synonymously with immunization*.

VAGINITIS: Inflammation of the vagina.

Aetiology and risk factors
Vaginitis can be caused principally by *Candida* (see Candidiasis) or by *Trichomonas vaginalis*, a flagellate protozoon. The latter is a sexually transmitted disease. The protozoa may be found in asymptomatic females and are often asymptomatic in males.

Pathology
Adhesion of *T. vaginalis* to the vaginal epithelial cells is an important first step in pathogenesis of disease. The trophozoite can engulf bacteria and erythrocytes and appears to lyse vaginal epithelial cells by direct contact, giving rise to micro-ulceration. Vaginitis due to *T. vaginalis* is characterized by a frothy vaginal discharge and pruritus. Laboratory diagnosis is by microscopy and culture. It is treated with metronidazole.

 Bacterial vaginosis

VARICELLA: An exanthem caused by the varicella-zoster virus.

 Chickenpox

VASCULITIS: Primary inflammation of blood vessels.

Aetiology and risk factors
The vasculitides form a large group of diseases caused by a variety of mechanisms. In some cases, vasculitis is caused by infectious agents such as bacteria, rickettsia, fungi or viruses. However, in most instances vasculitis is immunologically mediated. The pathogenesis varies according to the inducing process. Deposition of immune complexes to the vessel wall, direct antibody attack, and cell-mediated immunity have all been shown to play a role. In some cases, vasculitis is associated with circulating antineutrophil antibodies.

Pathology
The pathological findings vary depending on the cause of the vasculitis and the size and site of the vessels involved. Vasculitis can be classified into three groups according the size of the vessels involved:

Large vessel vasculitis
- Giant cell arteritis: see separate entry.
- Takayasu arteritis: a rare granulomatous vasculitis involving the aorta and other large vessels, predominantly affecting young adult females.
- Temporal arteritis

Medium-sized vessel vasculitis
- Polyarteritis nodosa: see separate entry.

Small vessel vasculitis
- Microscopic polyarteritis: necrotizing vasculitis involving medium- to small-sized vessels in the skin, mucosa, lungs, kidneys, heart or brain. Microscopically there is fibrinoid necrosis of the vessel wall with accumulation of neutrophils. In most instances fragmentation of neutrophils (leucocytoclasis) is seen. This histological finding is described as leukocytoclastic vasculitis. The disease usually develops secondary to immune reaction against foreign material such as drugs, infectious agents or heterologous proteins. Elimination of the offending agent results in resolution in many cases.
- Wegener granulomatosis: see separate entry.
- Henoch–Schönlein purpura: see separate entry.
- Cold agglutinin disease: see separate entry.
- Churg–Strauss syndrome: see separate entry.

Management
Vasculitis resulting from infection is treated with appropriate antimicrobial therapy. Immune-based vasculitis is treated with steroids.

VENO-OCCLUSIVE DISEASE: A disease of the liver characterized by endothelial swelling and perivenular fibrosis in the hepatic vein branches, usually secondary to toxic damage. In the long term, obliteration of hepatic vein branches and outflow obstruction develop.

VINCENT ANGINA: A severe necrotizing gingivitis with a characteristic overgrowth of *Fusobacterium* sp. and oral spirochaetes, presenting with bleeding gums, pain and halitosis.

VIRAL HAEMORRHAGIC FEVER: Infection caused by a number of different viruses, in which haemorrhagic manifestations are prominent features in the clinical presentation.

Table V1 Major viral haemorrhagic diseases

Virus	Vector	Geography
Yellow fever virus	Mosquito	S. America, Africa
Dengue types 1–4	Mosquito	Asia, S. America, S. Africa, India
Kyasanur forest virus	Mosquito	India
Omsk HF virus	Tick	Former Soviet Union
Crimean-Congo virus	Tick	Africa and former Soviet Union
Hantaan virus	Rodent excreta	USA, Far East
Lassa fever virus	Mouse excreta	Africa
Argentinian and Bolivian	Mouse excreta	S. America
Ebola virus	Unknown	Africa
Marburg disease	Unknown	Africa

Table V2 Aetiology of viral hepatitis

Virus	Route of infection	Incubation period (days)	Chronicity cirrhosis hepatoma
HVA	1 Faeco-oral 2 Food - shellfish	15–45	No
HVB	1 Parenteral – blood products, IVDU 2 Sexual contact 3 At birth	30–180	Yes
HVC	As HVB	15–150	Yes
HVD	As HVB	?	Yes
HVE	Faeco-oral	15–60	No

Aetiology and risk factors
Table V1 lists the major viral haemorrhagic diseases.

Pathology
These diseases usually present with fever, sometimes a pharyngitis, rash, myalgia and haemorrhagic manifestations of varying severity. There is usually a leucopenia and thrombocytopenia. In **yellow fever** there is a mid-zonal hepatic necrosis with eosinophilic degeneration of the hepatocytes, the patient developing jaundice and haemorrhages. There is an associated acute tubular necrosis and a myocarditis. Haemorrhagic manifestations occur in **dengue** in individuals who have already been infected previously with one of the other dengue virus types. The uptake of the virus into the macrophage-monocyte lineage is aided by the anti-dengue antibodies, which may lead to release of mediators of increased vascular permeability. There is hypovolaemia, disseminated intravascular coagulation and shock. In **Lassa fever** there is little evidence of hepatic damage, although an inhibitor of platelet function has been detected in patient's sera. There is no evidence of DIC. The patient shows hypovolaemia and CNS involvement. Less is known about the pathogenesis of the other haemorrhagic fever viruses.

There is a highly effective attenuated vaccine against yellow fever.

VIRAL HEPATITIS: Infection of the liver caused by a number of different viruses, some of which are specifically hepatotropic whilst others may cause hepatitis as part of a wider illness, e.g. yellow fever virus, EBV, CMV, Lassa fever virus.

Aetiology and risk factors
See Table V2.

Two more recently discovered hepatotropic viruses are hepatitis virus F (HVF) and hepatitis virus G (HVG or GB-C).

Pathology
Infection by the hepatitis viruses leads to disruption of the normal architecture of the liver sinusoids, ballooning of some cells, eosinophilic degeneration of others, leading to the formation of hyaline bodies, and hepatocellular necrosis. There is a lymphocytic cell infiltration with few polymorphs and evidence of cholestasis. The areas of necrosis can be few and widely scattered and there may be bridging necrosis between areas of necrosis in different portal zones or, in more severe cases, multilobular necrosis. The patient may complain of general malaise, anorexia, nausea, pain and tenderness over the liver, which may be slightly enlarged some days before the icteric phase starts, when the patient becomes jaundiced with dark urine and pale faeces. In some cases the infection can be anicteric and the patient has a non-specific flu-like illness whilst in others there may be immune-complex-type manifestations of fever, rash and arthralgia. Laboratory investigations show a large increase in serum alanine aminotransferase (ALT) and aspartate aminotransferase (AST) (markers of hepatocellular necrosis), milder elevation of serum alkaline phosphatase and γ-glutamyltransferase (markers of obstruction) and variable elevation of both conjugated and unconjugated bilirubin. The peripheral white cell count is usually normal to slight leucopenia and in the absence of complications the INR and platelet count are normal. Laboratory diagnosis is by serology and PCR.

Management

The management of acute viral hepatitis is supportive as specific antiviral agents do not exist. Prevention is by passive immunization or, in the case of hepatitis A and B, by vaccination.

 Hepatitis B infection

VIRAL MENINGITIS: The commonest cause of meningitis (adenoviruses, coxsackieviruses, enteroviruses). Clinically indistinguishable from bacterial meningitis (see Meningococcal meningitis) and characterized by a lymphocytic response in the CSF compared to a neutrophil response as occurs with bacterial meningitis. A lymphocytic response in the CSF can also be found with cryptococcal and tuberculous meningitis.

VISCERAL LARVA MIGRANS: An infection with the nematode *Toxocara* which migrates to all organs of the body including the CNS and eye and which may lead to blindness.

VITAMIN DEFICIENCIES: Vitamin deficiency is a consequence of inadequate fat-soluble (A, D, E, K) or water-soluble (B1, B2, niacin, B6, pantothenic acid, biotin, B12, folic acid, C) vitamin levels in the body.

Aetiology and risk factors

Vitamin deficiency is commonly seen in the developing world in patients with protein energy malnu-

Table V3 Clinical consequences of fat- and water-soluble vitamin deficiency

Vitamin	Clinical feature
A (retinol)	Xerophthalmia, night blindness, keratomalacia, follicular keratosis
D (cholecalciferol)	Rickets, osteomalacia
E (α-tocopherol)	Ataxia
K	Bleeding disorders
B1 (thiamine)	Beriberi
B2 (riboflavin)	Angular stomatitis
Niacin	Pellegra
B6 (pyridoxine)	Peripheral neuropathy
Pantothenic acid	
Biotin	Dermatitis
B12 (cobalamin)	Megaloblastic anaemia, neurological disorders
Folic acid	Megaloblastic anaemia
C (ascorbic acid)	Scurvy

trition. The following are some causes of vitamin deficiency in developed countries:
- decreased production: renal disease (vitamin D), drugs such as methotrexate (folic acid).
- decreased intake: alcohol abuse (vitamin B1), small bowel disease (folic acid, fat soluble vitamins), vegans (vitamin D, B12), elderly (vitamin D, folic acid), long-term parenteral nutrition (all vitamins).
- decreased absorption: liver and biliary tract disease (vitamins A, D, E, K), ileal disease/resection (vitamin B12).

Pathology

The clinical consequences of deficiency of the fat- and water-soluble vitamins are shown in Table V3.

Management

Management is by the correction of predisposing factors and/or vitamin replacement.

VON HIPPLE–LINDAU DISEASE: An autosomal dominant inherited disease. Affected individuals develop tumours of the cerebellum (haemangioblastoma) and retina and cysts in pancreas, liver and kidneys.

VON RECKLINGHAUSEN DISEASE: See Neurofibromatosis.

VON WILLEBRAND DISEASE (VWD): A bleeding disorder due to quantitative or qualitative deficiency of von Willebrand factor (vWF), usually inherited as an autosomal dominant disorder. It is the commonest inherited bleeding disorder in the UK.

Pathology

vWF is coded for by a gene on chromosome 12 and is produced in endothelial cells and megakaryocytes. vWF has two functions in haemostasis. It is a protective carrier for coagulation factor VIII, without which factor VIII is continually being subjected to degradation. Coagulation factor VIII levels are therefore reduced in vWD, though not usually to the low levels found in classical haemophilia. vWF also provides the link between platelets and vascular subendothelium by bridging between platelet membrane glycoprotein I and collagen. Thus the clinical manifestations of von Willebrand disease are platelet-type bleeding with purpura, nosebleeds, and menorrhagia rather than deep muscular haematoma and haemarthrosis seen in clotting factor deficiencies such as haemophilia* and Christmas disease.

vWF circulates as variable-sized polymers or multimers. von Willebrand disease may be subdivided into three types. Type 1 is a modest quantitative deficiency of vWF. Type 2 is a qualitative deficiency with various subtypes depending on the size of the circulating multimers and their functional characteristics. Type 3 is a rare severe deficiency of vWF and is autosomal recessive in inheritance.

Investigations in vWD will usually show a moderately reduced level of coagulation factor VIII, a low vWF (usually measured by an immunological assay, hence called vWF antigen) and a prolonged bleeding time. The platelet count is usually normal except in the rare type 2B disease where the abnormal vWF structure gives it increased affinity for platelets, resulting in formation of platelet aggregates *in vivo*.

Management

Mild types of vWD respond to desmopressin (DDAVP), a synthetic ADH analogue which causes release of stored vWF and factor VIII from endothelial cells. Repeated injections of DDAVP are less effective as stores of vWF are depleted.

As factor VIII is carried by vWF, most low and intermediate purity preparations of factor VIII concentrate contain useful amounts of vWF and can be used in the treatment of vWD. High purity and recombinant factor VIII concentrates do not contain vWF.

Cryoprecipitate contains vWF, but this blood product is not subjected to heat-detergent viral inactivation during its production.

V

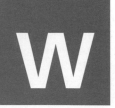

WAGR SYNDROME: A syndrome characterized by development of Wilms tumour, aniridia, genital abnormalities and mental retardation. Most of the affected individuals have a sporadic chromosomal deletion of genetic material from 11p13 which involves a gene for aniridia as well as the nearby Wilms tumour associated gene, *WT-1*.

 Wilms tumour.

WALDENSTRÖM DISEASE: A disorder lying half-way between chronic lymphocytic leukaemia* and myeloma*. The blood and bone marrow contain B-lymphocytes resembling plasma cells (lymphoplasmacytoid lymphocytes) (Fig. W1) and a paraprotein is produced which is usually of IgM type (in myeloma the paraprotein is most commonly of IgG type). As in chronic lymphocytic leukaemia, a generalized lymphadenopathy is usual, but hypercalcaemia and bone pain are rarely seen. Plasma hyperviscosity syndrome is common.

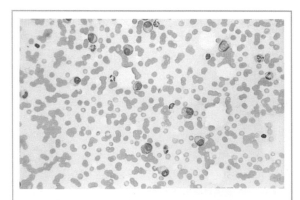

Fig. W1 Blood film showing lymphoplasmacytoid lymphocytes in Waldenström disease.

WARM AUTOIMMUNE HAEMOLYTIC ANAEMIA (WAIHA): Antibody-mediated destruction of red cells by an autoantibody that works best at body temperature (cf. cold agglutinins* which work best at lower temperatures). All the general features of haemolytic anaemia* may be present.

The anaemia may be macrocytic, reflecting the increased numbers of young red cells present, and the reticulocyte count increased. When the anaemia is severe, nucleated red cells may be present in the peripheral blood. Spherocytes are commonly found on the blood film. The spleen, a principal site of red cell destruction, may be palpably enlarged.

The red cells are coated with an antibody that is most commonly IgG and the direct antiglobulin (Coombs') test is positive. *In vivo*, this antibody opsonizes the red cells, making them attractive to the phagocytes of the reticuloendothelial system. Free antibody may be present in the plasma, making compatibility tests for blood transfusion difficult as all red cells will be incompatible with the patient's plasma, including the patient's own red cells. It is often necessary to set up many blood donations of the correct blood group and select those that are least incompatible for transfusion. When free antibody is not present in the patient's plasma it may still be obtained for investigation by displacing it from the red cell surface by a process known as elution. The autoantibody is usually directed against a core antigen of the Rhesus system present on all normal red cells, but absent on the very rare Rhesus null red cells that are devoid of Rhesus antigens.

Occasionally, a specificity may be established for the autoantibody, that is to say, the antibody will react with cells carrying a particular antigen such as c or D. In these cases, there is the possibility of selecting blood units for transfusion that may be destroyed less readily than the patient's own red cells that bear that antigen.

Causes of WAIHA
- Idiopathic: about 50% of cases.
- Drugs. The commonest offenders are α-methyl-dopa, mefenamic acid and high doses of benzylpenicillin. Sometimes the drug is absorbed onto the red cell surface to form a new antigen against which an immune attack is mounted; sometimes antibodies react directly with the drug and immune complexes are absorbed onto the red cell resulting in its destruction. Occasionally there is a modification of the body's immune reactivity by the drug.
- Associated with other autoimmune diseases such as systemic lupus erythematosus and rheumatoid arthritis.
- Associated with low-grade B-cell lymphoproliferative disorders such as chronic lymphocytic leukaemia*, non-Hodgkin lymphoma*.
Treatment with the cytotoxic agent fludarabine may predispose to the development of WAIHA

in chronic lymphocytic leukaemia by affecting the balance of helper and suppressor T-cells.

Management of WAIHA

For drug-induced WAIHA, the offending drug should be withdrawn. Immunosuppression with steroids such as prednisolone is the mainstay of treatment in idiopathic WAIHA. As the spleen forms the main site of red cell destruction in most cases, splenectomy may be beneficial in WAIHA resistant to steroids. In patients unfit for splenectomy, other immunosuppressive agents such as azathioprine or cyclosporin may be useful. Blood transfusion should be avoided if possible, because of the problems alluded to above. As in any case of haemolytic anaemia, folate supplements may help maintain haemoglobin levels.

WARTS: Infection of squamous epithelium by papilloma virus, e.g. types 1, 2, 3, 4 and 7. Other papilloma viruses (e.g. 6, 11, 16, 18 and 57) are associated with genital warts and cervical carcinoma (see Cervical carcinoma). The viral DNA is found in the basal cells of the epithelium and whole viruses in the terminally differentiated keratinocyte.

Pathology

The wart virus causes hypertrophy of all layers of the dermis, vacuolation of cells, which also have enlarged nuclei (koilocytes), elongation of the rete and hyperkeratosis of the stratum corneum, resulting in the formation of a papilloma with a horny surface. The patient can exhibit raised verrucous or flat lesions usually on the hands (common and planar warts), finger-like lesions usually on the eyelids (filiform warts), flat non-raised lesions on the soles (plantar warts), or moist, reddish cauliflower-like lesions on the genitals (condyloma acuminatum). The plantar warts are often painful. Immunosuppressed patients, e.g. renal transplant recipients, commonly develop warts during immunosuppression. Rarely, multiple warts (HPV 6 and 11) may develop in the respiratory mucosa, usually the larynx; this may occur in children (acquired during childbirth from an infected mother) or an adult (acquired sexually) and is called recurrent respiratory papillomatosis. The patients present with stridor. Laboratory diagnosis is by histology, electron microscopy, PCR or DNA hybridization. Treatment is with topical keratolytics, e.g. podophyllin, electrodiathermy, or cryotherapy.

WATERHOUSE–FRIDERICHSEN SYNDROME: Acute adrenal failure occurring in septic shock.

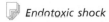 *Endotoxic shock*

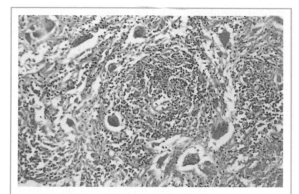

Fig. W2 A characteristic necrotizing granuloma in the lung of a patient with WG.

WEGENER GRANULOMATOSIS: A disease with characteristic necrotizing vasculitis within granulomas of the lung (Fig. W2), necrotizing glomerulonephritis and variable small vessel vasculitis. Autoantibodies to cytoplasmic antigens in neutrophils (c-ANCA, classical antineutrophil cytoplasmic antibodies) are present in 90% of cases and are of diagnostic value. Staining with ANCA shows two different cytoplasmic patterns by immunofluorescence: a cytoplasmic pattern (cANCA) or a 'peripheral' pattern (pANCA). These autoantibodies bind mainly to serine protease II and myeloperoxidase, respectively.

This is one of several forms of vasculitis involving the lung and is fatal if untreated (usually with steroids and cyclophosphamide, which appears to cure 90% of patients). Churg–Strauss syndrome or allergic granulomatosis is a related but rare multisystem disorder in young adults, in which asthma and systemic vasculitis are associated with eosinophilia.

WEIL DISEASE: A severe form of leptospirosis with hepatic and renal failure.

 Leptospirosis

WERNICKE–KORSAKOFF SYNDROME: A clinical syndrome characterized by psychotic symptoms and memory disturbances.

The syndrome is caused by an encephalopathy which develops secondary to thiamine deficiency. It is seen most commonly in chronic alcoholism. Histologically there is haemorrhage and necrosis in the mamillary bodies and damage in the thalamus.

WHIPPLE DISEASE: An uncommon condition affecting principally the small intestine, although any organ can be involved. The condition is characterized by fatty deposits in the affected organ and

W

regional lymph nodes. The intestine is thickened with blunting of the villi and dilated lymphatics, and infiltrated with characteristic foamy macrophages that stain a bright purple with PAS. A Gram-positive bacterium, phylogenically related to *Actinomyces* and called *Tropheryma whippelii*, can be found in the affected tissue, although its relationship to pathogenesis is uncertain. The patient presents with fever, diarrhoea, weight loss, hyperpigmentation of the skin and arthralgia, which is migratory and affects peripheral joints. There may be generalized lymphadenopathy and an iron- or folate-deficiency anaemia. Eosinophilia and thrombocytosis may occur. Complications include neurological, pulmonary, ocular and cardiac involvement and a protein-losing enteropathy. Laboratory diagnosis is by histology or the polymerase chain reaction. Treatment is with penicillin, streptomycin, tetracycline or co-trimoxazole.

WHOOPING COUGH: Infection caused by *Bordetella pertussis* and transmitted by the respiratory route. The infection typically affects children. The organism binds to respiratory ciliated epithelium and inhibits cilial action by the action of a toxin. The main toxin is an ADP-ribosyl transferase similar to diphtheria* toxin. Loss of cilial action allows mucus accumulation and prevents removal of the bacteria which multiply on the epithelial lining There is subepithelial inflammation and, in prolonged infection, loss of ciliated epithelium. Clinically, the patient presents with conjunctivitis, coryza, fever and malaise, which develops into a characteristic cough, followed by a forced inspiration against blocked bronchioles, producing the 'whoop'. There is a peripheral lymphocytosis. Complications can include convulsions due to cerebral haemorrhage or encephalopathy and pneumothorax. Diagnosis is by isolation of the organism and serology. Management includes erythromycin. The disease is preventable by a killed vaccine, which has, however, been blamed, without convincing proof, for fits and permanent brain damage.

WILMS TUMOUR: A malignant tumour of the kidney seen mostly in early childhood; also known as nephroblastoma. It is one of the commonest tumours before the age of 10 years.

Wilms tumour is thought to arise from primitive cells which differentiate to form the kidney in the fetus. Histologically, the tumour mimics the fetal kidney, forming structures similar to primitive glomeruli, which are surrounded by blastema and connective tissue. The *WT-1* gene located on chromosome 11 has been associated with Wilms tumour development. It is a tumour suppressor gene, regulating transcription of some growth factors. In Wilms tumour the gene is lost as a result of deletion or mutation. If untreated, Wilms tumour is an aggressive neoplasm; however, with the development of combination therapy (surgery, radiotherapy, chemotherapy), over 90% of the patients now survive beyond 5 years.

WILSON DISEASE: An inherited disorder of copper metabolism resulting in the deposition of toxic concentrations of copper in various organs. It is also known as hepatolenticular degeneration.

Aetiology and risk factors
Wilson disease is inherited in an autosomal recessive pattern. It manifests itself in young adult life, and is slightly commoner in males.

Pathology
Copper is normally absorbed from the stomach and small intestine; it is bound to ceruloplasmin in the liver and carried in the blood. It is disposed of in bile. In Wilson disease, there is defective excretion of copper into bile, which results in an increase in total body copper, which is deposited in the liver (progressive microvacuolar fatty change and focal necrosis and focal liver cell necrosis, progressing to fibrosis and finally cirrhosis*), in basal ganglia of the brain (lenticular degeneration, producing clinical features of extrapyramidal dysfunction), and in the cornea of the eye (Kayser–Fleischer rings).

The laboratory findings include a low serum ceruloplasmin concentration, increased liver copper (liver biopsy) and an increased urinary copper excretion.

Management
Wilson disease is treated with penicillamine or other chelating agents. In severe cases, liver transplantation has been used successfully.

WISCOTT–ALDRICH SYNDROME: An X-linked disease characterized by thrombocytopenia, eczema and recurrent infections.

Affected males have low numbers of small platelets and develop pyogenic and opportunistic infections. They have increased levels of both IgA and IgE, normal levels of IgG but decreased IgM (and hence blood group isohaemagglutinins are absent). The immune response to polysaccharide antigens is poor. T-cell-mediated immunity is defective and gets worse with disease progression. T-cells have an abnormal appearance and do not form normal interactions with other cells of the immune system.

 Immunodeficiency

XANTHOMA: A benign tumour of the skin composed of collections of macrophages with foamy cytoplasm.

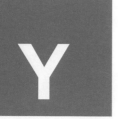

YAWS: A non-venereal treponemal disease of the skin caused by *Treponema pertenue*.

 Treponematosis

YELLOW FEVER: A viral infection affecting the liver.

 Viral haemorrhagic fever

YERSINIOSIS: Infection with *Yersinia* spp.

Aetiology and risk factors

The principal organisms causing infection are *Yersinia enterocolitica* or *Yersinia pseudotuberculosis* (see also Plague, caused by *Yersinia pestis*). The organisms are found widely in the animal kingdom: in farm animals, birds and rodents. Infections are zoonoses, acquired by eating contaminated food or by direct contact with an infected animal.

Pathology

Yersiniae produce proteins associated with invasion into eukaryotic cells, which are expressed when the organism is in the gastrointestinal tract. In addition both species have the Yop virulence cassette carrying the same toxins, affecting cell signalling and the cell cytoskeleton. The organisms show a tropism for lymphoid tissue in the intestine, invading the intestinal cells and causing mucosal ulceration and mesenteric adenitis. In the lymph nodes there is hyperplasia of the lymphoid tissue, the formation of epithelioid granulomas with giant cells with coagulative necrosis in the centre infiltrated by neutrophils. Occasionally septicaemia may occur and the organisms cause abscesses in many organs. There are several different clinical presentations. In the young, *Y. enterocolitica* presents as a dysentery-like illness with fever, diarrhoea, abdominal pain and bloody diarrhoea. Alternatively, the patient may present with an illness resembling acute appendicitis, with fever and right lower quadrant pain. This is a terminal ileitis and mesenteric adenitis and is mostly caused by *Y. pseudotuberculosis*. Focal infections with *Y. enterocolitica* may occur (e.g. skin abscess, pharyngitis) and septicaemia may occur, particularly in association with iron overload (e.g. thalassaemia), cirrhosis or immunosuppression. Complications of *Yersinia* infections include reactive arthritis*, Reiter syndrome* (both more common in HLA-B27 individuals) and erythema nodosum*. Laboratory diagnosis is by serology and isolation of the organism and treatment is usually not required unless there is septicaemia or the patient is immunocompromised, when an aminoglycoside, tetracycline, a quinolone, or a third-generation cephalosporin can be used.

ZOLLINGER–ELLISON SYNDROME: A clinical syndrome comprising peptic ulcer, steatorrhoea and diarrhoea as a result of high serum gastrin.

Aetiology and risk factors
The high gastrin levels are derived from gastrin-secreting tumours, arising mainly from G cells in the pancreas. Sixty per cent of these tumours are malignant. The syndrome is also seen in MEN syndrome*.

Pathology
The overproduction of gastrin causes peptic ulceration and the patients present with recurrent or atypical peptic ulceration, steatorrhoea (due to inhibition of pancreatic lipase by excess gastric acid), diarrhoea (as a result of low pH in the upper gastrointestinal tract) and glucose intolerance. The ulcers occur in the stomach, duodenum and jejunum and are often large and deep. Confirmatory tests of the diagnosis are the presence of a high serum gastrin and a high acid output. Another biochemical abnormality associated with this syndrome is a hypokalaemic metabolic alkalosis.

Management
The treatment is usually a combination of surgical and medical. Where possible, the tumour is resected. Otherwise vagotomy and long-term treatment with H2-receptor antagonists are employed.

ZOONOSIS: Infection acquired from an animal source either directly or via a vector such as an insect. Examples are given in Table Z1.

Table Z1 Examples of zoonoses

Organism	Animal reservoir	Vector
Viruses		
Rabies	Dogs, foxes	
Yellow fever	Monkeys	Mosquito
Encephalitic arbovirus		Mosquito, tick
Lassa fever virus	Mice	
Bacteria		
Bacillus anthracis	Cattle, horses	
Brucella	Cattle, sheep, goats	
Borrelia recurrentis		Tick, louse
Borrelia burgdorferi	Deer	Tick
Chlamydia psittaci	Birds	
Coxiella	Sheep	
Campylobacter	Poultry	
Listeria	Many	
Leptospira	Rats	
Rickettsia		Tick, mite, louse, flea
Salmonella	Poultry	
Streptobacillus	Rats	
Yersinia	Rats	Flea
Fungi		
Microsporium	Dogs	
Parasites		
Leishmania	Dogs, gerbils	Sandfly
Taenia	Cattle, pigs	
Toxoplasma	Cats	
Trichinella	Pigs	
Toxocara	Dogs	
Trypanosoma cruzi		Tsetse fly

APPENDIX 1: ORGANISMS CAUSING THE PRINCIPAL HUMAN INFECTIONS

VIRUSES

DNA

Herpes viruses	1, 2	Herpes simplex
	3	Varicella-zoster
	4	Epstein–Barr virus
	5	Cytomegalovirus
	6, 7, 8	
Poxviruses		(Smallpox)
		Cowpox
		Molluscum contagiosum
		Orf
Hepadnaviruses		Hepatitis B
Adenoviruses		
Parvoviruses		B19
Papovaviruses		Papillomaviruses
		Wart virus
		Polyomavirus

RNA

Retroviruses	HIV-1, 2; HTLV-1, 2
Orthomyxoviruses	Influenza A, B, C
Paramyxoviruses	Measles
	Mumps
	Respiratory syncytial virus
	Parainfluenza
Rhabdoviruses	Rabies
Arboviruses	Togaviruses
	Rubella
	Reoviruses
	Rotavirus
	Bunyavirus
	Hantaan virus
Flaviviruses	Yellow fever, dengue
Coronaviruses	
Arenaviruses	Lassa fever
	Lymphocytic choriomeningitis
Filoviruses	Ebola virus
Picornaviruses	Rhinoviruses
	Enteroviruses
	Polio
	Coxsackie
	ECHO
	Hepatitis A
Calicivirus	

Prions
CJD
Kuru

BACTERIA

Cocci

Gram-positive	Staphylococci
	Streptococci
	Enterococcus
Gram-negative	Neisseria
	meningitides
	gonorrhoeae
	Moraxella

Bacilli

Gram-positive	Clostridia
	Cl. tetani
	Cl. perfringens
	Cl. botulinum
	Corynebacteria
	C. diphtheriae
	Bacillus
	B. anthracis
	B. cereus
	Listeria
	Erysipelothrix
	Gardnerella
	Nocardia
	Actinomyces
	Streptomyces
	Tropheryma
(Ziehl–Neelsen positive)	Mycobacteria
	M. tuberculosis
	M. leprae
	M. avium
	M. ulcerans
Gram-negative	Escherichia
	Salmonella
	Shigella
	Yersinia
	Proteus
	Klebsiella
	Vibrio cholerae
	Campylobacter
	Helicobacter
	Pseudomonas
	Burkholderia
	Stenotrophomonas
	Anaerobic
	Bacteroides
	Fusobacterium
	Mobiluncus
	Porphyromonas
	Prevotella
	Miscellaneous
	Actinobacillus
	Bartonella
	Bordetella
	Brucella
	Eikenella
	Francisella
	Haemophilus
	Legionella
	Pasteurella
	Spirillum
	Streptobacillus

Spiral

Spirochaetes	*Borrelia*
	Leptospira
	Treponema

Obligate intracellular

Chlamydia
Coxiella
Ehrlichia
Rickettsia

Lacking cell wall

Mycoplasma

FUNGI

Yeasts (single-celled)

Cryptococcus
Malassezia
Candida
Pneumocystis

Dimorphic (single-celled or mycelial)

Blastomyces
Candida
Coccidioides
Histoplasma
Paracoccidioides
Sporothrix

Mycelial (filamentous)

Aspergillus
Epidermophyton
Fusarium
Madurella
Microsporum
Mucor
Penicillium
Pseudallescheria
Scopulariopsis
Scytalidium
Trichophyton

PROTOZOA

Insect-borne (blood/tissues)

Leishmania
Plasmodium
Toxoplasma
Trypanosoma

Water-borne (intestinal/urinogenital)

Balantidium
Cryptosporidium
Cyclospora
Entamoeba
Encephalitozoon
Enterocytozoon
Giardia
Isospora
Nosema
Pleistophora
Trichomonas

HELMINTHS (WORMS)

Nematodes (roundworms)

Ancylostoma
Ascaris
Brugia
Dracunculus
Enterobius
Loa loa
Onchocerca
Strongyloides
Toxocara
Trichinella
Trichuris
Wuchereria

Trematodes (flukes)

Clonorchis
Fasciola
Fasciolopsis
Metagonymus
Opisthorcis
Paragonimus
Schistosoma

Cestodes (tapeworms)

Diphyllobothrium
Echinococcus
Hymenolepsis
Spirometra
Taenia saginata
Taenia solium

APPENDIX 2: COMMON LABORATORY TESTS AND THEIR NORMAL VALUES

The following provide an approximate guide only. Every laboratory will establish its own normal ranges.

BLOOD COUNT (EDTA BLOOD)

Haematocrit (PCV)	
Male	0.37–0.5
Female	0.33–0.45
Haemoglobin	
Male	13–17 g/dl
Female	11.5–15.5 g/dl
Mean corpuscular haemoglobin (MCH)	26–33.5 pg
Mean corpuscular Hb concentration (MCHC)	32–34.9 g/dl
Mean corpuscular volume (MCV)	80–99 fl
Mean platelet volume	7–11 fl
Platelet count	150–450 × 10⁹/l
Red cell count	
Male	4.4–5.8 × 10¹²/l
Female	3.95–5.15 × 10¹²/l
Red cell distribution width (RDW)	11.5–15
Reticulocytes	<2%
Total white cell count	4–11 × 10⁹/l
Differential	
neutrophils	2–7.5 × 10⁹/l (40–75%)
monocytes	0.2–1 × 10⁹/l (2–10%)
eosinophils	0–0.4 × 10⁹/l (0–6%)
basophils	0–0.1 × 10⁹/l (0–2%)
lymphocytes	1.5–4 × 10⁹/l (20–45%)
T	1.1–1.7 × 10⁹/l (67–76% of ly)
B	0.2–0.4 × 10⁹/l (11–16% of ly)
NK	0.2–0.4 × 10⁹/l (10–19% of ly)
CD2+	0.68–3.28 × 10⁹/l
CD4+	0.35–2.2 × 10⁹/l
CD8+	0.2–1.5 × 10⁹/l
CD19+	0.05–0.6 × 10⁹/l

BLOOD GASES (HEPARIN BLOOD)

Ammonia	19–62 μmol/l
Base excess	–3 to +2 mmol/l
Carbon monoxide	7%
Total CO_2	20–30 mmol/l
pH	7.36–7.43
P_{CO_2}	4.66–6.1 kPa
P_{O_2}	10.7–13.9 kPa

COAGULATION TESTS

Activated partial thrombo-plastin time (APTT)	22–36 s
Antithrombin III	0.8–1.3 iu/ml
Factors II, V, VII, IX, X, XI and XII	0.5–1.5 u/ml
Heparin cofactor II	0.65–1.45 u/ml
International prothrombin ratio (INR)	0.8–1.2
Plasminogen	0.7–1.4 u/ml
Prothrombin time	10–13 s
Template bleeding time	<10 min
Thrombin time	12–16 s
von Willebrand factor Ag,	0.5–2 iu/ml
von Willebrand factor RiCof	0.5–2 iu/ml

ELECTROLYTES (PLASMA)

Bicarbonate	20–30 mmol/l
Calcium	2.2–2.6 mmol/l
Chloride	99–108 mmol/l
Osmolality	280–300 mmol/kg
Phosphate	0.65–1.5 mmol/l
Potassium	3.3–4.8 mmol/l
Sodium	137–145 mmol/l

ENZYMES (SERUM; PLASMA)

Acid phosphatase (prostatic)	≤1.6 u/l
Alanine aminotransferase	5–50 u/l
Alkaline phosphatase	100–280 u/l
Alpha-2 antiplasmin	0.8–1.2 u/ml
Alpha-1 antitrypsin	1.2–2.6 g/l
Amylase	70–300 u/l
Angiotensin converting enzyme	25–105 u/l
Aspartate aminotransferase	11–55 u/l
Cholinesterase	3–9 ku/l
Creatine kinase	
Male	24–195 u/l
Female	24–170 u/l
Gammaglutamyltransferase	5–37 u/l
Glucose-6-phosphate dehydrogenase	5.9–11.8 u/g Hb
Hydroxybutyrate dehydrogenase	55–140 u/l (at 25°C)
Lactate dehydrogenase	230–460 u/l
Lipase	7–60 u/l
Transketolase	34–90 u/l

HORMONES (PLASMA; SERUM)

Adrenaline	0.1–1.2 nmol/l
Aldosterone	100–500 pmol/l
Androstenedione	2–10 mmol/l
Calcitonin	≤80 ng/l
Cortisol	
Day	140–700 nmol/l
Night	≤140 nmol/l
Dehydroepiandrosterone (DHEA)	10 μmol/l
Follicle-stimulating hormone (FSH)	
Male	≤6 u/l
Female	1–20 u/l
Growth hormone (after glucose)	0.002 u/l
Gut hormones	
VIP	30 pmol/l
PP	300 pmol/l
Glucagon	50 pmol/l
Gastrin	40 pmol/l
Neurotensin	100 pmol/l
Hydroxyprogesterone	12 nmol/l
Insulin level (fasting)	<15 mU/l
Luteinizing hormone (LH)	
Male	6 u/l
Female	1–60 u/l
Noradrenaline	0.5–3.5 nmol/l

contd

HORMONES (PLASMA; SERUM) CONTD

Oestradiol	
Child	7–37 pmol/l
Male	37–130 pmol/l
Female, follicular	110–440 pmol/l
Female, luteal	370–770 pmol/l
Female, pre-ovulation	550–1290 pmol/l
Female, postmenopause	37–130 pmol/l
Parathyroid hormone	1–5.5 pmol/l
Progesterone (luteal phase)	32 nmol/l if pregnant
Prolactin	≤0.36 u/l
Renin	
Recumbent	1.14–2.65 nmol/h/l
Standing	2.82–4.49 nmol/h/l
Sex-hormone-binding globulin	40–137 nmol/l
Testosterone	
Male	11–33 nmol/l
Female	0.5–2.5 nmol/l
Thyroid hormones	
Tri-iodothyronine (T3)	
Adult	3–8.6 pmol/l
<20 years	4.2–10.4 pmol/l
Thyroxine (T4)	
Total	60–160 nmol/l
Free	9–23 pmol/l
Thyroid-stimulating hormone (TSH)	0.5–5 mU/l
Thyroglobulin	5 μg/l

METALS (SERUM)

Aluminium	2.2 μmol/l (on dialysis)
Copper	11–22 μmol/l
Ferritin	
Male	25–240 μg/l
Female	12–190 μg/l
Gold (therapeutic)	7.5–15 μmol/l
Iron	7–45 μmol/l
Iron-binding capacity (TIBC)	45–73 μmol/l
Lead	1.2 μmol/l
Magnesium	0.7–1 mmol/l
Zinc	11–18 μmol/l

PROTEINS (SERUM; PLASMA)

Albumin	35–53 g/l
Alpha-fetoprotein	
Adult	Up to 10 kU/l
Hepatoma	500 kU/l
Beta-2 microglobulin	0–3 mg/l
Carcinoembryonic antigen (CEA)	0–9 μg/l
Complement components	
C3	0.75–1.75 g/l
C4	0.1–0.35 g/l
C1 esterase inhibitor	0.18–0.26 g/l
C-reactive protein (CRP)	12 mg/l
Creatinine	50–125 μmol/l

Fibrinogen	1.5–4 g/l
Haptoglobin	0.3–1.9 g/l
Immunoglobulins	
IgG	8–18 g/l
IgA	0.9–4.5 g/l
IgM	0.6–2.8 g/l
IgE	0–120 kU/l
Protein C	0.7–1.3 iu/ml
Protein S	
Total	0.45–1.41 u/ml
Free	0.39–1.43 u/ml
Transferrin	2.5–4.3 g/l

VITAMINS

A (carotene)	0.9–3.7 μmol/l
B12	180–700 ng/l
D	3.2–30 μg/l
E	11.5–35 μmol/l
Red cell folate	150–650 mg/l

OTHER (PLASMA; SERUM)

Alcohol (RTA limit)	17.4 mmol/l
Bilirubin	
Adult	3–17 μmol/l
Neonate	Up to 70 μmol/l
Cholesterol	2.3–6.9 mmol/l
High density lipid (HDL)	
Male	0.7–1.6 mmol/l
Female	1–2 mmol/l
Glucose (fasting)	3.3–5.6 mmol/l
Prostate specific antigen	Up to 4 μg/l
Triglyceride (fasting)	0.5–1.8 mmol/l
Urate	150–500 μmol/l
Urea	3–8 mmol/l

URINE

Ascorbic acid saturation	0.28 mmol in 2 h
Beta-2 microglobulin	0.03–0.37 mg/24 h
Calcium	2–9 mmol/24 h
Citrate	
Male	0.6–4.8 mmol/24 h
Female	1.36 mmol/24 h
Cortisol	Up to 400 nmol/24 h
Creatinine	7–18 mmol/24 h
Cystine	42–420 μmol/24 h
Glucose	None
Glycollate	0.1–0.33 mmol/24 h
5HIAA	Up to 45 μmol/24 h
Hydroxyproline	Up to 0.4 mmol/24 h
Magnesium	2–8.2 mmol/24 h
Phosphate	15–50 mmol/24 h
Potassium	35–80 mmol/24 h
Protein (total)	Up to 0.05 g/24 h
Sodium	100–240 mmol/24 h
Urate	2–7 mmol/24 h
Urea	220–600 mmol/24 h
VMA (HMMA)	9–35 μmol/24 h

APPENDIX 3: MAJOR BOOK ENTRIES CLASSIFIED BY BODY SYSTEM

BONES, MUSCLES AND JOINTS

Achondroplasia
Ankylosing spondylitis
Arthritis
Botulism
Brittle bone disease
Brodie abscess
Duchenne muscular dystrophy
Dwarfism
Felty syndrome
Fracture
Gout
Juvenile arthritis
Lupus erythematosus
Mixed connective tissue disease
Myositis
Osteitis deformans
Osteoarthritis
Osteomalacia
Osteomyelitis
Osteoporosis
Paget disease of bone
Psoriatic arthritis
Reactive arthritis
Reiter disease
Rheumatic fever
Rheumatoid arthritis
Septic arthritis
Seronegative arthritis
Spina bifida
Still disease
Systemic lupus erythematosus
Tetanus

CARDIOVASCULAR SYSTEM

Aneurysm
Angioma
Arteriolosclerosis
Arteritis
Atheroma
Cardiac tamponade
Cardiogenic shock
Cardiomyopathy
Cerebrovascular disease
Coarctation
Congenital heart disease
Endocarditis
Endomyocardial fibrosis
Fallot tetralogy
Giant cell arteritis
Heart failure
Hypertension
Ischaemia

Myocardial infarction
Myocarditis
Pericarditis
Pre-eclampsia
Polyarteritis nodosa
Pulmonary hypertension
Raynaud disease
Septic shock
Temporal arteritis
Thromboembolism
Thrombosis
Vasculitis
Veno-occlusive disease

CENTRAL NERVOUS SYSTEM AND EYES

Acoustic neurofibroma
Alzheimer disease
Anencephaly
Arnold–Chiari malformation
Botulism
Cataract
Cerebrovascular disease
Chlamydial disease
Conjunctivitis
Creutzfeldt–Jakob disease
Dementia
Encephalitis
Encephalopathy
Guillain–Barré syndrome
Huntingdon disease
Intracranial haemorrhage
Meningioma
Meningocele
Meningococcal meningitis
Meningoencephalitis
Multiple sclerosis
Myasthenia gravis
Neuroblastoma
Neurofibromatosis
Neuropathy
Neurosyphilis
Parkinson disease
Poliomyelitis
Porphyria
Prion diseases
Progressive multifocal leucoencephalopathy
Rabies
Retinoblastoma
Retinopathy
Schwannoma
Spina bifida
Spongiform encephalopathy
Subacute sclerosing panencephalitis

Sympathetic ophthalmia
Tetanus
Trachoma
Trypanosomiasis
Uveitis
Viral meningitis

EAR, NOSE AND THROAT
Acoustic neurofibroma
Allergy
Anaphylaxis
Candidiasis
Diphtheria
Epiglottitis
Gingivitis
Hand-foot-and-mouth disease
Hay fever
Infectious mononucleosis
Laryngeal carcinoma
Leucoplakia
Mastoiditis
Measles
Mumps
Nasopharyngeal carcinoma
Otitis
Periodontitis
Quinsy
Reiter disease
Sarcoidosis
Sinusitis
Sjögren syndrome
Tonsillitis
Vincent angina

ENDOCRINE SYSTEM
Acromegaly
Addison disease
Cushing syndrome
De Quervain thyroiditis
Diabetes insipidus
Diabetes mellitus
Ectopic hormone production
Goitre
Graves disease
Gynaecomastia
Hormone-secreting tumours
Hypercalcaemia
Hyperparathyroidism
Hyperthyroidism
Hypoparathyroidism
Hypothyroidism
Myxoedema
Obesity
Phaeochromocytoma
Polycystic ovary
Thyrotoxicosis

GASTROINTESTINAL SYSTEM
Achalasia
Adenomatous polyposis coli
Amoebiasis
Appendicitis
Ascariasis
Barrett oesophagus
Cholera
Coeliac disease
Colitis
Colorectal carcinoma
Crohn disease
Diverticulitis
Diverticulosis
Dysentery
Enteric fever
Gastric carcinoma
Gastritis
Gastroenteritis
Giardiasis
Gluten-sensitive enteropathy
Hirschsprung disease
Hookworm
Inflammatory bowel disease
Malabsorption
Melanosis coli
Oesophageal carcinoma
Pancreatic carcinoma
Pancreatitis
Peptic ulcer
Peritonitis
Polyp; polyposis
Pseudomembranous colitis
Sprue
Strongyloidiasis
Tapeworm infection
Traveller's diarrhoea
Typhoid fever
Ulcerative colitis

GENITAL SYSTEM
Bacterial vaginosis
Candidiasis
Dysgerminoma
Endometrial carcinoma
Endometriosis
Epididymitis
Fibroids
Germ cell tumours
Gestational hypertensive disease
Hydatidiform mole
Hydrops fetalis
Ovarian cancer
Ovarian cyst
Pelvic inflammatory disease

Polycystic ovary
Pre-eclampsia
Prostatic carcinoma
Prostatic hyperplasia
Prostatitis
Salpingitis
Seminoma
Syphilis
Teratoma
Testicular tumours
Treponematosis
Vaginitis

HAEMOPOIETIC SYSTEM

Acute lymphoblastic leukaemia
Acute myeloid leukaemia
Agranulocytosis
Anaemia
Aplastic anaemia
Blood transfusion reactions
Bone marrow failure
Bone marrow transplantation
Chediak–Higashi syndrome
Chromosomal abnormalities
Chronic granulomatous disease
Chronic lymphocytic leukaemia
Chronic myeloid leukaemia
Disseminated intravascular coagulation
Essential thrombocythaemia
Glandular fever
Graft-versus-host disease
Haemolytic anaemia
Haemolytic disease of the newborn
Haemolytic uraemic syndrome
Haemophilia
Haemorrhagic anaemia
Haemorrhagic disease of the newborn
Haemosiderosis
Hairy cell leukaemia
Henoch–Schönlein purpura
Herditary haemorrhagic telangiectasia
Hereditary spherocytosis
Hodgkin disease
Hyperviscosity syndrome
Idiopathic thrombocytopenic purpura
Infectious mononucleosis
Iron deficiency anaemia
Leukaemia
Leucocytosis
Megaloblastic anaemia
Microangiopathic haemolytic anaemia
Myeloma
Myeloproliferative disorders
Neutropenia
Non-Hodgkin lymphoma

Paroxysmal nocturnal haemoglobulinaemia
Pernicious anaemia
Plasmacytoma
Polycythaemia
Purpura
Rhesus incompatibility
Sickle cell disease
Sideroblastic anaemia
Stem cell transplantation
Thalassaemia
Thrombocytopenia
Thrombocytosis
Thrombophilia
Thrombotic thrombocytopenic purpura
Waldenström disease
Warm autoimmune haemolytic anaemia

IMMUNE SYSTEM

Acquired immunodeficiencies
Acquired immunodeficiency syndrome
Adenosine deaminase deficiency
Agranulocytosis
Anaphylaxis
Antibody deficiency
Asthma
Autoimmunity
Blood transfusion reactions
Bruton disease
Bullous skin disease
Burkitt lymphoma
Complement deficiencies
Contact dermatitis
Dermatitis
Di George syndrome
Endotoxic shock
Extrinsic allergic alveolitis
Farmer's lung
Graft-versus-host disease
Haemolytic disease of the newborn
Hashimoto thyroiditis
Hay fever
Hyper-IgE syndrome
Hypersensitivity
Hyperthyroidism
Hypogammaglobulinaemia
Immune complex disease
Immunization
Immunodeficiency
Lupus erythematosus
Lymphoma
Myasthenia gravis
Myxoedema
Neutropenia
Paraproteinaemia
Reactive arthritis

Reiter disease
Renal transplant
Rheumatoid arthritis
Seronegative arthritis
Severe combined immunodeficiency
Sjögren syndrome
Sympathetic ophthalmia
Systemic lupus erythematosus
Thyrotoxicosis
Transplant rejection
Vaccination

KIDNEY AND BLADDER

Acute tubular necrosis
Berger disease
Bladder carcinoma
Glomerulonephritis
Goodpasture syndrome
IgA nephropathy
Medullary sponge kidney
Nephritis
Nephrotic syndrome
Polycystic kidney
Prostatic carcinoma
Prostatitis
Pyelonephritis
Renal cell carcinoma
Renal cyst
Renal failure
Renal transplantation
Uraemia
Urethritis
Urate nephropathy
Wilms tumour

LIVER AND GALLBLADDER

Alcoholic liver disease
Bilharzia
Biliary atresia
Cholangiocarcinoma
Cholangitis
Cholecystitis
Cholestasis
Cirrhosis
Fatty liver
Gallstones
Haemochromatosis
Hepatic (liver) failure
Hepatitis B infection
Hepatocellular carcinoma
Hydatid disease
Jaundice
Liver fluke disease
Primary biliary cirrhosis
Schistosomiasis
Viral hepatitis

Wilson disease
Yellow fever

RESPIRATORY SYSTEM

Acute bronchitis
Adult respiratory distress syndrome
Allergy
Alveolitis
Anaphylaxis
Asbestosis
Asthma
Atypical pneumonia
Bronchial carcinoma
Bronchiectasis
Bronchiolitis
Bronchopneumonia
Chronic obstructive airways disease
Cystic fibrosis
Emphysema
Extrinsic allergic alveolitis
Farmer's lung
Hay fever
Influenza
Laryngeal carcinoma
Lung carcinoma
Mycobacteriosis
Nasopharyngeal carcinoma
Oat cell carcinoma
Occupational lung disease
Otitis externa/media
Pancoast tumour
Pleurisy
Pneumonoconiosis
Pneumococcal pneumonia
Pneumocystis pneumonia
Sarcoidosis
Silicosis
Sudden infant death syndrome
Tuberculosis
Whooping cough

SKIN

Abscess
Acanthosis nigricans
Anthrax
Atopy/atopic
Basal cell carcinoma
Bullous skin diseases
Buruli ulcer
Candidiasis
Cat-scratch disease
Cellulitis
Chancroid
Cutaneous larva migrans
Dermatitis
Dermatitis herpetiformis

Dermatomyositis
Dermatophytosis
Discoid lupus erythematosus
Dracunculiasis
Ecthyma gangrenosum
Ecthyma infectiosum
Eczema
Elephantiasis
Erysipelas
Erysipeloid
Erythema chronicum migrans
Erythema multiforme
Erythema nodosum
Exanthema
Gangrene
Gumma
Hidradenitis
Hypersensitivity
Kaposi sarcoma
Keloid
Leishmaniasis
Leprosy
Lipoma

Liposarcoma
Lupus erythematosus/vulgaris
Lymphogranuloma venereum
Malignant melanoma
Melanoma
Molluscum contagiosum
Mycosis fungoides
Naevus
Necrotizing fasciitis
Paget disease of breast
Pemphigus; pemphigoid
Pityriasis versicolor
Purpura
Pyomyositis
Ringworm
Scabies
Scarlet fever
Scleroderma
Shingles
Systemic lupus erythematosus
von Recklinghausen disease
Warts
Xanthoma